The Changing Role of the Hospital in European Health Systems

Hospitals today face a huge number of challenges, including new patterns of disease, rapidly evolving medical technologies, ageing populations and continuing budget constraints. This book is written by clinicians for clinicians and hospital managers, as well as those who design and operate hospitals. It sets out why hospitals need to change as the patients they treat and the technology to treat them change. In a series of chapters by leading authorities in their field, it challenges existing models, reviews best practice from many countries and presents clear policy recommendations for policy-makers and hospital administrators. It covers the main patient groups and conditions as well as those departments that make modern effective care possible, in imaging and laboratory medicine. Each chapter looks at patient pathways, aspects of workforce, required levels of specialization and technology, and the opportunities and challenges for optimizing the delivery of services in the hospital of the future.

MARTIN MCKEE CBE is Professor of European Public Health at the London School of Hygiene & Tropical Medicine, Research Director of the European Observatory on Health Systems and Policies, and Past President of the European Public Health Association. His contributions have been recognized by election to the UK Academy of Medical Sciences, Academia Europeae, and the US National Academy of Medicine, and by six honorary doctorates. He was awarded the 2003 Andrija Stampar medal, the 2014 Alwyn Smith Prize, and the 2015 Donabedian International Award.

SHERRY MERKUR is a Research Fellow and Health Policy Analyst at the European Observatory on Health Systems and Policies, based at the London School of Economics and Political Science. She is Editor-in-Chief of *Eurohealth* and author and editor of *HiT: Health system reviews*. Recent books include *Promoting Health, Preventing Disease: The conomic Case* (2015) and with Ellen Nolte and Anders Anell, she is co-editor of *Achieving Person-Centred Health Systems* (Cambridge, 2020).

NIGEL EDWARDS is Chief Executive at The Nuffield Trust, a research and policy foundation based in London. Prior to this he was a senior fellow at the King's Fund and the Policy Director of the NHS Confederation. He is honorary visiting professor at the London School of Hygiene & Tropical Medicine and was awarded an honorary DSc by the University of Westminster.

ELLEN NOLTE is Professor of Health Services and Systems Research at the London School of Hygiene & Tropical Medicine. Her expertise is in health systems research, international health care comparisons and performance assessment. She has published widely on health systems, integrated care, European health policy and population health assessments. She is co-editor of the *Journal of Health Services Research & Policy*. With Anders Anell and Sherry Merkur, she is co-editor of *Achieving Person-Centred Health Systems* (Cambridge, 2020).

European Observatory on Health Systems and Policies

The volumes in this series focus on topical issues around the transformation of health systems in Europe, a process being driven by a changing environment, increasing pressures and evolving needs.

Drawing on available evidence, existing experience and conceptual thinking, these studies aim to provide both practical and policy-relevant information and lessons on how to implement change to make health systems more equitable, effective and efficient. They are designed to promote and support evidence-informed policy-making in the health sector and will be a valuable resource for all those involved in developing, assessing or analysing health systems and policies.

In addition to policy-makers, stakeholders and researchers in the field of health policy, key audiences outside the health sector will also find this series invaluable for understanding the complex choices and challenges that health systems face today.

LIST OF TITLES

Challenges to Tackling Antimicrobial Resistance: Economic and Policy Responses
Edited by MICHAEL ANDERSON, MICHELE CECCHINI, ELIAS MOSSIALOS

Achieving Person-Centred Health systems: Evidence, Strategies and Challenges
Edited by ELLEN NOLTE, SHERRY MERKUR, ANDERS ANELL

Series Editors

JOSEP FIGUERAS Director, European Observatory on Health Systems and Policies

MARTIN MCKEE Co-Director, European Observatory on Health Systems and Policies, and Professor of European Public Health at the London School of Hygiene & Tropical Medicine

ELIAS MOSSIALOS Co-Director, European Observatory on Health Systems and Policies, and Brian Abel-Smith Professor of Health Policy, London School of Economics and Political Science

REINHARD BUSSE Co-Director, European Observatory on Health Systems and Policies, and Head of the Department of Health Care Management, Berlin University of Technology

The Changing Role of the Hospital in European Health Systems

Edited by

MARTIN MCKEE
European Observatory on Health Systems and Policies;
London School of Hygiene & Tropical Medicine

SHERRY MERKUR
European Observatory on Health Systems and Policies

NIGEL EDWARDS
The Nuffield Trust

ELLEN NOLTE
London School of Hygiene & Tropical Medicine

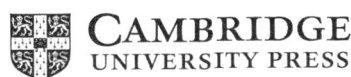

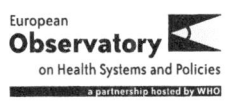

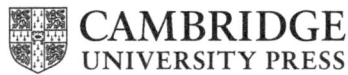

CAMBRIDGE
UNIVERSITY PRESS

Shaftesbury Road, Cambridge CB2 8EA, United Kingdom

One Liberty Plaza, 20th Floor, New York, NY 10006, USA

477 Williamstown Road, Port Melbourne, VIC 3207, Australia

314–321, 3rd Floor, Plot 3, Splendor Forum, Jasola District Centre, New Delhi – 110025, India

103 Penang Road, #05–06/07, Visioncrest Commercial, Singapore 238467

Cambridge University Press is part of Cambridge University Press & Assessment, a department of the University of Cambridge.

We share the University's mission to contribute to society through the pursuit of education, learning and research at the highest international levels of excellence.

www.cambridge.org
Information on this title: www.cambridge.org/9781108790055

DOI: 10.1017/9781108855440

First published 2020

A catalogue record for this publication is available from the British Library

ISBN   978-1-108-79005-5   Paperback

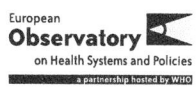 European Observatory on Health Systems and Policies

European Observatory
on Health Systems
and Policies

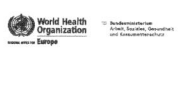 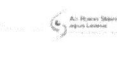

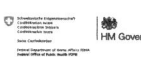

The European Observatory on Health Systems and Policies supports and promotes evidence-based health policy-making through comprehensive and rigorous analysis of health systems in Europe. It brings together a wide range of policy-makers, academics and practitioners to analyse trends in health reform, drawing on experience from across Europe to illuminate policy issues.

The European Observatory on Health Systems and Policies is a partnership hosted by the World Health Organization Regional Office for Europe which includes the Governments of Austria, Belgium, Finland, Ireland, Norway, Slovenia, Spain, Sweden, Switzerland, the United Kingdom, and the Veneto Region of Italy; the European Commission; the World Bank; UNCAM (French National Union of Health Insurance Funds); the Health Foundation; the London School of Economics and Political Science; and the London School of Hygiene & Tropical Medicine. The Observatory has a secretariat in Brussels and it has hubs in London (at LSE and LSHTM) and at the Berlin University of Technology.

Contents

Figures

Tables

Boxes

Contributors

Benjamin Bray, Research Director, Sentinel Stroke National Audit Programme, Royal College of Physicians, London, United Kingdom

Robab Breyer-Kohansal, Department of Respiratory and Critical Care Medicine, Otto Wagner Hospital, Vienna, Austria

Peter Cavanagh, former Vice-President and Dean, Faculty of Clinical Radiology, Royal College of Radiologists, United Kingdom

Matthew Cooke, Professor Clinical Systems Design, Warwick Medical School; Visiting Professor, Department of Engineering, Brunel University, United Kingdom

Alison Cracknell, Consultant Medicine for Older People and Honorary Clinical Associate Professor, Leeds Teaching Hospitals NHS Trust, United Kingdom

Nigel Edwards, Chief Executive, Nuffield Trust, United Kingdom

Jochen Ehrich, European Paediatric Association – Union of National Paediatric Societies and Associations (EPA-UNEPSA), Berlin, Germany; Children's Hospital, Hannover Medical School, Hannover, Germany

Michael Grocott, Professor of Anaesthesia and Critical Care Medicine, University of Southampton, United Kingdom

Wim Groen, Netherlands Cancer Institute

Zachi Grossman, Paediatric Clinic, Maccabi Health Services, Tel Aviv, Israel

Adamos Hadjipanayis, Faculty of Medicine, European University, Nikosia, Cyprus

Wim van Harten, Rijnstate Hospital, Netherlands Cancer Institute

Digby Ingle, Regional Coordination Manager, Royal College of Pathologists, United Kingdom

Reinhold Kerbl, European Paediatric Association – Union of National Paediatric Societies and Associations (EPA-UNEPSA), Berlin, Germany; General Hospital Leoben, Department of Paediatrics and Adolescent Medicine, Leoben, Austria

Simon Lenton, European Paediatric Association – Union of National Paediatric Societies and Associations (EPA-UNEPSA), Berlin, Germany

Rachael Liebmann, Consultant Histopathologist, Queen Victoria Hospital NHS Foundation Trust; Vice President, Royal College of Pathologists, United Kingdom

Jose Luis López-Campos, Unidad Médico-Quirúrgica de Enfermedades Respiratorias, Instituto de Biomedicina de Sevilla (IBiS), Hospital Universitario Virgen del Rocío/Universidad de Sevilla, Seville, Spain; Centro de Investigación Biomédica en Red de Enfermedades Respiratorias (CIBERES), Instituto de Salud Carlos III, Madrid, Spain

Clifford Mann, National Clinical Adviser, NHS England (A&E), United Kingdom

Martin McKee, Professor of European Public Health, London School of Hygiene & Tropical Medicine; Research Director, European Observatory on Health Systems and Policies, United Kingdom

Sherry Merkur, Research Fellow and Health Policy Analyst, European Observatory on Health Systems and Policies, London School of Economics and Political Science, United Kingdom

Eleanor Molloy, Trinity College, University of Dublin, Tallaght Hospital, Coombe Women's and Infants Hospital and Our Lady's Children's Hospital, Dublin, Ireland

Sherena Nair, Elderly Medicine Registrar, Leeds Teaching Hospitals NHS Trust, United Kingdom

Ellen Nolte, Professor of Health Services and Systems Research, London School of Hygiene & Tropical Medicine, United Kingdom

Bo Norrving, Professor of Neurology, Department of Clinical Sciences, Neurology, Lund University, Lund, Sweden

David Oliver, Elderly Care Consultant Physician, Royal Berkshire NHS Foundation Trust, United Kingdom

Massimo Pettoello-Mantovani, European Paediatric Association – Union of National Paediatric Societies and Associations (EPA-UNEPSA), Berlin, Germany; Institute of Paediatrics, University of Foggia, Istituto di Ricovero e Cura a Carattere Scientifico "Casa Sollievo", Foggia, Italy

Lucia da Pieve, Centro di Riferimento Oncologico (CRO), IRCCS, National Cancer Institute, Aviano

C. Michael Roberts, Managing Director of UCL Partners Academic Health Sciences Network; Professor of Medical Education for Clinical Practice, Queen Mary University of London; Associate Director, Clinical Effectiveness Unit, Royal College of Physicians; Consultant, Integrated Respiratory Care the, Princess Alexandra NHS Trust, United Kingdom

Anthony Rudd, Professor of Stroke Medicine, King's College London, United Kingdom

Sigbjørn Smeland, Oslo University Hospital and University of Oslo

Harry Thirkettle, Honorary Fellow, Medtech Campus, Anglia Ruskin University, United Kingdom

Stefano del Torso, Studio Pediatrico, Vecellio 33 ULSS16, Padova, Italy

Mehmet Vural, European Paediatric Association – Union of National Paediatric Societies and Associations (EPA-UNEPSA), Berlin, Germany; Istanbul University, Cerrahpaşa Medical Faculty, Neonatology Unit, Istanbul, Turkey

Björn Wettergren, Paediatric Department Region Gävleborg, Gävle, Sweden

Phil White, Professor of Interventional and Diagnostic Neuroradiology, Institute of Neuroscience, Newcastle University and Newcastle upon Tyne Hospital NHS Foundation Trust, United Kingdom

Anke Wind, Netherlands Cancer Institute – Antoni van Leeuwenhoek

Marc Wittenberg, Consultant in Anaesthesia & Perioperative Medicine, Royal Free London NHS Foundation Trust

Charles Wolfe, Professor of Public Health, School of Population Health & Environmental Sciences, Faculty of Life Sciences and Medicine, King's College London, United Kingdom

Foreword

Our world is volatile, uncertain, complex and ambiguous. Some might say that this is threatening and destabilizing, while others might say it is a world full of opportunities. But one thing is clear: we cannot ignore the constant change, whether technological or societal. This is also true for us as health policy-makers. But what stance should we take towards change: Accept? Adapt? Embrace? Or maybe actively shape and promote?

What if we ask "What kind of model of care do we want?" rather than "What model of health care does the technological advance impose on us?" And: "How can we include technology in a smarter, more effective and efficient organization of health care?". What if we ask ourselves what kind of health care providers we want and which role we want to give to insurers in the future?

The hospital has always been key in the delivery of health care. What do we expect of the hospital of the future? How do we see its impact and role in the health system, in society and regarding the wider environment? We know that its role is changing. It is faced with challenges regarding integrated care for chronic patients, the concentration of medico-technical capacity and medical expertise, patient expectations concerning their care process, etc. The way we see the institution "hospital" will need to adapt to these evolutions.

As policy-makers, we should actively engage in this reflection, linking evidence, vision, strategy and action. The present study by the European Observatory on Health Systems and Policies will provide important contributions to this reflection. The study takes a unique perspective by observing different patient groups seen in modern hospitals: from young to old, from acute to chronic. Each chapter considers the provision of services for these patients and how these will need to change.

This book has the ambition to guide readers in their thinking about how care can be optimized in hospitals of the future. It wants to help in the understanding of care pathways, bottlenecks to care optimization, workforce issues and future trends. Health policy-makers will benefit from gaining insights from the clinician's perspective on the current service landscape, ongoing change, and the need for further change. Likewise, the authors consider recent technological developments and address issues of changes in patient management – impacting hospitals, professionals and patient experience.

We would like to invite the reader to use this study as a basis for further reflection and to encourage this reflection to go beyond the existing; to think bold, transversal, across disciplines and diseases.

We wish you an interesting read!

Tom Auwers, President of the Executive Committee, Federal Public Service Health, Food Chain Safety and Environment, Belgium

Pedro Facon, Director-General Healthcare, Federal Public Service Health, Food Chain Safety and Environment, Belgium

Acknowledgements

This study, which was finalised before the COVID-19 pandemic, was produced by multiple experts over a period of time up to and including 2019. We would like to thank the following people for peer reviewing each of the core chapters: Matteo Cesari, Specialist in Geriatrics and Gerontology, Professor at the University of Toulouse, France; Ruth Gilbert, Professor of Clinical Epidemiology, UCL Great Ormond Street Institute of Child Health, England; Chris Harrison, National Clinical Director for Cancer, NHS England; Nicholas Hopkinson, Reader in Respiratory Medicine and Honorary Consultant Physician, National Heart and Lung Institute, Royal Brompton Hospital, England; Gavin Lavery, Clinical Director, HSC Safety Forum, Belfast, Northern Ireland; Kenneth Fleming, Senior Adviser for Pathology, Centre for Global Health, NCI, USA and Emeritus Fellow, Green Templeton College, University of Oxford, England; Martin O'Donnell, Professor of Translational Medicine, NUI Galway, Ireland; and Jane Young, Consultant Radiologist, Whittington Hospital, England.

We gratefully acknowledge the very helpful and insightful comments provided by Antonio Duran and Patrick Jeurissen on the full volume.

We would like to thank Sarah Cook for copy-editing and Jonathan North and Caroline White for the production of this book.

1 Introduction – The changing nature of care provided in the hospital

MARTIN MCKEE, SHERRY MERKUR, NIGEL EDWARDS, ELLEN NOLTE

The emergence of the modern hospital

Sometimes it seems that the hospital *is* the health system. Whether in popular culture, such as the American television series *ER*, in political and popular discourse, with its focus on opening and closing of hospitals, in statistical databases that give prominence to numbers of hospital beds, or in budgetary breakdowns, showing that the bulk of health service spending is concentrated in hospitals, it is clear that the hospital is seen as being at the heart of the health system (McKee & Healy, 2002). Even when the many other components of the health system are recognized, the hospital typically sits at the top of the pyramid. This is perhaps inevitable. Hospitals are highly visible. They are large buildings, well signposted, and adorned with the symbols of health care, such as red crosses. When politicians wish to make a statement on health services, they typically find a convenient hospital as a backdrop. Hospitals are also important for the public, not just when they are ill, but by providing reassurance that they will be cared for nearby if they become ill in the future. They play other roles too, as settings for the education of the next generation of health workers and through their contribution to the local economy. So even though they are only one part of the overall health system, they are an important part, and are recognized as such by almost everyone.

Yet the concept of the hospital is a relatively recent one. Before the 18th century most people were cared for in their own homes, usually by family members or traditional healers. Institutionalized care, to the extent that it existed at all, was often in the hands of religious orders, providing somewhere that those with incurable illnesses could spend their last days in peace and tranquillity (Porter, 1999). What changed was the scientific revolution. Advances in a number of different areas brought new opportunities. In physics, the discovery of X-rays made it possible to look inside the human body as never before (Reed, 2011). Advances in optics paved the way for microscopes, and thus the development of histopathology (Wollman et al., 2015). In chemistry and biology, technical advances made it possible to gain new insights into a patient's condition from samples of their bodily fluids (Moodley et al., 2015). Acceptance of the germ theory led to the emergence of bacteriology (Roll-Hansen, 1979). Meanwhile, the development of safe anaesthetics and an understanding of the importance of asepsis made possible surgical procedures inside bodily cavities (Jessney, 2012).

The technology required to exploit these developments was rudimentary and there were few with the necessary skills to take advantage of it. There was a need to concentrate resources. The hospital was an obvious setting to bring together laboratories, operating theatres, and X-ray departments. It was also the obvious place to train people in their use.

Throughout the 20th century the opportunities to intervene to save lives and reduce suffering advanced rapidly. Paradoxically, it was from the death and destruction of war that many of the most important developments arose, such as the mass production of penicillin (Neushul, 1993) and advances in plastic surgery (Geomelas et al., 2011), the management of burns, and orthopaedic surgery (Dougherty et al., 2004) during the Second World War, as well as new approaches to major trauma in the Korean and Vietnam Wars (Eiseman, 1967; Molnar et al., 2004). The earliest treatments for cancer were derived from chemical weapons, such as mustard gas (Mukherjee, 2010).

All of these expanded the scope of work of the acute hospital. Yet there were also changes that were reducing the work of some hospitals. From the 19th century onwards public bodies in many countries had invested in large hospital facilities, typically away from urban centres, in which they could place those with infectious diseases, especially tuberculosis, as well as mental illness. By the early 1950s the introduction of streptomycin had transformed the management of tuberculosis. Death rates in many countries were falling year on year and it was no longer necessary to incarcerate patients for long periods of time in the hope of spontaneous recovery (Daniel, 2006). By the early 1960s new antipsychotics had transformed the management of schizophrenia. Coupled with new models of care in the community, the days of the large psychiatric hospital were numbered (Clifford et al., 1991). Similar changes were happening within the acute hospital. Improvements in hygiene, linked to better living conditions, brought about a dramatic reduction in the number of children requiring admission for infectious jaundice, gastroenteritis, and respiratory infections (Wolfe & McKee, 2014).

But much more was happening in the hospital. Populations were ageing, benefiting from a remarkable increase in our ability to control many common chronic diseases. The consequence was that patients who would have died in previous years, were now surviving but with growing numbers of clinical conditions, a phenomenon termed multimorbidity (Barnett et al., 2012). Ultimately, many experienced what has been termed frailty, involving decline in a wide range of bodily functions (Nicholson, Gordon & Tinker, 2016). When they became seriously ill, they could require inputs from a wide range of health professionals, working together. But it was not just changes in the characteristics of patients. New opportunities to intervene also required new models of working based on teamwork, whether the problem was cancer (Prades et al., 2015), gastro-intestinal haemorrhage (Lu et al., 2014), or major trauma (McCullough et al., 2014). The evidence was accumulating that a multidisciplinary team (MDT), using shared protocols, achieves the best results.

Sometimes, changes in patterns of disease have even more profound consequences. The epidemic of HIV infection that began in the 1980s led to widespread changes in some of the fundamental elements of health care. These ranged from new approaches to infection control, in particular the risk of transmission of infection through surgical and medical procedures, to a new way of thinking about patient confidentiality and informed consent (Hayter, 1997). Similarly, the growth of antimicrobial resistance has major consequences for many aspects of care delivered in hospitals and, in the future, is likely to have even greater impact, potentially threatening the fundamental principles on which hospitals are organized (Goff et al., 2017).

At the same time it became increasingly apparent that what was important in achieving the best outcomes was not *where* treatment was provided but *how*. In particular, waiting for the patient to arrive at hospital often meant missing important opportunities. Innovative treatments, such as thrombolysis for patients with myocardial infarction, could be initiated in an ambulance on the way to hospital, thereby reducing delays in this time-critical treatment (McCaul, Lourens & Kredo, 2014). The use of advanced techniques to stabilize patients at the scene of major trauma meant that they arrived at the hospital in much better condition (Wilson et al., 2015).

It is not, however, only those things that happen before the patient gets to hospital that are important. Changes in family structure and in labour mobility mean that growing numbers of older people, including those with multiple disabilities, are living alone. Once they have completed active treatment in hospital they may have inadequate support at home, reflecting both the breakdown of traditional extended family structures and reductions in services, exacerbated since 2008 in countries that have imposed austerity policies leading to cuts in social care (Loopstra et al., 2016). The result in some countries is that much-needed hospital beds are occupied by patients who would be much more appropriately cared for elsewhere, if only appropriate accommodation and support structures existed (Turner, Nikolova & Sutton, 2016).

Other technological changes have challenged some aspects of the rationale for the hospital. The original justification for concentrating resources in hospitals stemmed from the need to avoid duplication of three sets of resources: imaging equipment, laboratories, and operating theatres. However, the advent of portable ultrasound machines, coupled with mobile magnetic resonance imaging (MRI), offered new means of seeing inside the human body. Advances in near-patient testing, from the first simple test strips to complex micro-arrays (Voswinckel, 1994), have challenged the role of the laboratory. Injectable anaesthetics, endoscopic procedures, and minimally invasive surgery have enabled what were once major procedures to be undertaken outside hospital. Many treatments that still need to take place in hospital can be completed in hours rather than days, and the pace and intensity of hospital work has changed beyond recognition; however, many processes, ways of working, and individual professional roles have struggled to keep pace.

In summary, the challenges facing hospitals have changed enormously in recent decades. The factors involved are extremely complex and interlinked. However, in broad terms, they can be divided into: changes in technology, including diagnostics and treatments; changes in patients, who have become older, frailer, and often more socially isolated; changes in models of care, involving networks and integrated pathways; and changes in staffing, affecting the need for both specialists and generalists.

The changing policy context within which hospitals operate

The preceding paragraphs have outlined the clinical changes that have driven developments in hospitals. However, there have also been many changes in the broader policy context within which they operate.

The first of these changes is in relation to accountability. For most of the 20th century what a hospital did, and how it did it, was determined largely by the medical profession (Freidson, 1974). Typically, each department was headed by a specialist physician or surgeon whose rule was absolute. Each department was largely autonomous, maintaining strict control over staff and resources. There was a tacit assumption that the senior physicians knew best, drawing on their long experience and status. It was inconceivable that their decisions would be questioned, no matter how idiosyncratic they seemed. Their relations with other health professionals, their junior staff, and patients were characterized by deference and, in some elite hospitals, their ward rounds could assume the trappings of a royal visit (Osterberg, 1990).

This situation reflected the prevailing approach to the professions. Professions were granted certain rights, in particular that of self-regulation, and high status. Members of professions had accumulated knowledge through a long process of apprenticeship. They were expected to exercise complex judgement, often in the face of uncertainty. It was not clear how anyone from outside the profession could second-guess them. In return, they were expected to maintain high ethical standards and obligations to the public (Freidson, 1988).

In all but a few places such situations are no more. There are many reasons. One is a wider societal rejection of deference to authority of all sorts. Another is a recognition that sometimes the professions fail to live up to the high standards they are expected to adhere to, whether in terms of competence or probity (Kaplan, 2007). A third relates to the growing commercialization of health care in some countries, whereby professional knowledge and status are seen as a barrier to the operation of the free market. Although health professionals remain among the most trusted groups in society (Appleby & Robertson, 2016), politicians and the media are unwilling to countenance the high level of professional autonomy that once existed (Rao et al., 2017). The extent to which this has happened varies enormously among countries and in some the concept of the liberal profession still holds sway. In others, however, health professionals are finding their work increasingly subject to high levels of regulation and monitoring, impacting adversely on morale and levels of burnout (Chamberlain, 2016; Rao et al., 2017).

A second development relates to the explosion in data for monitoring. Health professionals have been monitoring outcomes of patients at least since the days of Florence Nightingale, albeit in very basic ways

(Caelleigh, 1997). Advances in information technology, psychometrics, and health services research more generally have led to new ways of monitoring health outcomes, often using linked data, for example, to the deaths occurring after discharge from hospital, as well as a wide range of patient-related outcome measures (Black, 2013).

These developments have facilitated a revolution in methods for assessing quality of care since the 1980s. However, this brings both opportunities and risks. In particular, publication of outcomes by individual health professionals has proven highly controversial, for several reasons. One is the challenge of adjusting adequately for case-mix or attributing an outcome to the action of an individual when the care is provided by a team (Jacobson, Mindell & McKee, 2003). A second is the potential for opportunistic behaviour, which can range from changes in recording of patient characteristics to avoidance of those patients at greatest risk of an adverse outcome (Burns et al., 2016). Finally, there are questions about whether publication accelerates or slows improvements in outcomes (Joynt et al., 2016). Notwithstanding these concerns, it is clear that hospitals now and in the future will increasingly be evaluated in terms of the health gain that they bring about and not just the money they spend and the patients that flow through their wards.

A third issue, also related to the first two, has been the emergence of what has been termed "patient safety" on the policy agenda (Longo et al., 2005). While overlapping to some extent with the concept of quality of care, this explicitly reflects a recognition that hospitals may, on occasions, damage health. This can happen in many ways (Institute of Medicine, 2001). Failures to put in place appropriate procedures can lead to patients receiving the wrong treatment, for example, an incompatible blood transfusion, a drug to which they are allergic, or even a surgical procedure on the wrong patient or on the wrong side of the right patient. Recognition that this is a problem has led to new organizational structures, to ensure that problems are identified early and dealt with effectively. Lessons have been learnt from other sectors, such as the system used by airline pilots experiencing near-misses (Nicholson & Tait, 2002).

A fourth issue is a change to the way in which hospitals are funded. Traditionally, hospitals receive their funding in a number of ways, including historical budgets and payments per patient or per bed day (McKee & Healy, 2002). However, the recognition that patients with different conditions incurred very different levels of expenditure created pressure for a much more differentiated system. The result in many countries has been the implementation of some form of activity-based system, typically based on the diagnosis of the patient and the procedures they undergo, with the best-known being versions of the American Diagnosis Related Groups (Busse, Geissler & Quentin, 2011). These systems are designed to incentivize hospitals to increase their efficiency, treating each patient with the minimum necessary resources. One consequence has been to bring about reductions, often substantial, in length of stay. Often this is a good thing, given the risks associated with being in hospital for prolonged periods (Asher, 1947). However, it presupposes that patients have somewhere safe and supportive to go to.

A final set of issues facing hospitals relates to the broader political context and, specifically, whether health care is seen as a tradable or a public service (Starr, 2008). In some countries, where the latter view has so far prevailed, hospitals are increasingly being seen as corporate entities and profit centres. This creates a powerful incentive to work in isolation, notwithstanding the importance of collaboration across the entire patient journey. Elsewhere, there is an increasing emphasis on networks, allowing patients to move freely within a system, obtaining routine care close to home when needed, but also access to advanced specialized services and specialized facilities if required. In a number of countries there has also been a significant growth in the number of hospitals that are part of groups, partly as a way of responding to some of the challenges detailed here but also as a method of reducing costs and improving quality through standardization and a greater role for professional management.

As with the changing clinical context, these issues are well recognized by those working in hospitals, but less often by those elsewhere who may be responsible for decisions that have profound consequences for hospitals and those who work in them. We believe that there is a need to bring all of these issues together: something that we have attempted to do in this book.

Rather than seeing hospitals as discrete entities within the health system that are often viewed in a mechanistic way through metrics such as numbers of beds or physicians, we view hospitals as complex adaptive systems, each containing a multiplicity of subsystems, some dealing with patients with particular conditions, such as a surgical department for example, while others provide resources that are shared among many of the other systems, such as operating theatres and pharmacies.

All of these systems interact with each other and are shaped by these interactions (Checkland, 1981).

We can only understand how they operate by looking at all levels, from the individual interaction between the patient and health professional through to the design and operation of the facility. However, this approach also recognizes that hospitals are situated within a broader health system, the optimal functioning of which depends on the linkage of many parts. This includes prehospital and post-discharge care. It also includes linkages to the training of health professionals, and the research and development that generates the knowledge on which effective care should be based. All of these systems and subsystems are operating in a rapidly changing environment, involving: the patients and their conditions; the opportunities to intervene, including technological advances and evidence on innovative models of care; and the broader policy and political context in which health care is delivered.

Consistent with the wider discourse in health policy, we have chosen to take a patient-centred approach. Pragmatically, this creates a problem. On the one hand, as we have noted, growing numbers of patients have multiple, complex needs and cannot easily be placed into individual categories. On the other hand, it is necessary to simplify our approach to make sense of the complexity. Consequently, in this book we have focused primarily on the acute general hospital rather than single speciality or specialized hospitals, long-stay facilities, and those providing restricted services or mainly convalescence (although in some chapters we do consider specialist hospitals too). We have looked at a number of the most important activities in which hospitals engage, defined by the conditions of their patients.

Meeting the needs of patients

We now look at the areas of hospital activity that are discussed in this volume. It is impossible to cover everything that is done within the hospital. Nor is it easy to create a simple taxonomy of the areas we could have covered. Consequently, we have selected a series of examples, looking at different patient groups, defined variously by age, disease process, and type of treatment, as well as some other areas where scientific advances have led to changes in patient management, such as imaging and laboratory science. While each contains a number of issues specific to the topic of the chapter, collectively they highlight many issues that have applicability more widely.

We start with children, the subject of Chapter 2 in this book. As noted above, the population of children in hospital has changed beyond all recognition in the last four decades. The wards that were once filled with children with common infectious diseases have gone. So has the generic paediatrician who once would have cared for children from birth to adolescence. Instead, there has been a remarkable diversification, of necessity given the high level of specialist skills required in many of the new areas that have emerged. This is perhaps most apparent with neonatal care. In 1975 one in every two premature newborns with a birthweight of less than 1500g died in the perinatal period. By 2009 this had fallen to one in eight. Moreover, an increasing proportion of births in some countries are at low birthweight, as a consequence of multiple pregnancies related to in vitro fertilization. This has had enormous implications for both obstetrics and neonatal paediatrics, although not without controversy, as it has brought into sharp relief the tension between centralization, specialization, and medicalization on the one hand and a vision of birth as a natural event, involving a partnership between the mother and her midwife that is usually free from complications. Clearly there is a challenge in getting the balance right. However, this can only be done by close coordination between the different facilities providing obstetric and neonatal care. It illustrates perfectly the need for clinical networks of hospitals and other settings for childbirth working together collaboratively.

The chapter also looks at developments in care for older children. This is also an area that has been transformed by the creation of new knowledge (Wolfe et al., 2013), although there is enormous diversity among European countries (Ehrich et al., 2015). One result is increasing specialization. As with adults, it is not possible to expect a single physician to be an expert in the many body systems in which problems may arise. Moreover, as is frequently pointed out, children are not simply small adults. Consequently, there is a need for the specialist knowledge that paediatricians bring to these areas. The difficulty is that many of these diseases are relatively uncommon. Services must be concentrated to be viable, leading to the growth of highly specialized paediatric centres. This can be a major challenge for many small countries, in this case calling for networks that extend beyond national frontiers (Saliba et al., 2014). Finally, it should never be forgotten that children should be kept out of hospitals as much as possible. Their physical, mental, and social development is best achieved at home with their families. As the chapter shows, there is much that can be done to make the hospital as friendly as possible for children (Lenton & Ehrich, 2015). However, although it may sometimes be needed, admission of children to hospital should always be a last resort.

The third chapter moves to the opposite end of the age spectrum, looking at one of the most common afflictions of middle and old age: stroke. Fortunately, the incidence of stroke has been falling dramatically in many high and middle income countries, largely as a result of improvements in the detection and management of hypertension (Lackland et al., 2014). However, as populations age, the absolute number of people affected by stroke is rising. The management of stroke has been transformed in recent years. Even as recently as the 1990s, many patients with stroke would simply be admitted to hospital to await a hopefully spontaneous recovery. Now, the focus is on early recognition of symptoms and signs, rapid transfer to hospital, early diagnosis using brain imaging, and definitive treatment. All of this must be achieved within a few hours and, if it can be, levels of disability can be reduced greatly. In a number of places, stroke services are organized on a population basis, reaching outside the hospital to begin the process of restoring blood supply to the affected part of the brain as soon as possible (Alonso de Lecinana et al., 2016; Turner et al., 2016), in some cases using ambulances with computerized tomography (CT) scanners linked by telemedicine to specialist centres (Ebinger et al., 2014). However, this is only the beginning of the process, with subsequent management seeking to tackle the reasons why the stroke occurred, to prevent it recurring, and to provide the rehabilitation necessary to make as full a recovery as possible.

Once again, this chapter makes a very strong argument for a comprehensive approach to, in this case, a particular condition. This involves measures that address all of the building blocks of the health system, including a trained workforce, appropriate technology, and high levels of training. Yet, as it also shows, there are many barriers to achieving this and – still – great variation in the outcomes of treatment. This is an area where there are many opportunities for shared learning and comparisons of policies and practices.

The fourth chapter looks at a group of people whose numbers are growing rapidly but who often fall through the gaps in the hospital system (Oliver, Foot & Humphries, 2014). These are frail elderly people. Successes of modern medicine have allowed many more people to live into old age, albeit while experiencing the consequences of multiple disorders and declining bodily functions. Yet, with appropriate support, they can still live a fulfilling and satisfying life. The loss of functional reserve does, however, mean that they will require specialist advice in hospital outpatient clinics from time to time, and are prone to episodes of illness when they will require treatment in hospital. The challenge, in an increasingly specialized hospital system, is how best to design hospitals that are appropriate to their often complex needs (Crews & Zavotka, 2006) and how to manage individuals who may have disorders of four or five different body systems, drawing on evidence such as that showing how procedures like comprehensive geriatric assessment can improve management and outcomes (Ellis et al., 2011).

This chapter looks at some of the more innovative approaches to responding to the needs of this vulnerable group of people. It includes the creation of care coordination mechanisms, whereby they are helped to navigate through the complexities of the health care system, and in particular, avoiding the risk of falling through the gaps. It also includes the availability of rapid access and response teams, located either in hospitals or in the community, but able to provide assessment and treatment wherever it is needed (Wright et al., 2014). In some ways, the process of ageing is the mirror image of development in childhood. Just as with children, frail elderly and, especially, confused people can find hospitals unfamiliar and disorientating. Yet, as with children, there is much that can be done to ensure that hospitals are friendly to older people when they do need to be admitted. One solution is the creation of dedicated frailty units, where patients can be cared for by specialized nurses with experience in issues such as falls, dementia, and incontinence (Conroy et al., 2014). And finally, it involves attention to hospital design, to ensure that the accommodation in which frail elderly people find themselves can meet their needs and expectations as effectively as possible.

The fifth chapter looks at another complex problem: cancer. This is an area that has been in the forefront of developing networks and multidisciplinary teams, recognizing the need for patients to be able to move seamlessly through a complex system from diagnosis to treatment and, if this is unsuccessful, to palliation. Often the management of cancer is straightforward, with surgery or radiotherapy achieving high levels of cure. But in many cases it is extremely complex. There have been remarkable advances in our understanding of the biology of cancer cells, leading to innovative new treatments that target them precisely. However, this can only be achieved with close working between a wide range of specialists. As with many of the other areas considered in this book, this increased knowledge has brought about a high level of specialization, with oncologists, or in some cases teams of surgeons, interventional radiologists, oncologists and others working together, now increasingly specializing in cancer of a single organ.

Cancer care has also been at the forefront of monitoring and evaluation, with most countries having well-functioning cancer registries. This has made it possible to identify, and in many cases explain, variations in outcomes. In some countries this knowledge has contributed to major reorganizations of cancer services, and in particular the creation of integrated networks. Yet again, cancer reveals the importance of organization, with collaboration rather than competition among hospitals.

The burden of disease in high income countries is dominated by chronic disorders. Increasingly, these are managed out of hospital. This was not always the case, and even now in many countries people with diabetes spend long periods in hospital, especially if they have complications. To illustrate the challenges involved in the hospital management of chronic diseases, we have selected, for the sixth chapter, one condition: chronic obstructive pulmonary disease (COPD). In most cases, those affected will be managed outside hospital, but they will, from time to time, often experience exacerbations that require admission. As with stroke, in the past such patients were often admitted, treated, and discharged. Many of them would return frequently, especially in winter, so they became well known to the hospital staff. As this chapter shows, treatment has been revolutionized by new approaches to the active management of this condition, and in particular a major focus on prevention, involving measures to improve lung function. Yet, as with stroke and cancer, there are still large variations across and within industrialized countries in the extent to which services for these people have moved from a reactive model to one that actively seeks to restore them to as good health as possible.

The seventh chapter deals with that part of the hospital that has come, in the popular imagination, to represent acute health care. This is the case of emergency medicine. As with all of the other areas, this has changed remarkably. Traditionally, the emergency department functioned as the front door of the hospital, through which an undifferentiated mass of people, with problems ranging from the trivial to the life-threatening, would pass. Those in the emergency department were confronted with the challenge of sorting them out, deciding which required immediate treatment and which could wait. Mixed among them were children, often exposed to sights that they would be forbidden from watching in a movie theatre. Now, however, the management of the acutely ill patient often begins before they ever reach the hospital, with trained paramedics commencing treatment in the patient's home, at the roadside, or in the ambulance. Once they reach the hospital, they are triaged rapidly, their needs prioritized, and appropriate treatment begun as rapidly as possible. As with the conditions discussed in the other chapters, technological advances have transformed many aspects of emergency medicine. There has been a growing recognition of the importance of early stabilization and resuscitation and in many cases definitive treatment. Yet again, this demands a high level of organization. Teams need to be brought together, they need shared protocols, and they need to be present, with the appropriate equipment and facilities, at all times.

The eighth chapter looks at another aspect of the work of the hospital that, for many people, characterizes it. This is what happens in operating theatres, but now increasingly also what happens before patients get to theatre and how they recover afterwards. Technological advances, for example in intravenous anaesthesia, allowing people to recover rapidly, as well as in minimally invasive surgery and interventional radiology, have transformed surgery. For many people, especially if they are young and healthy, this means that a procedure that would once have required an admission over several days can now be completed within hours, allowing them to return home that evening. However, these advances have also lowered the threshold for intervention, especially with regard to those whose conditions might once have precluded surgery (Moug et al., 2016). This, coupled with new opportunities for the more complex types of surgery, means that there is an increasing need for post-operative care, which has developed into a specialty in its own right. Again, this is something that requires careful planning, not just to put the systems in place, but to ensure the flow of patients through the hospital.

The final two chapters look at two of the reasons why the modern hospital developed in the first place: laboratories and imaging. As noted earlier, these are areas that have changed remarkably, in many different ways. Once, an imaging department depended on X-rays to look inside the body. Now, it can call upon ultrasound and MRI, with the bodily organs highlighted using a multiplicity of contrast agents and, in some cases, radioactive tracers. It can do so with a precision undreamt of in the past, allowing the radiologist to view the patient in three dimensions and creating a form of virtual reality. In parallel, a new specialization has emerged. This is interventional radiology, where endoscopic instruments are manipulated under radiographic guidance, making it possible to undertake major proceedings without actually opening the body cavities. However, this has created tensions in some countries, with demarcation disputes between this new group of interventional radiologists and surgeons (Baerlocher & Detsky, 2009).

Laboratory medicine has also changed, again driven by advances in technology. There has been a remarkable growth in opportunities for near-patient and self-testing (Larsson, Greig-Pylypczuk & Huisman, 2015) but this has also created challenges as the results must frequently be interpreted by those with the expertise and ability to make an assessment of the whole patient. Increasingly, this means that pathologists are moving out of the laboratory, becoming part of the MDT caring for the patient, advising on the most appropriate tests that should be done and how their results should be interpreted, especially in patients that have multiple disease processes simultaneously.

Conclusion

As this introduction shows, the work of the hospital has changed beyond all recognition in a few decades. Yet its design has often failed to keep pace with these developments. In the final chapter, we will look at some of the challenges that face the hospital in the future. These include the growth of antimicrobial resistance, a problem that has largely been created by hospitals in the way that they operate. Yet there is now extensive evidence that the design and function of hospitals can do much to prevent its emergence. They also include the need to design hospitals in ways that take account of the needs of different groups of patients (Rechel, Wright & Edwards, 2009). As discussed already, these include children and frail elderly people. There are already many examples of good practice, with designs that address their needs, but too often there is a sense that the hospital has been assembled with no thought about those who will use it, whether this involves the use of materials that amplify noise at night, thereby preventing people from sleeping (DuBose & Hadi, 2016), or the lack of signposting that allows people to get lost (Wright, Hull & Lickorish, 1993). Finally, it is often forgotten that those who spend the most time in hospitals are not the patients but the staff. At a time when many countries are facing acute shortages of health workers, it is essential that the hospital is configured in a way that is welcoming to them and allows them to do their work as effectively and efficiently as possible.

Above all, the pace of change is so rapid that it is essential that those facilities being designed today are built in a manner that is flexible, and allows them to adapt to these changing circumstances. We hope that this book will assist those who, in whatever role, are interested in hospitals and, in particular, how they can best meet the needs of patients and staff in the future.

References

Alonso de Lecinana M et al. (2016). A collaborative system for endovascular treatment of acute ischaemic stroke: the Madrid Stroke Network experience. *Eur J Neurol*, 23:297–303.

Appleby J, Robertson R (2016). *Public satisfaction with the NHS in 2015*. London, King's Fund.

Asher RA (1947). Dangers of going to bed. *BMJ*, 2:967.

Baerlocher MO, Detsky AS (2009). Professional monopolies in medicine. *JAMA*, 301:858–60.

Barnett K et al. (2012). Epidemiology of multimorbidity and implications for health care, research, and medical education: a cross-sectional study. *Lancet*, 380:37–43.

Black N (2013). Patient reported outcome measures could help transform healthcare. *BMJ*, 346:f167.

Burns EM et al. (2016). Understanding the Strengths and Weaknesses of Public Reporting of Surgeon-Specific Outcome Data. *Health Aff (Millwood)*, 35, 415–21.

Busse R, Geissler A, Quentin W (2011). *Diagnosis-related groups in Europe: moving towards transparency, efficiency and quality in hospitals*. Buckingham, McGraw-Hill.

Caelleigh AS (1997). Florence Nightingale and medical statistics. *Acad Med*, 72:668.

Chamberlain JM (2016). Risk-based regulation and reforms to fitness to practise tribunals in the United Kingdom: Serving the public interest? *Health, Risk & Society*, 18:318–34.

Checkland P (1981). *Systems thinking, systems practice.* Chichester, Wiley.

Clifford P et al. (1991). Planning for community care. Long-stay populations of hospitals scheduled for rundown or closure. *Br J Psychiatry,* 158:190–6.

Conroy SP et al. (2014). A controlled evaluation of comprehensive geriatric assessment in the emergency department: the "Emergency Frailty Unit". *Age Ageing,* 43:109–14.

Crews DE, Zavotka S (2006). Aging, disability, and frailty: implications for universal design. *J Physiol Anthropol,* 25:113–18.

Daniel TM (2006). The history of tuberculosis. *Respir Med,* 100:1862–70.

Dougherty PJ et al. (2004). Orthopaedic surgery advances resulting from World War II. *J Bone Joint Surg Am,* 86:176–81.

DuBose JR, Hadi K (2016). Improving inpatient environments to support patient sleep. *Int J Qual Health Care,* 28:540–53.

Ebinger M et al. (2014). Effect of the use of ambulance-based thrombolysis on time to thrombolysis in acute ischemic stroke: a randomized clinical trial. *JAMA,* 311:1622–31.

Ehrich JH et al. (2015). Diversity of Pediatric Workforce and Education in 2012 in Europe: A Need for Unifying Concepts or Accepting Enjoyable Differences? *J Pediatr,* 167:471–6.e4.

Eiseman B (1967). Combat casualty management in Vietnam. *J Trauma,* 7:53–63.

Ellis G et al. (2011). Comprehensive geriatric assessment for older adults admitted to hospital: meta-analysis of randomised controlled trials. *BMJ,* 343:d6553.

Freidson E (1974). *Professional dominance: The social structure of medical care.* Livingston, NJ, Transaction Publishers.

Freidson E (1988). *Profession of medicine: A study of the sociology of applied knowledge.* Chicago, University of Chicago Press.

Geomelas M et al. (2011). "The Maestro": a pioneering plastic surgeon – Sir Archibald McIndoe and his innovating work on patients with burn injury during World War II. *J Burn Care Res,* 32:363–8.

Goff DA et al. (2017). A global call from five countries to collaborate in antibiotic stewardship: united we succeed, divided we might fail. *Lancet Infect Dis,* 17:e56–e63.

Hayter M (1997). Confidentiality and the acquired immune deficiency syndrome (AIDS): an analysis of the legal and professional issues. *J Adv Nurs,* 25:1162–6.

Institute of Medicine (2001). *Crossing the quality chasm: a new health system for the 21st century.* Washington, DC, National Academy Press.

Jacobson B, Mindell J, McKee M (2003). Hospital mortality league tables. *BMJ*, 326:777–8.

Jessney B (2012). Joseph Lister (1827–1912): a pioneer of antiseptic surgery remembered a century after his death. *J Med Biogr*, 20:107–10.

Joynt KE et al. (2016). Public Reporting of Mortality Rates for Hospitalized Medicare Patients and Trends in Mortality for Reported Conditions. *Ann Intern Med*, 165:153–60.

Kaplan R (2007). The clinicide phenomenon: an exploration of medical murder. *Australas Psychiatry*, 15:299–304.

Lackland DT et al. (2014). Factors influencing the decline in stroke mortality: a statement from the American Heart Association/American Stroke Association. *Stroke*, 45:315–53.

Larsson A, Greig-Pylypczuk R, Huisman A (2015). The state of point-of-care testing: a European perspective. *Ups J Med Sci*, 120:1–10.

Lenton S, Ehrich J (2015). Approach to Child-Friendly Health Care – The Council of Europe. *J Pediatr*, 167:216–18.

Longo DR et al. (2005). The long road to patient safety: a status report on patient safety systems. *JAMA*, 294:2858–65.

Loopstra R et al. (2016). Austerity and old-age mortality in England: a longitudinal cross-local area analysis, 2007–2013. *J R Soc Med*, 109:109–16.

Lu Y et al. (2014). Multidisciplinary management strategies for acute non-variceal upper gastrointestinal bleeding. *Br J Surg*, 101:e34–50.

McCaul M, Lourens A, Kredo T (2014). Pre-hospital versus in-hospital thrombolysis for ST-elevation myocardial infarction. *Cochrane Database Syst Rev*, 9:Cd010191.

McCullough AL et al. (2014). Early management of the severely injured major trauma patient. *Br J Anaesth*, 113:234–41.

McKee M, Healy J (2002). *Hospitals in a changing Europe*. Citeseer.

Molnar TF et al. (2004). Changing dogmas: history of development in treatment modalities of traumatic pneumothorax, hemothorax, and posttraumatic empyema thoracis. *Ann Thorac Surg*, 77:372–8.

Moodley N et al. (2015). Historical perspectives in clinical pathology: a history of glucose measurement. *J Clin Pathol*, 68:258–64.

Moug SJ et al. (2016). Frailty and cognitive impairment: Unique challenges in the older emergency surgical patient. *Ann R Coll Surg Engl*, 98:165–9.

Mukherjee S (2010). *The emperor of all maladies: a biography of cancer*. New York, Simon & Schuster.

Neushul P (1993). Science, government, and the mass production of penicillin. *Journal of the history of medicine and allied sciences*, 48:371.

Nicholson AN, Tait PC (2002). Confidential reporting: from aviation to clinical medicine. *Clin Med (Lond)*, 2:234–6.

Nicholson C, Gordon AL, Tinker A (2016). Changing the way "we" view and talk about frailty. *Age Ageing,* 46:349–51.

Oliver D, Foot C, Humphries R (2014). *Making our health and care systems fit for an ageing population.* London, King's Fund.

Osterberg P (1990). The lure and lore of surgery. *Ulster Med J*, 59:11.

Porter R (1999). *The Greatest Benefit to Mankind: A Medical History of Humanity.* London, WW Norton & Company.

Prades J et al. (2015). Is it worth reorganising cancer services on the basis of multidisciplinary teams (MDTs)? A systematic review of the objectives and organisation of MDTs and their impact on patient outcomes. *Health Policy*, 119:464–74.

Rao SK et al. (2017). The Impact of Administrative Burden on Academic Physicians: Results of a Hospital-Wide Physician Survey. *Acad Med*, 92:237–43.

Rechel B, Wright S, Edwards N (2009). *Investing in hospitals of the future.* Copenhagen, WHO Regional Office for Europe on behalf of the European Observatory for Health Systems and Policies.

Reed AB (2011). The history of radiation use in medicine. *J Vasc Surg*, 53:3s–5s.

Roll-Hansen N (1979). Experimental method and spontaneous generation: the controversy between Pasteur and Pouchet, 1859–64. *Journal of the History of Medicine and Allied Sciences*, 34:273.

Saliba V et al. (2014). Clinicians', policy makers' and patients' views of pediatric cross-border care between Malta and the UK. *J Health Serv Res Policy*, 19:153–60.

Starr P (2008). *The social transformation of American medicine: The rise of a sovereign profession and the making of a vast industry.* New York, Basic Books.

Turner AJ, Nikolova S, Sutton M (2016). The effect of living alone on the costs and benefits of surgery amongst older people. *Social Science & Medicine*, 150:95–103.

Turner S et al. (2016). Lessons for major system change: centralization of stroke services in two metropolitan areas of England. *J Health Serv Res Policy*, 21:156–65.

Voswinckel P (1994). A marvel of colors and ingredients. The story of urine test strip. *Kidney Int Suppl*, 47:S3–7.

Wilson MH et al. (2015). Pre-hospital emergency medicine. *Lancet*, 386:2526–34.

Wolfe I, McKee M (2014). *European Child Health Services and Systems: Lessons Without Borders*. Buckingham, McGraw-Hill.

Wolfe I et al. (2013). Health services for children in western Europe. *Lancet*, 381:1224–34.

Wollman AJ et al. (2015). From Animaculum to single molecules: 300 years of the light microscope. *Open Biol*, 5:150019.

Wright P, Hull AJ, Lickorish A (1993). Navigating in a hospital outpatients' department: the merits of maps and wall signs. *Journal of Architectural and Planning Research*, 10:76–89.

Wright PN et al. (2014). The impact of a new emergency admission avoidance system for older people on length of stay and same-day discharges. *Age Ageing*, 43:116–21.

2 | *The challenges of adapting hospital care for children*

JOCHEN EHRICH[1,2], MASSIMO PETTOELLO-MANTOVANI [1,3], ELEANOR MOLLOY[4], REINHOLD KERBL[1,5], MEHMET VURAL[1,6], SIMON LENTON[1,7], STEFANO DEL TORSO[8], ADAMOS HADJIPANAYIS[9], BJÖRN WETTERGREN[10], ZACHI GROSSMAN[11]

[1] European Paediatric Association – Union of National Paediatric Societies and Associations (EPA-UNEPSA), Berlin, Germany
[2] Children's Hospital, Hannover Medical School, Hannover, Germany
[3] Institute of Pediatrics, University of Foggia, Istituto di Ricovero e Cura a Carattere Scientifico "Casa Sollievo", Foggia, Italy
[4] Trinity College, University of Dublin, Tallaght Hospital, Coombe Women's and Infants Hospital and Our Lady's Children's Hospital, Dublin, Ireland
[5] General Hospital Leoben, Department of Paediatrics and Adolescent Medicine, Leoben, Austria
[6] Istanbul University, Cerrahpaşa Medical Faculty, Neonatology Unit, Istanbul, Turkey
[7] Child Health Department, Bath, United Kingdom
[8] Studio Pediatrico, Vecellio 33 ULSS16, Padova, Italy
[9] Faculty of Medicine, European University, Nikosia, Cyprus
[10] Paediatric Department, Region Gävleborg, Gävle, Sweden
[11] Paediatric Clinic, Maccabi Health Services, Tel Aviv, Israel

Acknowledgement: The authors gratefully acknowledge the discussions with the presidents of national paediatric societies and associations in Europe.

Child health care in Europe

The role of the hospital in caring for children has changed beyond recognition in the past five decades. On the one hand, the conditions that were once responsible for most bed occupancy, such as respiratory tract infections, gastroenteritis, and hepatitis A, are now far less common and, when they occur, are managed at home in all but the most severe cases. On the other hand, advances in medicine and technology, coupled with better understanding of genetics, metabolic and neonatal medicine, new treatments for cancer and acute/chronic organ failure, advances in surgical techniques, and new ways of managing severe mental disorders, have created a need for services that did not previously exist (Wolfe et al., 2013). Consequently, the hospital continues to play a key role in the health care of children, albeit one that is rapidly adapting to the changing needs of sick foetuses, newborns, infants, children, and adolescents. Hospital services for children must also be able to work closely with other parts of the health system and beyond, reaching out to wider services for children including education, prevention, long-term outpatient care for children with rare diseases, and primary care out of normal hours. Yet a survey conducted in 2015 revealed great diversity in hospital services for children in the 53 countries of the World Health Organization's European region (Ehrich, Namazova-Baranova & Pettoello-Mantovani, 2016). Differences are apparent even at the most basic level: the definition of a child. The age at which young people are no longer managed in children's hospital services varies among countries. In 53% of countries childhood is defined as up to 18 years of age, but in one country it is up to 11, in three up to 14, in four up to 15, in six up to 16, and in one up to 17 years of age. Two countries reported the upper age limit for children in paediatric services to be 19 and in one country it is 26 years (Ehrich et al., 2015a).

There are also considerable variations in the settings in which children receive hospital care. A 2009 survey conducted by the European Paediatric Association identified four different types of children's hospital in Europe: 1) general children's hospitals and paediatric units (or paediatric wards) within larger hospitals for adults; 2) stand-alone children's hospitals; 3) university children's hospitals; and 4) mother and child centres. Day clinics and neonatal intensive care units (NICUs) were found in all four types of hospital. There are also major differences in infrastructure, such as diagnostics and therapeutics, especially high technology equipment, as well as organizational arrangements and markers of quality.

As with every other aspect of medicine, health services for children must adapt to a rapidly changing landscape. One way in which this landscape is changing is the demography of Europe. With a falling birth rate, Europe is facing a declining child population. The mean shares of the total population aged 0–14 years and 0–4 years in Europe were 21.2% and 6.4% respectively in 1982 but these figures had fallen to

15.2% and 5.0% in 2014. The scale of the change can be seen from looking at three countries, Belgium, Ireland, and Portugal, where the fertility rate decreased from 2.54, 3.78 and 3.16 respectively in 1960 to 1.75, 1.96 and 1.21 in 2013 respectively (Eurostat, 2016).

This demographic change, coupled with changes in disease patterns and treatment settings, has contributed to a large reduction of hospital beds and to the closure or merging of children's hospital facilities and thus is challenging conventional ways of thinking about hospital facilities for children. Traditionally based on a division between primary, secondary, and tertiary care, new models of care seek ways to innovate and improve the whole system. The changes are complex and do not simply involve crude reductions in hospital capacity. For example, on the one hand, the decline in the incidence of communicable diseases through immunization programmes, as well as injuries through injury prevention programmes, has caused a decrease in the need for care and consequently hospital admissions. On the other hand, medical and surgical advances, in areas such as neonatal surgery and intensive care, oncology, and interventions for inherited diseases, are increasing the need for highly specialized care that can only be provided in tertiary hospitals. At the same time, there is a continuing burden of chronic diseases – some attributable to increasing risk factors, such as childhood obesity, and some to improved survival of previously fatal conditions, such as malignancies and certain inherited disabilities. This has created a greater need for specialist care that transcends the hospital and the community (Wolfe & McKee, 2014), a need that is also increasing because of the improved survival of very low birthweight babies, some of whom are living with long-term disabilities. These children require sophisticated diagnostic and therapeutic interventions delivered by well-trained personnel using technologically advanced infrastructure.

In addition to the complications created by the increasing specialization of care provided for children in hospitals, there is a growing recognition of the importance of designing systems from the perspective of the user rather than the provider of services. This is exemplified by the call to design "a hospital that does not feel like a hospital". This thinking has been captured in the Council of Europe's "Child-Friendly Health Care" approach, which was endorsed by 47 ministers representing the nations of Europe (Lenton & Ehrich, 2015) (Box 2.1). This approach brought systems thinking and values based on the United Nations Convention on the Rights of the Child together into a practical framework to plan, deliver and improve services for children and families. The child-friendly health care approach builds on patient-centred care and patient pathways. The responsibility of the health system is to ensure that all the component parts are in place and working well together to achieve the best possible outcomes. This can only happen if appropriate child health care networks, based on collaboration (Future Ho . This spital Commission, 2013), can work together to improve quality continuously. Crucially, the hospital is a key element of these networks. Despite the shift from inpatient to outpatient care and the fall in the mean duration of stay in hospital the hospital is still very important. Although their work often extends beyond the walls of the hospital into the community, it is still the case that in many European countries about half of all paediatricians are still hospital-based (Ehrich et al., 2015a).

Box 2.1 Extract from the terms of reference of the Council of Europe on child-friendly health care

Five principles are particularly relevant to the child-friendly health care approach:

1. Participation

Participation means that children have the right to be informed, consulted, and heard, to give their opinions independently from their parents, and to have their opinions considered. It implies the recognition of children as active stakeholders and describes the process by which they take part in decision-making. The level of child participation depends both on his or her age, evolving capacities, maturity, and on the importance of the decision to be taken.

Parents and families should encourage children to participate in family, community and society decision-making – encouraging increasing independence and reducing their support as the child's capacity for autonomy and independence develops.

2. Promotion

Health promotion is "the process of enabling people to increase control over their health and its determinants and thereby improve their health". Promotion therefore includes all actions that allow

Box 2.1 (cont.)

children to become more involved in their own health and increase their exposure to positive determinants of health (defined as factors which will improve health or well-being). Health promotion covers not only activities in families and communities, directed at health determinants or lifestyles, but also factors in health care services and settings which will improve outcomes.

3. Protection

Health protection includes all actions that either limit or avoid children's exposure to any hazard which can be defined as a factor that has the potential to cause harm. Hazards can occur in families, communities and health services. Medical interventions can cause harm and patient safety perspectives highlight the fact that children are particularly vulnerable to medication errors and hospital-acquired infections.

4. Prevention

Prevention is an active process the aim of which is to avoid future health, social or emotional problems to enable the fullest realisation of human potential. This includes action to reduce adverse health determinants, to prevent the development of a disease or condition, to avoid complications of a disease or condition, to prevent the impact of a disease or condition on the lifestyle or aspirations of an individual, and to prevent harm caused by a service or intervention.

5. Provision

Provision refers to any service which contributes to the health and well-being of children and families, and therefore includes more than just traditional health services. "Pathway-based provision" is a concept that describes all the component parts that need to be in place and working well together to achieve an excellent patient experience which brings about optimal outcomes for children and families in their journey through services.

Source: Lenton & Ehrich, 2015

Clearly, in the light of the preceding discussion, there is no simple way to structure a chapter on the care of children in hospital. Consequently, we have taken a pragmatic approach, looking first at the highly-specialized care of newborn infants, followed by the care of older children with common conditions requiring hospitalization, and then the provision of highly specialized care in tertiary hospitals. We then review some common patient pathways, illustrating the inter-linkages between the different elements of the system before looking to emerging developments that may impact on the health system response to children in the future.

Maternal, neonatal and follow-up care in specialized facilities

Trends in obstetric and neonatal care

The management of pregnancy and childbirth has been transformed in recent decades, both organizationally and in terms of the technology and knowledge base required to achieve improved outcomes. These changes have been accompanied by a marked improvement in outcomes. Neonatal mortality has improved substantially during the last four decades. In 1975 the 28 current European Union Members (EU28) experienced 12.84 neonatal deaths per 1000 live births, yet by 2014 this had fallen to 2.52 per 1000 live births. This reflects several factors, including a reduction in low birthweight babies, and especially, survival among those born prematurely. Consequently, in 1975 half of all premature newborns with a birthweight less than 1500g died during the postnatal period but this fell to 14.3% and 12.4%, in 2000 and 2009 respectively (European Society for Neonatology, 2015). Maternal morbidity and mortality have also improved significantly.

These changes have been accompanied by several, often conflicting, trends taking place in the organization of services during childbirth in European countries that have implications for the future role of the hospital. In the past, many deliveries took place in small local hospitals, close to where people lived. These hospitals often had limited facilities but had the advantage of convenience for the mother and her family. However, the falling birth rate in many countries and the subsequent reduction in demand for delivery facilities threatens the viability of these hospitals, many of which have closed for other reasons, such as the inability to provide comprehensive, 24-hour, advanced medical and surgical services. Moreover, the smaller hospitals were unable to provide the facilities required when complications arose during childbirth. Yet, while many of the other services that these hospitals once provided have been transferred to larger hospitals with more sophisticated equipment, there is also pressure to de-medicalize childbirth, leading either to increased home births or to the development of stand-alone family friendly facilities, separate from acute hospitals.

Such facilities clearly meet the needs of the majority of expectant mothers. However, there are some who have other conditions that place them at high risk, such as advanced cystic fibrosis or cardiac insufficiency, or who are post-transplant, who require careful monitoring by a MDT that brings together adult medical, obstetric, and neonatal care. In the past, many of these mothers would not have survived into adulthood, and those who did would have been advised against becoming pregnant. With individualized care planning for delivery, coupled with advances in intra-partum care, they can now expect to have a healthy baby. However, this intensity of management, and especially the involvement of multidisciplinary teams, can only be undertaken from a well staffed and equipped hospital facility, even though those expectant mothers that do require specialized medical or surgical intervention can often receive it on an ambulatory basis. An added complication is that in some countries there have been increases in the number of infants who require intensive care and specialist intervention, in part reflecting later pregnancies and multiple births following in vitro fertilization. Finally, as often noted, a normal delivery can only be assessed as such in retrospect.

For these reasons, there is a need to ensure close coordination between facilities undertaking deliveries, whether stand-alone or within acute general hospitals, and those facilities providing specialized neonatal care. Ideally, any pregnancy identified as high-risk should be delivered in a setting where the delivery suite and the NICU are adjacent, or at least on the same site, but it is also important to recognize that, while unanticipated complications of delivery are fortunately rare, they do happen, so there should also be mechanisms in place to enable early referral and rapid intervention to save the life of the mother and baby in stand-alone facilities.

There are other reasons for close collaboration between obstetric and neonatal services, including shared training and participation in research, especially that responding to the needs of mothers and babies with complications. Obstetrician involvement in postnatal NICU ward rounds and discussions with parents can improve the knowledge base for antenatal counselling, which should also ideally involve the MDT, including the obstetrician, neonatologist, and, where appropriate, teams providing surgical and highly specialized paediatric expertise.

This is, however, an area where technology and knowledge continue to advance rapidly. New resuscitation guidelines have recently been published by ILCOR/ERC/AHA in 2015 (Wyllie et al., 2015), including changes in resuscitation practice, such as resuscitation closer to the mother to allow delayed cord clamping, but requiring greater involvement of specialist neonatal care in the delivery suite. At the same time, advances in remote monitoring are making it possible for senior staff to provide input remotely during resuscitation. Other advances include greater use of point-of-care testing (POCT), discussed further in Chapter 10, but this will require adaptation, including the use of nanotechnology, to take account of the very small volumes of blood that can be taken from extremely premature infants.

Provision of NICU

Existing guidance suggests that in a typical western European country, based on contemporary practice, there is a need for 0.75 cots per 1000 births for intensive care, 0.75 cots per 1000 births for high dependency care, and 4.4 cots per 1000 births for special care (Laing et al., 2004). However, this must also take account of changes in the frequency of preterm births, such as the increases in several countries including the USA, Canada, Australia, Sweden, Scotland, and Wales (Hallsworth et al., 2008). In Europe, in countries with comparable levels of development and health care systems, preterm birth rates vary markedly, ranging from 5% to 10% among live births. A second question relates to the distribution of facilities. A German population-based study found that 28-day mortality was more closely associated with the numbers of neonates looked after in a NICU than with the number of births in the hospital, with the effect greatest for infants of less than 29 weeks' gestation (Heller et al., 2007), although a study in the USA found that, while both the number of very low birthweight babies and the numbers treated in NICUs were important determinants of good outcomes, the former was more important. Other researchers found that mortality in small NICUs is significantly increased (Bartels et al., 2006). This evidence has led the American Academy of Pediatrics, in its Committee on Fetus and Newborn report on Levels of Neonatal Care, to support larger-volume NICUs.

NICU design and environment

As survival of preterm infants has improved dramatically during recent decades, there has been a marked increase in the number of children treated in NICUs. Initially, in the late 1970s and 1980s, NICUs were designed as multipatient wards with some private rooms to isolate infants with infections. In the 1990s, as survival became commonplace, new ideas began to emerge about possible effects of the physical environment on the fragile, growing brain of newborns. In 1992 White and Whitman (1992) recommended some private rooms for neonates. Many studies have now found that preterm infants are influenced by the physical conditions in NICUs, such as noise (Long, Lucey & Philip, 1980) and lighting (Mann et al., 1986). Box 2.2 sets out suggested environmental and building standards.

The first all-private room NICU in Europe was built in Brest, France, for the express purpose of minimizing nosocomial infection (White, 2011), although no study has yet found that private rooms in NICUs enhance infection control. A study from the Karolinska group of hospitals in Stockholm compared the results of two different types of NICU: those with private rooms versus those with four-bed open rooms (Ortenstrand et al., 2010). Premature newborns cared for in private rooms showed marked reduction in ICU and total hospital days, as well as a reduction of bronchopulmonary dysplasia. However, recent research has highlighted the need for greater attention to the sound in the NICU as infants nursed in single rooms had significantly altered MRI findings compared to those in an open ward (Smith et al., 2011).

Guidelines developed within the WHO/UNICEF Baby-friendly Hospital Initiative (BFHI) (World Health Organization, 2016) propose that newborns who do not need NICU facilities should be cared for in their mother's room, with the support of specialized nurses to encourage and support bonding and support breastfeeding. Family rooms that allow parents to "room-in" and care for their infants also offer a means for siblings to meet and bond with the new baby without creating infection-control issues for the NICU.

Box 2.2 Environmental and building standards for NICUs

Noise: Sound levels should be kept at less than 40dB. Private rooms provide a decrease in the number of adults in the room, and a study by Robertson, Cooper-Peel & Vos (1999) showed clearly that decreasing conversation had the greatest effect on decreasing noise levels in a NICU.

Light: Adjustable lighting between 0.5 and 60ft-candles (5–600 lux) is appropriate for general lighting levels in NICUs and an indirect room lightening should be preferred. A circadian lighting scheme should be used in the patient care area.

Air quality: NICUs should be air-conditioned to the highest standards, with air temperature at 22–26 degrees Celsius, 30–60% relative humidity, and a minimum of six air-changes per hour.

Design: Careful design is needed, with extensive additional space for family, overnight stays, privacy and staff.

Private rooms: Single-family rooms (private rooms) allow infants to be cared for in a room where they are shielded from medical or social activity at a neighbouring bed. The risk of cross-contamination may also be reduced.

Levels of newborn care

Newborns need different levels of care in NICUs. The 2012 classification developed by the American Academy of Paediatrics is used widely (American Academy of Pediatrics, 2012). These facilities are divided among those providing basic care (level I), specialty care (level II), and subspecialty intensive care (level III, level IV). Level I facilities (well newborn nurseries) provide a basic level of care to neonates who are low risk. Neonatal resuscitation can be undertaken if required for every delivery in these units and healthy newborns can be evaluated and receive routine postnatal care. In addition, Level I units can care for preterm infants at 35 to 37 weeks' gestation who are physiologically stable, and can stabilize newborn infants who are less than 35 weeks' gestation or who are ill until they can be transferred to a facility at which specialty neonatal care is provided. Care is provided by paediatricians, family physicians, and nurse practitioners. The recommended ratio of nurses to babies is 1:4. Interestingly, a study of NICUs in California found no difference in quality across levels of NICU (Profit et al., 2016).

The British Association of Perinatal Medicine (BAPM) has published guidelines suggesting that units with fewer than 50 infants with birth-weight less than 1500g should plan to amalgamate with other units to ensure clinical skills and expertise are retained (British Association of Perinatal Medicine, 2010). The BAPM guidelines also highlight the importance of hand-washing facilities for parents and staff, as well as adequate space to prevent cross-infection between babies and isolation facilities for infected infants.

Care in a specialty-level facility (level II) should be reserved for stable or moderately ill newborn infants who are born at ≥32 weeks' gestation or who weigh ≥1500g at birth but have problems that are expected to resolve rapidly and who would not be anticipated to need subspecialty-level services on an urgent basis. Level II nurseries may provide assisted ventilation until the infant's condition either soon improves or the infant can be transferred to a higher-level facility. Care is provided by neonatologist and neonatal nurse practitioners (NNPs) in addition to level I staff. The recommended ratio of nurses to babies is 1:2.

Infants who are born at less than 32 weeks' gestation, weigh less than 1500g at birth, or have major medical or surgical conditions, regardless of gestational age, should be cared for at a level III facility. Level III facilities should be able to provide ongoing assisted ventilation for 24 hours or more, which may include conventional ventilation, high-frequency ventilation, and inhaled nitric oxide. A broad range of paediatric medical subspecialists and paediatric surgical specialists should be readily accessible on site or by prearranged agreements. Level III facilities should have the capability to perform advanced imaging with interpretation on an urgent basis, including CT, MRI, and echo-cardiography. Care is provided by paediatric medical subspecialists, paediatric anaesthesiologists, paediatric surgeons, and paediatric oph-thalmologists in addition to level II staff. The recommended ratio of nurses to babies is 1:1.

Level IV units include everything that is available at level III with additional ability to care for the most complex and critically ill newborn infants. Such units should have specialist paediatric medical and surgical consultants continuously available 24 hours a day. Level IV facilities also include the capability for surgical repair of complex conditions (such as congenital cardiac malformations that require cardiopulmonary bypass with or without extracorporeal membrane oxygenation). Care is provided by level III staff plus paediatric surgical subspecialists.

Good outcomes for neonates in the NICU are dependent on the availability of sufficient numbers of skilled neonatal nurses. Developing NNPs can help maintain skills and continuity of care as medical staff change frequently. In many countries NNPs are expanding into roles such as neonatal transport and NNP-led clinics. Clinical nurse specialists provide vital services in the areas of discharge planning, support for lactation, and resuscitation. In some areas community neonatal nurses provide pre- and post-discharge care and visits. Clinical nurses and midwives specializing in bereavement play an important and expanding role in maternity hospitals, supporting parents faced with an antenatal diagnosis of a potentially lethal condition or who have newborns who die in the first few weeks of life. The United Kingdom's Royal College of Paediatrics and Child Health (RCPCH) framework on withholding or withdrawing life-sustaining treatment in children and the neonatal palliative care guidelines offer guidance to health care providers in these situations. These health professionals can also address issues such as neonatal organ donation.

Speech and language therapists, dieticians, physiotherapists, psychologists, medical social workers and occupational therapists are all essential to the operation of a level III NICU. Neonatal dieticians are playing an increasing role in optimizing nutrition. The extended role pharmacist will become more important in contributing to staff and parental education on medication use and prevention of prescribing errors, as well as new pharmaceutical agent use in the NICU. The role of clinical engineers has expanded with newer devices with a broader range of uses, such as neonatal ventilators and monitoring equipment for transport and care of infants with neuro-critical conditions. Neonatal transport is an essential part of an integrated neonatal network. This service needs to be available round-the-clock, including specialized equipment such as that required for hypothermia therapy.

Beyond the classification of NICUs set out above, there is a need to consider separately the provision of extracorporeal membrane oxygenation (ECMO), a life support mechanism which allows blood to be taken from the body, oxygenated outside the body and returned, and carbon dioxide and oxygen exchanged. A randomized controlled trial conducted in the United Kingdom showed a clear benefit for newborn infants with severe respiratory failure.

Education for staff and families

The European Society of Neonatology (ESN) Curriculum for Training in Neonatology in Europe (European Society for Neonatology, 2015) was developed to support national training programmes. The ESN has created a database of national training programmes to encourage transparency and harmonization of subspecialist training in neonatology.

Technological advances have enabled simulation to become a core element of training, with dedicated simulation laboratories equipped with high-fidelity mannequins in many new level III units. This development has been encouraged by the implementation of the European Union (EU) working time directive, designed to reduce the known risks associated with long working hours. However, despite the clear benefits for patient safety, it has posed problems in enabling medical trainees to obtain adequate practical experience. Simulation offers a means to deliver carefully designed, well supervised training experiences that are a significant improvement over the ad hoc approaches used previously. Simulation also offers a means to provide coordinated training for the multidisciplinary teams whose work is now so essential in NICUs, allowing them to develop their skills in a team setting where they can realistically model clinical scenarios.

Reflecting the important role that parents play in the care of newborn infants, it is important that training should not be limited to staff. Although parents are supported as they come to terms with the health of their newborn infants, there is considerable scope to develop this more formally in association with NICUs, including preparation for those expectant parents where it is anticipated that their babies are likely to require a stay in a NICU, as well as preparation for the post-discharge period.

Secondary care for children

While much childhood illness can be managed in primary care, there will inevitably be children who require hospitalization in secondary care facilities. Table 2.1 sets out some examples of such conditions. However, the numbers involved will depend not only on the burden of disease in the population but also on the scope and quality of primary care, which varies greatly around Europe. Policies in many countries have sought to reduce unnecessary admissions to hospital as they are distressing for children, cause problems for parents, and are usually a less cost-effective way of treating acute illness. On the other hand, delayed referral of severely sick children to hospital may lead to preventable complications and death. Closing the organizational gaps between primary and secondary care for children is therefore an important task.

Table 2.1 *Selected examples of indications for admission of children to hospitals*

Paediatric subspecialty care	Standard indications	Optional* indications
Neurology	developmental disorders, di-/tetraplegia, gait disorders, headache, neuropathies, seizures, etc.	myopathies, motor, hearing, visual, mental and skeletal disabilities, specific sleep disorders, etc.
Ear, nose and throat	tonsillitis, otitis, sinusitis, lymphadenopathies, etc.	cholesteatoma
Cardiology	arterial hypertension, arrhythmias, myocarditis	cardiomyopathy
Pulmonology	laryngitis, bronchi(oli)tis, asthma, pneumonia	cystic fibrosis
Hepato-gastroenterology-Nutrition	gastroenteritis, appendicitis, hepatopathies, abdominal pain, etc.	chronic inflammatory bowel disease, intussusception, cholestasis, etc.
Hematology/Hemostaseology	anaemia(s), leukopaenia, immune thrombocytopaenia (ITP), preoperative screening	coagulopathies
Infectious diseases	meningitis, encephalitis, upper airway infections, hepatitis, borreliosis, etc.	tuberculosis
Urology/Nephrology	urinary tract infection, hydronephrosis, glomerulonephritis, etc.	common nephritic and nephrotic syndrome
Dermatology	all kinds of rashes, atopic dermatitis	haemangioma
Mental disorders	somatoform disorders	ADHD, depression

It is important to see the hospital as only one element within the wider health system. However, the way in which the hospital interacts with the other elements of the health system will vary, influenced by the organizational characteristics of the system. Across Europe, the responsibilities of hospitals caring for children are not uniformly defined and vary between countries and even regions within countries. Furthermore, they may vary according to whether the hospital is publicly or privately owned, with the former typically responsible for providing a comprehensive range of services while the latter can select those areas that are most profitable and incur least risk to the provider. Figure 2.1 illustrates these relationships, with the hospital bringing together a range of specialist expertise.

Where in the system a child is treated will vary according to a range of factors. However, even within a single system, the boundaries are not necessarily clear. Decision-making processes relating to treatment and referral are subject to different rules and regulations of the health systems, but also policies about what services to offer in what facility, themselves influenced by the interests of the health care personnel involved. For instance, the management of many long-term conditions, such as asthma, diabetes, or coagulopathies, may be provided in different settings in different countries. Despite the existence of such variations, it is desirable that those responsible for managing and providing care in hospitals should find ways to achieve consensus with primary care physicians and tertiary care paediatricians on standards to be adopted for infrastructure, facilities, staff, and quality of medical treatment.

Recognizing that, where possible, children and adolescents should be managed in settings other than in hospitals, when they are admitted they are entitled to have certain expectations:

- To be welcomed by friendly staff, whether doctors, nurses or others
- To be adequately informed about what is to be done and when;
- To have the option to be accompanied by mother, father, and other relatives;
- To be treated according to modern standards of evidence-based medicine;
- To experience as little pain as possible;
- To receive age- and disease-appropriate treatment;
- To be treated by staff trained to communicate with children and parents;
- To experience a private and respectful atmosphere whenever possible;

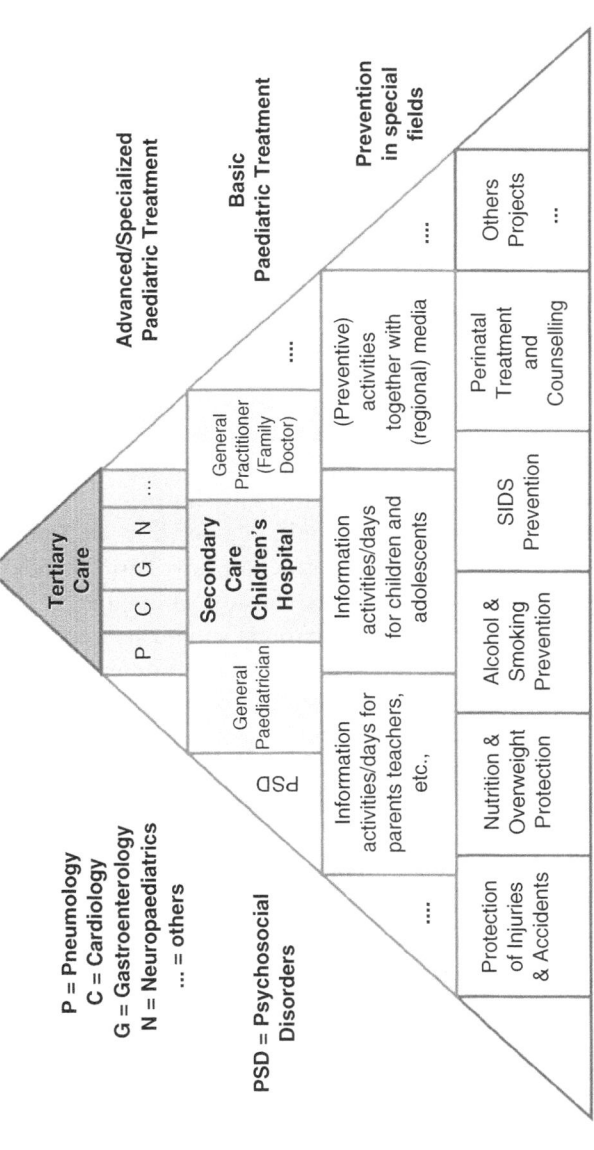

Figure 2.1 The position of hospital care for children within the health system

Source: Authors' compilation

- To be properly informed about all procedures and results of investigations;
- To stay in hospital for as short a time as possible;
- To receive adequate information about further treatment;
- To receive full treatment free of charge.

These expectations of patients and their care takers are consistent with the Charter of the European Association for Children in Hospital (EACH) (Box 2.3) (European Association for Children in Hospital, 2015).

Box 2.3 Charter of the European Association for Children in Hospital (EACH)

Article 1 Children shall be admitted to hospital only if the care they require cannot be equally well provided at home or on a day basis.

Article 2 Children in hospital shall have the right to have their parents or parent substitute with them at all times.

Article 3 Accommodation should be offered to all parents and they should be helped and encouraged to stay. Parents should not need to incur additional costs or suffer loss of income. In order to share in the care of their child, parents should be kept informed about ward routine and their active participation encouraged.

Article 4 Children and parents shall have the right to be informed in a manner appropriate to age and understanding. Steps should be taken to mitigate physical and emotional stress.

Article 5 Children and parents have the right to informed participation in all decisions involving their health care. Every child shall be protected from unnecessary medical treatment and investigation.

Article 6 Children shall be cared for together with children who have the same developmental needs and shall not be admitted to adult wards. There should be no age restrictions for visitors to children in hospital.

Article 7 Children shall have full opportunity for play, recreation and education suited to their age and condition and shall be in an environment designed, furnished, staffed and equipped to meet their needs.

Box 2.3 (cont.)

Article 8 Children shall be cared for by staff whose training and skills enable them to respond to the physical, emotional and developmental needs of children and families.

Article 9 Continuity of care should be ensured by the team caring for children.

Article 10 Children shall be treated with tact and understanding and their privacy shall be respected at all times.

Source: European Association for Children in Hospital, 2015

Highly specialized paediatric centres (tertiary care)

Expert specialist care is essential for the diagnosis and treatment of rare conditions and for children who require complex investigations and highly technical interventions, such as transplantation. This care typically requires sustained collaboration between different specialists and subspecialists to ensure optimal outcomes. However, while anecdotally it is known that there are different models of care, these have not, to our knowledge, been documented in detail.

Less well resourced countries in central and eastern Europe face the dilemma of how best to develop and fund specialist care in the future. Better resourced countries in western Europe face the problem of how best to rationalize and co-locate interdependent specialist services to improve outcomes. Small countries must find ways of developing effective cross-border care with larger countries, drawing on the many existing examples such as that between Malta and the United Kingdom (Saliba et al., 2014).

One of the key questions facing those organizing specialized paediatric services is how best to balance centralization and decentralization. There are various arguments for creating a small number of large centres that can concentrate expertise and equipment, can create multidisciplinary teams, and can provide 24-hour services where necessary. The last of these is particularly important as it typically requires about 10 individuals to provide round-the-clock service, a number that can only be justified if there is sufficient caseload. The question of whether concentration of services achieves better outcomes has been debated extensively. There is clear evidence to support this for some services, such as neonatal intensive care and cardiac surgery. However, the evidence is rather more limited in other areas. It is also important to recognize that concentration of services in large centres, especially in countries with low population densities, can create a significant barrier to access, although it may be possible to compensate for this by the development of outreach services, whereby specialists travel from tertiary centres to other facilities. These decisions about how to provide highly specialized services are complex and require many, often competing, objectives to be balanced (Ehrich et al., 2015a).

These decisions must also be informed by considerations of which specialties should be co-located. The current situation is characterized by significant differences in care across European countries. One fact is the absence of consistent European definitions of either specialist care or specialist centres. There are also differences in training programmes and assessment, both within and between specialties, with 38 different accredited paediatric subspecialties reported in a European Paediatric Association survey in 2014 (Table 2.2), which exceeded the 22 recognized in the USA in 2012. Individual European countries recognize between 0 and 20 separate paediatric subspecialties (Ehrich et al., 2015a). This also poses challenges to those organizing training programmes, especially where the numbers of physicians in particular subspecialties are very low. However, the situation is further complicated by the scarcity of data on the numbers and qualifications of specialists in most countries. There is also little information on scope of practice and required competencies.

While recognizing these difficulties, it is possible to suggest the most important interdependencies among specialties (Figure 2.2). Where possible, those services with clear interdependency should be co-located. For example, a centre undertaking organ transplantation should also have the expertise necessary to provide care in haemato-oncology, cardiology, nephrology, metabolic medicine, paediatric surgery, and a paediatric intensive care unit (grey squares), while subspecialties such as endocrinology (white squares) are not required. Tertiary care children's hospitals should have departments of child psychiatry and psychosomatic care in the same building. Transition and transfer of adolescents from paediatric to adult care should also take place in the same hospital, where possible (Crowley et al., 2011). Finally, the teams caring for children in hospital include teachers, who face particular challenges in meeting the needs of

Table 2.2 *Paediatric subspecialties in child health and the number of European countries in which each is recognized*

Adolescent medicine	1	**Neonatology**	16
Allergology	8	**Nephrology**	12
Anaesthesiology	2	**Neurology**	14
Cardiology	14	Neuro disability	1
Community paediatrics	1	Neuropsychiatry	5
Dermatology	2	**Oncology**	12
Developmental paediatrics	1	Ophthalmology	3
Emergency paediatrics	5	Orthopaedics	2
Endocrinology	13	Otorhinolaryngology	3
Gastroenterology	13	Palliative paediatrics	1
Genetics	2	Pharmacology	1
Gynaecology	2	**Pneumonology**	12
Haematology	8	Primary care paediatrics	5
Hepatology	2	Radiology	3
Immunology	3	Rehabilitation	3
Infectious diseases	4	**Rheumatology**	8
Intensive care	9	Stomatology	2
Mental health	1	Surgery	6
Metabolic diseases	5	Urology	5

Note: Those in **bold** are also recognized by the American Council of Pediatric Subspecialties in Pediatrics 2012.
Source: Ehrich et al., 2015a

children who may divide their time between hospital and home over a prolonged period.

The organization of services should be viewed from the perspective of both the child and their family and the health professionals working in the service. For the child and their family, it is important that all parts of the system should be in place and working well together with specialist advice easily accessible, but delivery should be as close to home as is safe and sustainable. This suggests the need to develop networked solutions where all those involved actively collaborate and constantly strive to improve safety and experienced outcomes. From the perspective

Subspecialty	H-O	CARD	NEPH	META	ENDO	HEPA	OTx	CHIR	PICU
Hemato-Oncology (H-O)									
Cardiology (CARD)									
Nephrology (NEPH)									
Metabolism (META)									
Endocrinology (ENDO)									
Hepatology (HEPA)									
Organ transplantation (OTx)									
Paediatric surgery (CHIR)									
Paediatric intensive care unit (PICU)									

Figure 2.2 Appropriate co-location of paediatric subspecialties

Source: Authors' compilation

of the health professional, the specialist centre should not be seen as a "stand-alone" institution but as part of a well managed clinical network that promptly refers the most appropriate children and simultaneously receives children back into the local system for rehabilitation after specialist care. Clinical leadership for specialist care resides with the centre which organizes shared care with clear clinical care plans, with training and joint clinics for local teams. The local team should organize routine health and social care and education as appropriate. This model, based on good two-way communication, has already been achieved in some cancer and neonatal networks. The ideal system can be summarized with the phrase "centralized specialization and decision-making, but decentralized provision of treatment whenever possible".

It is important to recognize that there is a risk that highly specialized paediatric subspecialty care may lead to fragmentation (Ehrich et al., 2015b). Consequently, especially where a child has multiple health problems, there is a strong argument for oversight of their care being undertaken by a general paediatrician, who can work closely with the child and their family. As Vohra et al. (2012) state, "paediatric integrative medicine should be the paediatricians' new subspecialty" to bring specialist care together.

In summary, there are many challenges in providing highly special-ized paediatric care in Europe but there is a limited evidence base to inform the decision-making process. The most urgent questions needing answers include:

- how best to plan an adequate number of specialist centres, where appropriate, taking account of possibilities created by the European Union Directive on Cross Border Care, so as to avoid both under-provision and over-supply;
- how to develop a sustainable workforce to meet the medical needs of children; many different factors must be taken into account, including geography, population distribution, transport links, and relationships between centres;
- how to balance any benefits from centralization with problems of access, recognizing that while most families will accept travelling long distances to receive episodes of specialist investigations or treatment, it is desirable that regular visits, for example for administration of treatment or follow-up, should take place as close to their homes as possible.

Typical patient pathways

We now look at the health system as seen through the eyes of the child. We do this by describing a series of journeys undertaken by children with four common conditions: an acute infectious disease, a chronic illness, a critical condition, and an illness requiring new technologies.

A child with acute infectious disease: acute lower respiratory tract infection (LRTI)

Acute LRTI in children – bronchiolitis and pneumonia – are normally managed in primary care by the first contact care giver. Should treatment fail, or in cases of atypical or recurrent pneumonias, the infant or child is referred to a secondary paediatric care setting (either ambulatory or inpatient facility) for further investigations, parenteral antibiotic therapy, oxygen and supportive treatment. Occasionally, a child with an LRTI might be found to have an underlying disorder, such as cystic fibrosis. In such cases, the child will be referred to a specialist team, normally at a tertiary care facility. The clinician treating the sick child must answer two questions. Is the infection due to a virus or bacteria? Antibiotic treatment is only indicated for the latter and unnecessary prescriptions increase the risk of antimicrobial resistance. Second, how likely is the child to respond to treatment, recognizing that small children in particular can deteriorate rapidly. On the one hand, it is necessary to ensure that further action is taken if there is such a deterioration. On the other hand, unnecessary admission to hospital should be avoided as far as possible. Advances in technology do, however, offer a possible solution as instruments based on evaluating gene expression profiles of leukocytes have demonstrated the ability to differentiate viral from bacterial infections, and scoring systems based on whole gene expression analyses may offer scope to assess severity in children with LRTI (Wallihan & Ramilo, 2014). In the future, these novel strategies may be able to identify rapidly those children who need antibiotics and those who should be promptly hospitalized.

A child with a chronic illness: asthma

If the asthma is moderate or severe, or if the diagnosis is uncertain, the child/adolescent is referred to a competent paediatric team either in an ambulatory paediatric setting or at the ambulatory clinic in a hospital paediatric department. Current recommendations are that such children should be referred to a specialist team at a regional centre if there are uncertainties about the diagnosis, or when children do not respond to recommended treatments. The paediatric teams should consist of specialized paediatricians and paediatric nurses. These teams will have access to lung function tests, blood tests and allergy testing. Ideally, the child will have a personalized treatment plan that is clearly documented, linked to a written asthma home management plan that is reviewed at every visit. Continued monitoring of asthma therapy is essential. Some centres offer group training (asthma schools). In case of an emergency, the child should be admitted to a paediatric department in a hospital. New biomarkers in blood, such as chitinases and periostin, as well as new means of diagnosing allergies, including component resolved diagnosis, which can identify the allergens involved, and basophil allergen threshold sensitivity, offer scope for more precise diagnosis of asthma and its triggers, and predict its severity. Novel treatment possibilities may include macrolide antibiotics and individualized cytokine antagonist therapies (Hedlin, 2014). In-home monitoring using telemedicine also offers future potential (Starmer et al., 2010).

A child in a critical condition

When a child has an overtly critical condition, such as foreign body aspiration or ingestion, head injury, poisoning, or serious respiratory or cardiac failure, then immediate provision of ambulance services, contactable by phone, must be guaranteed. Ideally, paramedics in the ambulance will be able to initiate immediate life-saving treatment, if that has not already been provided by first-aid. The ambulance should take the child to the emergency unit at the nearest hospital. Ideally, this will have separate provision for emergency care of children.

Countries should have poison control centres offering haemodialysis/adsorption, plasma exchange, and blood exchange at regional or national level, open for consultation by phone 24/7 for medical staff and the public.

Continuous medical education and professional development, including practical training of parents and care givers in emergency situations at both community and hospital level, are essential. It is also important that the equipment provided for emergency responses should cover the entire age spectrum of children. All those staff involved in the emergency response should also be trained in the specific health problems of children. This includes paramedical staff in ambulances but also those who staff emergency telephone services. Teleconsultations can facilitate the emergency care delivered to children in remote areas (Burke & Hall, 2015).

A child with a chronic illness requiring new technologies – type I diabetes mellitus (DM)

Immediate admission of children with diabetic ketoacidosis to hospital is warranted. Insulin, fluids and electrolytes are given while closely monitoring the patient. After stabilization is reached, a well planned preparation of the families for home treatment should be initiated in the paediatric department. Children with type 1 diabetes mellitus are increasingly utilizing continuous subcutaneous insulin infusions (insulin pumps) and continuous glucose monitoring systems (CGMS), both of which have been shown to improve glycaemic control and quality of life if the families are well trained. Proper education for families and providers should be provided to promote successful use of high-tech equipment and will reduce the number of adverse events (Ernst et al., 2016). These children should be closely followed in diabetes outpatient clinics of hospitals or in community centres providing appropriate staff and expertise. Future technology will focus on the new generation of pumps and monitoring (Carchidi et al., 2011). Telemedicine applications can facilitate monitoring and adherence to therapy (Burke & Hall, 2015).

Future trends

The care of children has changed remarkably in the past few decades and will continue to do so. Many of the same factors that drove changes in the past will remain important, including advances in technology, models of care, and professional roles. However, it is likely that there will be particularly important advances in information technology, enabling care to be coordinated across many different settings. A number of these key drivers for change are set out in Table 2.3. Beyond these individual drivers, it is clear that there will be a need for much greater integration of services, with child-oriented care delivered jointly by child health professionals working in different locations.

Conclusions and key messages

Existing systems providing secondary health care for children are facing several major challenges. First, there is enormous variation in the quality and nature of care provided for children across the European region, including differences in financial resources, organization of health care, and access to skilled health professionals and advanced technology. Second, the care of sick children has undergone a process of fragmentation, largely reflecting new opportunities to intervene, driven by scientific and technological advances. However, this fragmentation risks being exacerbated by organizational changes in some health systems. Third, although the sick child is on a journey that moves between different levels of care, they and their parents will often be challenged by structural and organizational barriers between primary, secondary, and tertiary care. Finally, all health systems are facing upward pressure on costs, with some aspects of paediatric care, including neonatal intensive care and highly specialized tertiary care, being especially vulnerable.

Table 2.3 *Future trends influencing the delivery of integrated care to children on five different levels*

Trend	Impact on the future hospital	Example	Challenges
Ongoing medical advances	New diagnostics supporting personalized medicine	e.g. Microarray in paediatric rheumatology (Punaro, 2014)	Funding of new devices and drugs
	New therapeutic interventions	e.g. Nanomedicines in acute lymphatic leukaemia (Sosnik & Carcaboso, 2014)	
Health information technology	Paper free children's hospital	e.g. One record for all health care providers caring for a child with type 1 diabetes mellitus: the primary care taker, hospital paediatric department, subspecialists and community services	Interoperability of electronic health recording systems in hospital and community
Innovative models of care (Starmer et al., 2010)	Inpatient – mostly medically complex cases and intensive care	e.g. A child with a neuro-developmental syndrome and epilepsy	Coordination of care across service settings
	Post-discharge treatment in ambulatory settings		
Telemedicine	Monitoring of medically complex patients	e.g. Monitoring a child with inflammatory bowel disease in a rural area (Burke & Hall, 2015)	Infrastructure
Skill mix	Task shifting	e.g. Nurse practitioners in intensive care units (Kotzer, 2005)	New professional hierarchies, team working, quality assurance

Many of these challenges apply equally to the provision of hospital care for adults. However, there are some specificities (Box 2.4). All hospitalized children should be admitted to children's wards and not to adult wards, and those caring for children in hospital face some additional challenges. For example, while it is the child who is being treated in hospital, it is important to find ways to include other members of the family in the process, for example by the creation of family-friendly facilities. It is also the case that children are not simply small adults and many can find the clinical environment frightening, so it is important to incorporate elements of design that create a child-friendly environment (Boxes 2.1 and 2.2). As with any patient with a complex chronic disease, care is increasingly being delivered by multidisciplinary teams but, in the case of children, these teams extend beyond the health sector to the education sector. There are many opportunities for learning from the different models of care seen in Europe but this will require considerable effort to overcome the scarcity of comparative information and of health services research focusing on children's services.

Box 2.4 Ten rules for the care of children in hospitals

1. The interests of the child should come first, with policies based on an understanding of the importance, and the life course model, of development.
2. Children should be cared for by a team of competent care givers who have been trained in communicating with children and in treating children of all ages.
3. Sick children should be treated in special age-appropriate units and not in adult units.
4. Priority should be given to non-invasive and ambulatory care for children as far as possible.
5. Care givers must have adequate time to communicate with children to strengthen their engagement in the clinical process. Hospital care for children includes support for patients, families and care givers, including the provision of relevant training, a process facilitated by enabling parents to stay with their children.
6. Hospital care for children must be adequately financed and staffed.

Box 2.4 (cont.)

7. Child care at all levels should be integrated, taking account of lessons from whole systems thinking.
8. Competition between different care givers and between different institutions is unhelpful and can create unnecessary barriers to the seamless provision of care for children with complex needs.
9. Those providing hospital care for children should participate in research that advances knowledge on the care of children, including both scientific and organizational interventions, and should develop mechanisms to ensure that these advances are incorporated into practice to continuously improve quality of care.
10. Hospital care means a combination of inpatient and outpatient care to avoid fragmented care.

We conclude with a series of challenges for those responsible for the organization and delivery of health care for Europe's children.

1. How can health systems prepare for the "unknown unknowns" in meeting the health needs of children? There are still many questions about how to translate the explosion in knowledge of the molecular basis of disease, including genomics, proteomics, and metabolomics, into practical solutions that can be applied widely and at scale, and in ways that are affordable.
2. Do stand-alone children's hospitals have any future? Ageing societies and reduced demands for inpatient care of children, coupled with payment systems that often fail to cover the costs of paediatric care, suggest that most will struggle to survive, with the possible exception of some highly specialized facilities, such as those linked to academic health centres. The challenge facing those stand-alone children's hospitals that are privately owned are especially great.
3. The motto "sick child in and healthy child out" simplifies the current problems of child health care. Prior to and following a stay in hospital there must be well developed pathways for long-term care, involving a wide range of child health care providers in a variety of settings.
4. How can models of care based on networks and integration across settings be delivered where there is choice of provider? Experience in Germany, for example, suggests that hospitals in such a setting have no incentive to develop initiatives designed to respond to the needs of chronically ill children in and outside hospitals (Busse, 2004).

References

American Academy of Pediatrics (2012). Levels of neonatal care. *Pediatrics*, 130:587–97.

Bartels DB et al. (2006). Hospital volume and neonatal mortality among very low birth weight infants. *Pediatrics*, 117:2206–14.

British Association of Perinatal Medicine (2010). *Service standards for hospitals providing neonatal care*. London, BAPM.

Burke BL Jr, Hall RW (2015). Telemedicine: Pediatric Applications. *Pediatrics*, 136:e293–308.

Busse R (2004). Disease management programs in Germany's statutory health insurance system. *Health Aff (Millwood)*, 23:56–67.

Carchidi C et al. (2011). New technologies in pediatric diabetes care. *MCN Am J Matern Child Nurs*, 36:32–9; quiz 40–1.

Crowley R et al. (2011). Improving the transition between paediatric and adult healthcare: a systematic review. *Arch Dis Child* 96(6):548–53.

Ehrich J, Namazova-Baranova L, Pettoello-Mantovani M (2016). Introduction to "Diversity of Child Health Care in Europe: A Study of the European Paediatric Association/Union of National European Paediatric Societies and Associations". *J Pediatr*, 177s:s1–s10.

Ehrich JH et al. (2015a). Diversity of Pediatric Workforce and Education in 2012 in Europe: A Need for Unifying Concepts or Accepting Enjoyable Differences? *J Pediatr*, 167:471–6.e4.

Ehrich JH et al. (2015b). Opening the Debate on Pediatric Subspecialties and Specialist Centers: Opportunities for Better Care or Risks of Care Fragmentation? *J Pediatr*, 167:1177–8.e2.

Ernst G et al. (2016). How to Train Families to Cope with Lifelong Health Problems? *J Pediatr*, 170:349–50.e1–2.

European Association for Children in Hospital (2015). *EACH Charter* (Online). Available at: https://www.each-for-sick-children.org/each-charter/introduction-each-charter-annotations.html (accessed 21 November 2016).

European Society for Neonatology (2015). *ESN Curriculum for in Neonatology (syllabus) in Europe* (Online). Available at: http://esn.espr.info/training-esn/national-programmes (accessed 21 November 2016).

Eurostat (2016). *Eurostat: your key to health statistics* (Online). Available at: http://ec.europa.eu/eurostat (accessed 21 November 2016).

Future Hospital Commission (2013). *Future hospital: caring for medical patients*. London, Royal College of Physicians.

Hallsworth M et al. (2008). *The provision of neonatal services: Data for international comparisons*. Cambridge, Rand Europe.

Hedlin G (2014). Management of severe asthma in childhood – state of the art and novel perspectives. *Pediatr Allergy Immunol*, 25:111–21.

Heller G et al. (2007). [Annual patient volume and survival of very low birth weight infants (VLBWs) in Germany – a nationwide analysis based on administrative data.] *Z Geburtshilfe Neonatol*, 211:123–31.

Kotzer AM (2005). Characteristics and role functions of advanced practice nurses in a tertiary pediatric setting. *J Spec Pediatr Nurs*, 10:20–8.

Laing I et al. (2004). *Designing a Neonatal Unit Report for the British Association of Perinatal Medicine*. London, British Association of Perinatal Medicine.

Lenton S, Ehrich J (2015). Approach to Child-Friendly Health Care – The Council of Europe. *J Pediatr*, 167:216–18.

Long JG, Lucey JF, Philip AG (1980). Noise and hypoxemia in the intensive care nursery. *Pediatrics*, 65:143–5.

Mann NP et al. (1986). Effect of night and day on preterm infants in a newborn nursery: randomised trial. *Br Med J (Clin Res Ed)*, 293:1265–7.

Ortenstrand A et al. (2010). The Stockholm Neonatal Family Centered Care Study: effects on length of stay and infant morbidity. *Pediatrics*, 125:e278–85.

Profit J et al. (2016). The Association of Level of Care With NICU Quality. *Pediatrics*, 137:e20144210.

Punaro M (2014). Use of microarrays in the clinical practice of pediatric rheumatology: the future is now? *Curr Opin Rheumatol*, 26:585–91.

Robertson A, Cooper-Peel C, Vos P (1999). Contribution of heating, ventilation, and air conditioning airflow and conversation to the ambient sound in a neonatal intensive care unit. *J Perinatol*, 19:362–6.

Saliba V et al. (2014). Clinicians', policy makers' and patients' views of pediatric cross-border care between Malta and the UK. *J Health Serv Res Policy*, 19:153–60.

Smith GC et al. (2011). Neonatal intensive care unit stress is associated with brain development in preterm infants. *Ann Neurol*, 70:541–9.

Sosnik A, Carcaboso AM (2014). Nanomedicines in the future of pediatric therapy. *Adv Drug Deliv Rev*, 73:140–61.

Starmer AJ et al. (2010). Pediatrics in the year 2020 and beyond: preparing for plausible futures. *Pediatrics*, 126:971–81.

Vohra S et al. (2012). Pediatric integrative medicine: pediatrics' newest subspecialty? *BMC Pediatr*, 12:123.

Wallihan R, Ramilo O (2014). Community-acquired pneumonia in children: current challenges and future directions. *J Infect*, 69 Suppl 1:S87–90.

White RD (2011). The newborn intensive care unit environment of care: how we got here, where we're headed, and why. *Semin Perinatol*, 35:2–7.

White R, Whitman T (1992). Design of ICUs. *Pediatrics*, 89:1267.

Wolfe I, McKee M (eds) (2014). *European Child Health Services and Systems: Lessons Without Borders*. Buckingham, Open University Press.

Wolfe I et al. (2013). Health services for children in western Europe. *Lancet*, 381:1224–34.

World Health Organization (2016). *Baby-friendly Hospital Initiative* (Online). Available at: http://www.who.int/nutrition/topics/bfhi/en/ (accessed 21 November 2016).

Wyllie J et al. (2015). Part 7: Neonatal resuscitation: 2015 International Consensus on Cardiopulmonary Resuscitation and Emergency Cardiovascular Care Science with Treatment Recommendations. *Resuscitation*, 95:e169–201.

3 | Patients with stroke

BENJAMIN BRAY, ANTHONY RUDD, PHIL WHITE,
BO NORRVING, CHARLES WOLFE

The burden of stroke

Stroke is one of the leading causes of acute medical admissions to hospitals. It is among the most common causes of death and is a major cause of disability and poor health outcomes (Box 3.1). Worldwide, 17 million people suffer a stroke each year and stroke is the third most common cause of death around the globe, accounting for 12% of all deaths, and exceeded only by heart disease and cancer (Feigin et al., 2009; Thrift et al., 2014; GBD 2013 Mortality and Causes of Death Collaborators, 2015). While its management involves a series of specific responses by the hospital, the principles underlying them – including the importance of coordinated multispeciality and multiprofessional care, speed of response in the acute episode, the importance of prevention (of both the initial episode and any recurrence), and a model of care that follows the patient along the entire pathway, from the onset of illness to recovery and rehabilitation – apply equally to many other common medical conditions, such as acute myocardial infarction, gastrointestinal haemorrhage, or the acute and chronic complications of diabetes.

Age-adjusted incidence and mortality rates for stroke have fallen significantly over recent decades, thought to be due to improvements in stroke prevention through improved management of risk factors for stroke, especially hypertension and tobacco control, and, in some places, improved acute care. Between 1990 and 2013 the age-adjusted mortality rate for stroke in developed countries fell from 113 to 67 per 100 000 (Feigin et al., 2015). However, because of increasing longevity and the strong association between stroke risk and age, the absolute numbers of people having stroke are rising year on year, from an estimated 4.3 million globally in 1990 to 6.9 million by 2013 (Feigin et al., 2015). This is leading to increasing numbers of people dying from stroke (2.1 million in 1990 to 3.3 million deaths in 2013 from ischaemic stroke), increasing disability adjusted life years and an almost doubling in the prevalence of stroke between 1990 and 2013, from 14 million

---

Box 3.1 What is stroke?

A stroke is an episode of neurological dysfunction caused by disruption of blood circulation (ischaemic stroke) or bleeding (haemorrhagic stroke) in an area of the central nervous system: the brain, spinal cord or retina. Approximately 90% of strokes are ischaemic and 10% are due to haemorrhage, although there is variation between populations in the relative proportions of ischaemic and haemorrhagic stroke. There are two main types of haemorrhagic stroke: primary intracerebral haemorrhage and subarachnoid haemorrhage. This chapter will address the health care needs of patients with the most frequent types of stroke: ischaemic stroke and primary intracerebral haemorrhage. Subarachnoid haemorrhage, although important in its own right, is less common and patients typically follow different patient pathways than those with ischaemic stroke or primary intracerebral haemorrhage – subarachnoid haemorrhage will therefore not be covered in this chapter.

A transient ischaemic attack (TIA) is caused by a temporary disruption of blood supply to the central nervous system – the symptoms are short-lived but it is a warning sign that an ischaemic stroke may be about to occur. The symptoms of stroke and TIA depend on the area of the nervous system affected, but commonly include muscular paralysis, loss of sensation, loss of vision and speech and language problems. The main risk factors for stroke and TIA are hypertension, physical inactivity, tobacco smoking, other cardiovascular disease (such as diabetes or ischaemic heart disease), atrial fibrillation (AF) and increasing age.

---

to 26 million (Feigin et al., 2015). Essentially, changes in population demographics are outpacing improvements in stroke prevention, resulting in an increasing burden of stroke on populations and health systems, particularly in lower and middle income countries.

In addition to mortality, stroke causes a wide range of disabilities and impairments and has long-term implications for the health and well-being of survivors. These include neurological impairments such as muscle weakness or paralysis, impaired vision and impairments of speech and language skills. Up to 50% of patients will develop major depression in the years after stroke (Ayerbe et al., 2013). Cognitive impairment is common and cerebrovascular disease is a major risk factor for dementia. More subtle cognitive problems, such as perceptual impairments, a change in personality, and profound fatigue are common, often lasting for years after the stroke (Wolfe et al., 2011). These problems are often referred to as "hidden deficits" but they account for a significant proportion of the suffering and costs that stroke causes. Effective risk reduction and high quality treatment should not only result in improvements in physical health but also reduce the future burden of dementia and mental health problems.

The financial costs of stroke are large and diverse: to the individual and their family in terms of health care and time off work; to governments in terms of medical and social care; and to wider society in terms of lost productivity. Other non-monetary costs are harder to calculate but are equally important – such as the emotional cost to family and friends of caring for a loved one who can no longer live independently.

Stroke accounts for between 2% and 4% of the total health care expenditure in developed countries. Moreover, stroke incurs substantial costs outside the health care system, reflecting survivors' high rates of disability and dependence. In 2008 the total direct and indirect costs associated with stroke were approximately £8.9 (€9.7) billion per year in the United Kingdom (Saka et al., 2009). Most costs are incurred in the initial months and years after the patient has been discharged from hospital (Saka et al., 2009). Studies from Italy (Bottachi et al., 2012), Denmark (Jennum et al., 2015) and France (Schmidt et al., 2015) have produced similar estimates of the costs of stroke in Europe, at €7000–20 000 per stroke. Almost any intervention that reduces the incidence of stroke or reduces the likelihood of long-term disability will be cost-effective in countries with expensive health and social care systems.

Evidence-based stroke care

Historically, stroke was considered a condition for which little could be done, but there is now an extensive evidence base for interventions that are effective in improving outcomes after stroke: reducing disability, improving survival and reducing the risk of stroke recurrence. Some of these interventions (such as stroke unit based care) are applicable to almost all patients with stroke, while others are limited to selected patient groups (Figure 3.1).

	Proportion of patients with ischaemic stroke applicable	Outcome	Number needed to treat to benefit	Estimated number with improved outcomes per 1000 patients with ischaemic stroke if intervention was given to all applicable patients
Stroke unit care	90–100%	Death or long-term institutionalization	19	50
Antiplatelet therapy	85–95%	Death or dependency	79	11
Early supported discharge	Up to 50%	Death or dependency	20	25
Thrombolysis	Up to 20%	Death or dependency	25	8
Thrombectomy	Up to 10%	Dependency	3	33

Figure 3.1 Number needed to treat for the main evidence-based interventions in acute ischaemic stroke

Source: Authors' compilation

Organized multidisciplinary stroke care

In the past 25 years the medical care of patients with stroke has changed enormously in high income countries. The central change has been the development of organized systems of stroke care, characterized by a move away from general medicine towards specialized multidisciplinary models of care based on the stroke unit model. Randomized controlled trials have shown that being admitted to a stroke unit improves survival and reduces long-term dependency: in the most recently updated Cochrane review of organized stroke care summarizing the results of 31 trials, the odds of death or death or dependency at one year were reduced by 14% and 18% respectively (Stroke Unit Triallists' Collaboration, 2007). Stroke units have been evaluated in many different countries and settings, and found to be effective in all types of stroke patient and in both high and middle/low income countries (Langhorne, de Villiers & Pandian, 2012). Organized models of rehabilitation care after stroke have also been found to improve outcomes. In particular, early supported discharge (ESD) services, where multidisciplinary care and therapy are provided in the patient's own home at a similar intensity to inpatient rehabilitation, improve long-term recovery and shorten length of hospital stay (discussed in detail later in this chapter) (Langhorne & Baylan, 2017).

Acute re-perfusion

For patients with ischaemic stroke, early treatment to restore blood flow to the affected area of the brain can limit the extent of damage and increase the patient's chance of making a recovery. Re-perfusion can be achieved either through administration of a clot-busting drug or through a procedure. The first landmark trial to demonstrate the effectiveness of thrombolysis was the National Institute of Neurological Disorders (NINDs) trial in 1995 (National Institute of Neurological Disorders, 1995), which found that the drug alteplase significantly reduced the rate of disability if given within 3 hours of stroke onset. As well as demonstrating the effectiveness of the therapy, the results also had the effect of highlighting the very poor quality of existing health care systems for patients with acute stroke, since the effectiveness of the drug was entirely dependent on very rapid recognition, triage and diagnosis. In the United States the results of this trial prompted in 1995 the first national effort to define standards about how to organize acute stroke care (National Institute of Neurological Disorders and Stroke rt-PA Stroke Study Group, 1995) and the subsequent development of the Joint Commission's Comprehensive Stroke Centre hospital certification scheme. Thrombolysis has since been evaluated in a number of trials, and has been shown to improve recovery if provided to suitable patients within 4.5 hours of stroke onset (Emberson, 2014).

More recently, evidence has emerged that early physical removal of the blood clot causing ischaemic stroke (a procedure called mechanical thrombectomy) improves outcomes. If provided within 6 hours to suitable patients, thrombectomy is very effective in increasing the chance of patients regaining functional independence after stroke (Goyal, 2016).

The impact of both these approaches is, however, limited by being suitable only for a minority of patients: up to 20% of patients with ischaemic stroke may be eligible for thrombolysis and approximately 10% (McMeekin, 2017) for thrombectomy.

Prevention of complications and stroke recurrence

Evidence-based secondary prevention for stroke includes antiplatelet therapy (Sandercock et al., 2008), anticoagulation in people with AF, blood pressure-lowering therapy, and treatment with statins to lower cholesterol (American Heart Association/American Stroke Association, 2014; Intercollegiate Stroke Working Party, 2016). The risk of recurrent stroke can also be reduced in some patients by early vascular surgery (carotid endarterectomy) to the carotid arteries (North American Symptomatic Carotid Endarterectomy Trial Collaborators, 1991). Early initiation of these therapies is also effective in reducing the risk of stroke in patients with TIA (Rothwell et al., 2007). Identifying the specific cause of the stroke for each patient is an important part of stroke care so that appropriate secondary prevention can be initiated, such as long-term treatment with anticoagulation in patients with AF. As discussed later in this chapter, this involves an increasingly sophisticated array of diagnostic tests and technologies.

Most patients dying of acute stroke do not die directly from brain injury, but from the complications of immobility and impairment. Preventing complications through, for example, screening patients for swallowing problems after stroke to reduce the risk of pneumonia, and using intermittent pneumatic compression (IPC) devices (CLOTS Trials Collaboration et al., 2013) to prevent venous thromboembolism, contribute to preventing the complications of acute stroke and improving survival after stroke.

The great majority of patients with stroke do not require any surgical intervention, but early neurosurgery can improve outcomes in selected patients with very extensive ischaemic strokes (Cruz-Flores, Berge & Whittle, 2012) and in patients with certain types of intracerebral haemorrhage (Mendelow et al., 2013).

Rehabilitation

Helping people to recover, regain function and return to doing the activities and work they were doing before their stroke is an essential component of stroke care. Compared to other areas of stroke care, however, there have been very few large clinical trials of stroke rehabilitation and a relatively weak evidence base exists. There is evidence that very early mobilization with high intensity therapy after stroke may actually lead to poorer outcomes (AVERT Trial Collaboration Group et al., 2015) than physiotherapy protocols that use more frequent but less intense spells of activity.

The stroke care pathway

Hospitals are central to stroke care but exist as components of a pathway of care that spans pre-hospital emergency medical services, acute hospital care, rehabilitation and primary care (Figure 3.2). For many of the elements of the patient pathway, there is now good quality evidence about how to organize health services to optimize patient outcomes. At the same time, we also know that in the real world there are wide variations both across Europe and within individual health economies in how stroke care is delivered.

Pre-hospital

Most people develop acute stroke out of hospital, although hospital inpatients are at high risk of stroke (particularly people undergoing cardiothoracic surgery or angioplasty) and approximately 5% of strokes

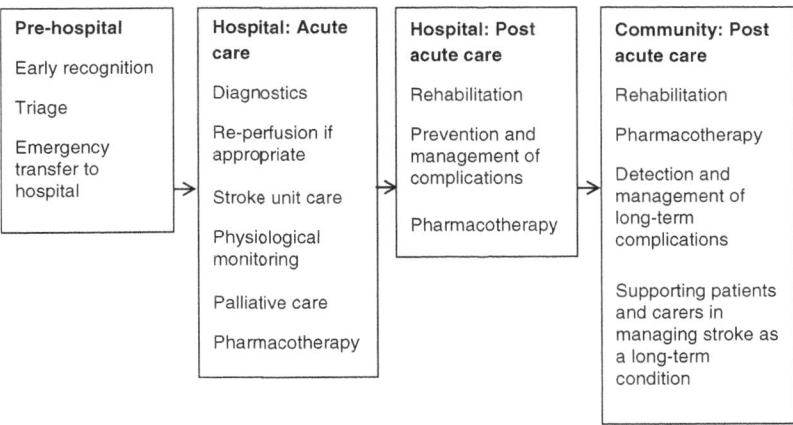

Figure 3.2 An example of a typical stroke care pathway in high income settings

Source: Authors' own

occur in people who are already in hospital for another reason. Both stroke and TIA are medical emergencies, and delays in presentation to hospital are associated with worse outcomes. Delays in the assessment and treatment of patients presenting with TIA increase the risk of their going on to have a stroke (Rothwell et al., 2007), while pre-hospital delays in patients with ischaemic stroke reduce the chance that they will benefit from re-perfusion therapy. Patients with acute stroke should be admitted directly to hospital and patients with TIA may be managed as outpatients provided that clinics provide urgent (e.g. within 24 hours) assessment, diagnostics (brain and vascular imaging, blood tests, cardiac tests) and treatment (Luengo-Fernandez, Gray & Rothwell, 2009).

Public awareness of stroke symptoms is poor (Reeves et al., 2008) and contributes to the significant number of people presenting late after stroke onset. The FAST (Face Arm Speech Time) test was developed to improve recognition of stroke by the general public and has now been adopted worldwide into public campaigns as part of efforts to inform the general population about how to respond to a stroke (Public Health England, 2015). Promotion of this test as part of a mass media campaign in the United Kingdom appeared to be successful in increasing the proportion of people attending hospital rather than primary care with stroke symptoms (Flynn et al., 2014), but evidence of effectiveness in other countries has been variable (Mellon et al., 2013).

Pre-hospital delays in care can also be reduced by having effective systems to triage patients with possible stroke and alert the receiving hospital that a patient with stroke is on their way to hospital (Fassbender et al., 2013). Tools have been developed (e.g. the ROSIER tool) that allow for the rapid triage of patients with probable stroke pre-hospital or in the emergency department (Nor, 2005).

Acute hospital care

Upon arrival at hospital, the key diagnostic test is brain imaging with CT and/or MRI. Most patients receive a CT scan acutely in order to distinguish between ischaemic stroke and primary intracerebral haemorrhage, and the main role of MRI is in follow-up imaging, in the assessment of patients with TIA or in cases of diagnostic uncertainty (Intercollegiate Stroke Working Party, 2016). For patients who are potentially eligible for thrombolysis or thrombectomy, more advanced types of imaging (such as CT angiography) may be used to identify appropriate patients and reducing the time from admission to brain imaging is critical in achieving delivery of these treatments quickly: co-location of scanning suites in or adjacent to the "front door" can help in reducing delays in scanning (Meretoja et al., 2013). With the development of thrombectomy as an established therapy, it is essential to rapidly develop robust stroke imaging protocols that include CT or MR angiography as well as CT (or MRI).

For patients suitable for thrombolysis, the sooner it is administered ("door to needle time"), the greater is the likely benefit. Some single centres routinely achieve extraordinarily fast times for treatment, with thrombolysis being administered in just 20 minutes after arrival at hospital (Meretoja et al., 2013), and there is evidence from the United Kingdom that treatment is fastest in larger/higher volume centres (Bray et al., 2013b). Typical door to needle times in Europe are approximately 1 hour, although there is significant international variation in times between countries (for example, a median door to needle time of 56 minutes in England and Wales compared to 45 minutes in Sweden (RiksStroke, 2018; Sentinel Stroke National Audit Programme, 2018).

Inpatient care for stroke patients should be on a specialist stroke unit (Intercollegiate Stroke Working Party, 2016). A stroke unit consists of a discrete area of a hospital ward that exclusively or nearly exclusively takes care of stroke patients and is staffed by a specialist MDT (Cochrane Stroke Group, 2013). A small proportion (less than 5%) of patients will require ICU care or surgical interventions as part of their stroke management – such as neurosurgical management of very large ischaemic strokes and intracerebral haemorrhages, or vascular surgery. However, most patients should spend the majority of their inpatient stay on either an acute stroke unit or a rehabilitation stroke unit.

Acute care in the stroke unit involves (Langhorne, Pollock & Stroke Unit Triallists' Collaboration, 2002):

- medical assessment and diagnosis
- early assessment of nursing and therapy needs
- monitoring of physiological and neurological status
- screening and prevention of complications
- mobilization
- rehabilitation therapy (physiotherapy, occupational therapy, speech and language therapy).

Priorities in the first few hours after admission are physiological monitoring, correction of problems such as dehydration, fever and high blood sugar, and managing the complications of stroke. For patients with primary intracerebral haemorrhage, there is some evidence that rapid blood pressure lowering may improve functional outcomes (Anderson et al., 2013). Swallowing problems are common after stroke and place patients at increased risk of pneumonia if they eat or drink; patients need to be screened for swallowing problems and may be temporarily fed through a feeding tube during this time to reduce the risk of pneumonia. Delivering these interventions as a care bundle has been shown to improve patient outcomes (Middleton et al., 2011) and delays in carrying out swallow screening are associated with higher rates of stroke-associated pneumonia (Bray et al., 2017). Careful nursing care in this early period is especially important in preventing complications of stroke (Middleton, Grimley & Alexandrov, 2015), since most of the early deaths after stroke are caused not directly by the stroke itself, but by complications such as pneumonia, sepsis or venous thromboembolism.

Many patients with stroke are immobile and so are at high risk of pressure ulcers and venous thromboembolism (VTE). Managing VTE risk is complicated in patients with stroke because the risk of intracranial bleeding is increased by the anticoagulants typically used for VTE prevention. VTE risk can, however, be reduced by the use of IPC devices in patients who are unable to mobilize (CLOTS Trial Collaboration et al., 2013).

End of life care

Approximately one in six patients admitted to hospital with stroke will die in the next 30 days, and the risk of death is particularly high in older people, those with more severe stroke and patients with intracerebral haemorrhage. Providing good quality palliative and end of life care is therefore an essential component of all stroke services. This requires health care professionals on stroke units to have the relevant knowledge and skills to provide palliative care, and the availability of specialist palliative care services for patients with complex or hard to manage symptoms. Palliative care for patients with stroke is complex, and requires not only the provision of symptom control and compassionate and dignified end of life care, but also complicated decision-making about treatment withdrawal, artificial nutrition and feeding, and goal setting (Holloway et al., 2014).

Rehabilitation

Most patients with stroke will require a period of rehabilitation and assessment of their impairments and needs. This usually involves physiotherapy, occupational therapy, and speech and language therapy. Care models for this vary considerably between health economies. In some settings the stroke unit will provide both acute care and rehabilitation, whereas in other settings these functions are separated, with patients being transferred to a dedicated rehabilitation ward. Models commonly used in Europe include:

- inpatient rehabilitation on a stroke unit which also provides acute care
- inpatient rehabilitation on a stroke unit dedicated to providing rehabilitation
- inpatient rehabilitation in a generic rehabilitation ward or facility
- discharge home, with community-based rehabilitation provided in outpatient facilities
- discharge home, with community-based rehabilitation provided in the patient's place of residence.

In contrast to the strong evidence base concerning the organization of acute stroke care (see Figure 3.2), there is relatively scant evidence about the clinical cost and cost-effectiveness of the later stages of the stroke care pathway. One of the models of care that has been well studied is ESD. In this model, stroke patients are discharged home when medically stable, and continue to receive rehabilitation in their own home at the same intensity as they would do as an inpatient. This has several potential advantages: patients recover and learn to adapt to impairments in their own environment, leave hospital sooner and may be less exposed to hospital-related harms.

A strong body of research has shown that ESD provides better outcomes in terms of mortality, disability, institutionalization, patient satisfaction, and length of hospital stay (Langhorne & Baylan, 2017). These improved outcomes are achieved at a reasonable additional cost. The incremental cost-effectiveness ratio of stroke unit care followed by early community rehabilitation is £10 661, compared with the general medical ward without such care, and £17 721 compared with the stroke unit without early community rehabilitation (Saka et al., 2009). Despite this evidence, there has been limited uptake of this model of care. For example, although the service is applicable to up to 40% of stroke discharges in the United Kingdom, 25% of the regions of the country have not commissioned an ESD service and overall only 20% of patients receive the services of a dedicated team (Sentinel Stroke National Audit Programme, 2018). ESD has also been slower to develop in other high income countries in Europe, which have traditionally focused more on inpatient or clinic-based models of rehabilitation (Douw, Nielsen & Pedersen, 2015).

Recovery and long-term management

The final stage of the pathway is long-term care, management and support. This includes maintaining and monitoring secondary prevention therapy, identifying and managing the longer-term consequences of stroke, and providing support and information provision to patients and their families. In contrast with the acute phase of this pathway, it is arguable that this is an area of stroke care that has been relatively neglected by health care systems. Certainly, many stroke survivors express dissatisfaction about the quality of this longer-term support and many patients have a high burden of unmet needs after stroke (McKevitt et al., 2011). An additional challenge comes from managing multimorbidity, which is common in people with stroke (Gallacher et al., 2014) and adds to disease burden, increases the complexity of treatment decisions, and places patients at risk of the harmful effects of polypharmacy.

Workforce

Optimal stroke care is highly multidisciplinary, with a core stroke service requiring specialist doctors, nurses, physiotherapists, occupational therapists, speech and language therapists, dieticians and psychologists. Coordinating the work of the team is essential and formal MDT working (such as regular MDT meetings to discuss individual cases) is one of the components of stroke unit care (Langhorne, Pollock & Stroke Unit Triallists Collaboration, 2002).

Stroke medicine has traditionally not existed as a medical speciality in its own right, and as a result there is variation between countries in the specialty background of the lead physician. In most countries acute stroke care is largely provided by neurologists, but in some countries (such as the United Kingdom) stroke care is mainly led by stroke specialist physicians with a background in geriatric medicine.

Other medical specialties with important roles in the stroke pathway include neuroradiology (both diagnostic and interventional), neurosurgery, vascular surgery, intensive care, emergency medicine, rehabilitation medicine, and primary care.

Nursing care is an essential aspect of acute stroke care and it is likely that good quality nursing is one of the key mechanisms for the beneficial effect of stroke units (Middleton, Grimley & Alexandrov, 2015). In addition to general nursing skills, nurses need specific skills and knowledge in managing patients with stroke, such as screening and managing dysphagia, the positioning and mobilization of patients with muscle weakness or paralysis, prevention of pressure sores, and communicating with patients with language impairment after stroke (aphasia). Because many patients with stroke die as inpatients, nurses also need skills in providing end of life and palliative care. In some countries (such as the United Kingdom) nurses have taken on extended roles in prescribing, diagnostics, and assessing patients for thrombolysis.

In addition to the general evidence concerning nurse staffing levels and patient outcome (Needleman et al., 2011), there is specific evidence in stroke care that nursing-to-patient staffing ratios are associated with patient outcomes, with higher mortality rates for patients admitted at weekends to units with lower numbers of trained nursing staff (Bray et al., 2014).

Rehabilitation is typically carried out by physiotherapists, occupational therapists, and speech and language therapists (speech pathologists). This includes carrying out assessments of the extent of a patient's impairments and the impact of these on functioning, and planning treatment goals. Describing the full range of assessments and therapies provided by stroke therapists is beyond the scope of this chapter, but a wide range of methods may be used, from relatively simple mobilization techniques to more sophisticated interventions requiring the use of specialized equipment and aids. Therapists may also carry out additional diagnostic tests requiring additional skills and equipment. Therapists are central in planning patients' discharge from hospital and implementing adaptations or the installation of equipment in patients' homes, and have a key role in communicating with and providing psychological support for patients and their families and carers.

Stroke services also involve a variety of other allied health professionals. Dietetics is a core component of an acute stroke service, since many patients require nutritional support or assisted feeding. Problems with cognition, memory, mood or executive functioning are common after stroke and access to a clinical psychologist enables more detailed neuropsychological assessments to be carried out and appropriate information, support and therapy to be provided. Some patients with persistent physical or visual impairments may also require the provision of support aids from prosthetics and orthoptics specialists. As most patients will be discharged home on new or changed medications, pharmacists have an important role in ensuring safe prescribing, medicines reconciliation and in providing information to patients and family members about medications and side effects.

Networks of stroke care

In parallel with the development of organized stroke care in individual hospitals, many health systems have developed regional and network models of stroke care. In much of Europe and the USA a distinction is made between primary stroke centres and comprehensive stroke centres. Primary stroke centres are those with the necessary staffing, infrastructure and expertise to provide treatment for most stroke patients, but which may not have the capability to manage patients with more complex problems. Comprehensive stroke centres provide the same core stroke service but also the high technology and resource-intensive elements of care, such as interventional neuroradiology or neurosurgery, and play a greater role as centres for research and education. The European Stroke Organisation has produced guidelines setting out in detail the facilities and staffing required by comprehensive stroke centres ("ESO Stroke Centre") in Europe (Ringelstein et al., 2013), which includes 24/7 provision of advanced imaging and interventional neuroradiology. In many countries these levels of care are formally accredited through certification schemes (for example, in the USA and Germany) or through quality registers (for example, in the United Kingdom and Sweden). There is evidence from the USA (Xian et al., 2011), Japan (Iihara et al., 2014), Finland (Meretoja et al., 2013) and the United Kingdom (Bray et al., 2013a) that hospitals with higher levels of organized stroke care provide better outcomes for patients, suggesting that formal mechanisms to ensure stroke quality standards are important.

Networks of hospitals are frequently used in stroke care to provide access to the higher technology care offered in comprehensive stroke centres. These may act as the central referral centre for "hub and spoke" networks of hospitals, taking referrals from a number of primary stroke centres. Such networks have become increasingly important with the advent of more sophisticated diagnostic and interventional innovations, such as advanced brain imaging and thrombectomy, which would not be feasible or cost-effective to provide in smaller hospitals. In the United Kingdom the concept of the comprehensive stroke centre and primary stroke centre is more frequently defined in terms of hyperacute stroke units (HASUs) (providing acute care for the first 72 hours after stroke) and stroke units (for post-72 hour care).

There is evidence that these types of network can lead to better patient outcomes. In 2010 health care providers in London carried out a major reorganization of stroke services, reducing the number of acute admitting hospitals from 28 to 8 centres, each serving a population of approximately 1–1.5 million people. These eight hospitals were designated as HASUs and formal pre-hospital protocols were established so that all patients with suspected stroke would be transferred to a HASU. These HASUs provide acute care for up to 72 hours, and patients requiring ongoing inpatient treatment and rehabilitation are then transferred to a stroke unit closer to their home. The network is supported by agreed protocols for patient transfers, minimum standards for training, facilities and staffing, a common framework for payment and reimbursement from funders, and regular audit of quality and performance. Since these changes were established, there have been large improvements in the quality of stroke care in London, with stroke case fatality rates falling faster in London than in other urban areas in England (Morris et al., 2014). One of the key aspects of stroke care in London that is different from many other "hub and spoke" models of care is the concept of providing higher level acute care to all patients and not just to selected patients; the majority of patients therefore have the opportunity to benefit from early intensive acute stroke care in an HASU.

Some models of care have emerged to help tackle the issue of providing specialist stroke care at scale by providing regional systems for transferring patients to specialist centres or providing specialist input remotely. Telemedicine is widely used in stroke care and many areas have implemented telemedicine systems to transmit video, audio and imaging data so that stroke specialists at home or working in another hospital can help in assessing patients presenting with acute stroke (Hess & Audebert, 2013). This has particular uses in delivering thrombolysis in rural areas where it may not be feasible to provide specialist stroke services in areas of low population density.

Telemedicine models may also be augmented by pathways that provide initial triage and assessment of patients in local hospitals, initiate thrombolysis if appropriate, and then transfer the patient to a hospital with specialist stroke care provision. These "drip and ship" models have been used particularly in the USA, where one in four patients treated with thrombolysis is now managed this way (Sheth et al., 2015).

Variation in quality

Within Europe there is wide variation in the organization of stroke services and in the use of policies aimed at increasing care quality, such as clinical audit, financial incentives, clinical guidelines, accreditation and regulations (Di Carlo et al., 2015). The quality of care delivery across Europe is hard to measure consistently, since even when data are available, differences in the choice and definition of quality indicators make comparisons difficult (Wiedmann et al., 2012). Nonetheless, wide variation exists even for aspects of stroke care with the strongest evidence base and most consistent inclusion in guidelines and audits, such as admission to a stroke unit or treatment with thrombolysis (Ayis et al., 2013). For example, in 2011 only 33% of stroke patients in France were admitted to a stroke unit (Schmidt et al., 2015), compared with 62% in Scotland (Turner et al., 2016). A survey of 25 European countries in 2005 found evidence of extremely wide variation in the provision of acute stroke care, with particularly poor provision of stroke unit care in Estonia, France, Greece and Portugal (Leys et al., 2007). Only 49% of the 886 hospitals included in the survey provided the minimum level of care to be considered a primary or comprehensive stroke centre. Stroke outcomes also vary significantly across Europe. For example, one comparative study of stroke outcomes between six European cities (in France, Italy, Lithuania, the United Kingdom, Spain and Poland) found three-fold variation in the risk of death after stroke (Heuschmann et al., 2011).

Poor provision of acute stroke care occurs even in higher income European countries. For example, a survey of neurology services in

Italian hospitals found that only 28% provided stroke unit based care, and large numbers of patients with stroke were admitted to hospitals without stroke units (de Falco, Leone & Beghi, 2009). Organized stroke care was also relatively slow to develop in France, with only two hospitals out of 121 surveyed in 2005 providing stroke unit care (Leys et al., 2009). Policy-makers in France have subsequently prioritized stroke care and developed a national strategy for improvements, with a particular focus on developing stroke care networks (Lebrun et al., 2011).

Information on stroke care quality is collected systematically in some European countries (Wiedmann et al., 2012), but most countries in Europe lack or have only fragmentary systems of data collection for quality improvement (Di Carlo et al., 2015). Where data are available, there is evidence of widespread variation in care quality within countries, not just between countries. For example, stroke care quality is measured in England and Wales by the Sentinel Stroke National Audit Programme (SSNAP) (Sentinel Stroke National Audit Programme, 2018) and there are wide geographical variations in a variety of care quality indicators (Figure 3.3). National clinical audits and registries in other countries show similar variation in stroke care quality, including Scotland (Scottish Stroke Care Audit; SSCA), Sweden (RiksStroke) and Germany (Wiedmann et al., 2014). Some of these variations reflect broader geographical inequalities in the provision of health care services, such as the relative under-provision of stroke units in southern Italy compared to northern Italy (Guidetti et al., 2013).

Specialist resources

The main essential component of a stroke service is a stroke unit (Figure 3.4), and stroke unit beds should be available 24 hours a day for new admissions. Stroke units are more defined by staffing than by physical infrastructure, but stroke units do have a few specialist environmental and equipment considerations. Acute stroke units need to have the equipment to provide continuous (or regular) physiological monitoring. There is evidence that care bundles of nursing interventions that focus on physiological monitoring and detecting complications are effective in improving outcomes after stroke (Middleton, Grimley & Alexandrov, 2015). Appropriate facilities and space need to be available to mobilize patients and provide rehabilitation. This might include a gym for physiotherapy and areas (such as a therapy kitchen) for occupational therapy assessments.

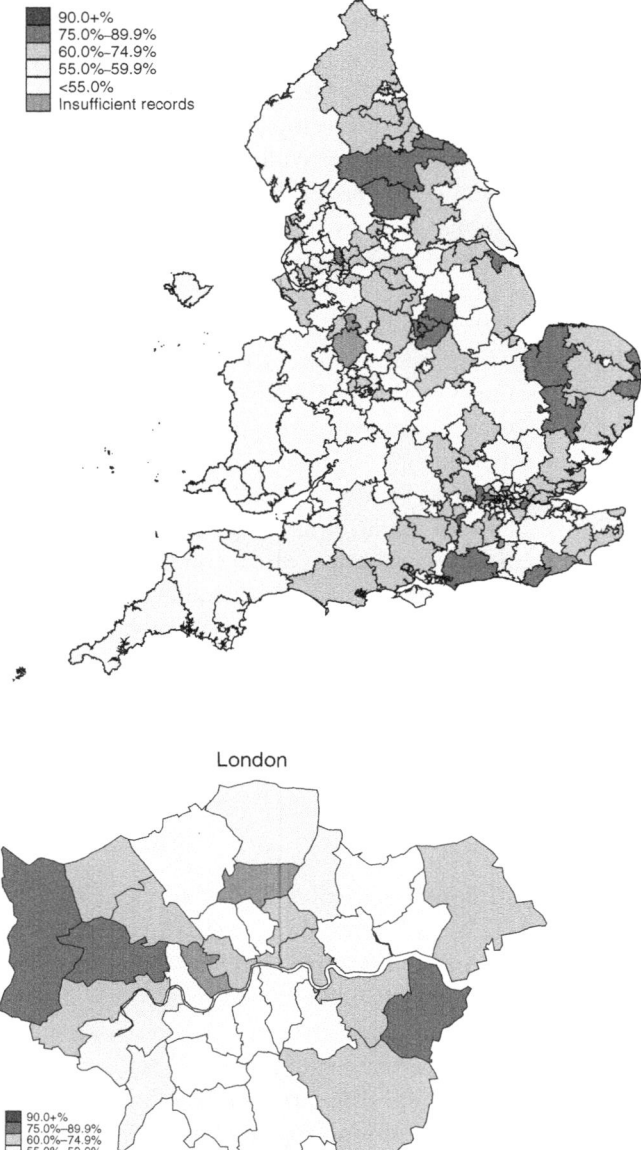

Figure 3.3 Geographical variation in admission to a stroke unit within four hours of admission in England and Wales

Source: January–March 2015, SSNAP

Specialist resources required for a core stroke service	Specialist resources required for subgroups of patients
Brain imaging	Specialist diagnostics
Stroke unit	Neuroradiology/thrombectomy
Diagnostics (blood tests, ECG)	Neurosurgery
Rehabilitation	Vascular surgery
Pharmacotherapy for secondary prevention & thrombolysis	Critical care
Long-term care (follow-up, primary care)	

Figure 3.4 Specialist resources for a stroke service

Source: Authors' compilation

Brain imaging is the core diagnostic requirement of a stroke service. CT imaging needs to be available 24 hours a day for the assessment of new patients and in carrying out imaging on patients who develop neurological deterioration after stroke. Although non-contrast CT imaging is adequate for most acute treatment decisions, increasing use is being made of more advanced CT imaging modalities (CT angiography and perfusion) and MRI.

A small proportion (less than 5%) of patients will require neurosurgical intervention (Vahedi et al., 2007). Managing these patients requires access to neurosurgical infrastructure (theatres, specialist surgical, anaesthetic and nurse staffing, critical care facilities) either on site or after transfer to a referral centre. Similarly, some patients with stroke or TIA require vascular surgery for carotid endarterectomy. Patients with strokes that result in reduced consciousness may need to be managed in an intensive care unit as part of their admission. As thrombectomy services become more widely available, stroke care in high income countries will increasingly require access to neurointerventional facilities and the staffing required to provide them for patients suitable for this treatment.

Vascular ultrasound and echocardiography are also recommended as part of the diagnostic work-up for many patients (European Stroke Organisation Guidelines). All of these investigations require appropriate equipment and staff skilled in carrying out and interpreting these tests.

The requirements from stroke services of laboratory and pathology services are limited largely to common blood tests and in the diagnostic work-up of rarer causes of stroke. POCT is widely used in the emergency room for patients being assessed for thrombolysis, where rapid results are important in achieving fast door to needle times (Rizos et al., 2009).

Stroke is not an area with a high use of specialist pharmaceuticals. The main pharmaceuticals that are required for an acute stroke service are alteplase (the only agent licensed for stroke thrombolysis in Europe) and secondary prevention agents (anticoagulants, antiplatelets, statins, anti-hypertensives).

Barriers to delivering optimal care

Training sufficient numbers of specialist staff has been a challenge in many countries. In the United Kingdom, for example, despite training pathways for physicians developing a specialty interest in stroke and the existence of stroke-specific professional organizations to support trainees and specialists, there is a shortage of physicians specialized in stroke medicine, with 25% of consultant posts remaining unfilled (Sentinel Stroke National Audit Programme, 2018). The reasons for this are unclear but might include the increasing requirement for out-of-office-hours working as stroke care has become higher in intensity. There are also fewer options for private practice for stroke specialist physicians than many other procedure-based or office-based specialties, which may affect its perceived attractiveness as a specialty. Lack of staffing resources, particularly of therapists and nursing home staff, was also identified as being one of the main barriers to improving stroke care in France (Gache et al., 2014). There is potential for tackling staff shortages by expanding the roles and skills of existing clinical staff, such as empowering nurses to manage thrombolysis calls and take on leadership roles in stroke services.

One of the key barriers to providing optimum care has been the difficulty of closing the gap between evidence and widespread implementation into practice. Here the barriers are not merely lack of financial or other resources, but also contextual and behavioural factors such as culture, organization and leadership. Indeed, implementation gaps in stroke care involve not only the high technology and resource-intensive elements of stroke care, but also the key evidence-based components of care (such as stroke units and secondary prevention): even "getting the basics right" can be difficult. For example, even 20 years after the publication of the first trial to demonstrate the effectiveness of thrombolysis for ischaemic stroke, rates of use of thrombolysis vary widely even in highly developed health economies. In particular, the uptake of thrombolysis was initially very poor in the United Kingdom: when the National Audit Office reported on the quality of stroke care in England in 2005 it found that fewer than 1% of stroke patients were receiving thrombolysis. By contrast, during the same period 3–4% of stroke patients were treated with thrombolysis in Sweden (Eriksson et al., 2010). The low rate of implementation in the United Kingdom occurred in the context of underdeveloped stroke services and highly variable care between centres, with only 60% of stroke patients being cared for in a stroke unit and many patients waiting more than two days for a brain scan (National Audit Office, 2005). This report prompted the development of a national improvement strategy, financial investment in stroke care, an expansion in training for stroke specialists and new resources allocated to quality improvement and audit. National clinical audits have since demonstrated significant improvements in the quality of stroke care in England and an acceleration in the uptake of thrombolysis, with 11–12% of patients (of all ages) now treated with thrombolysis: rates that are comparable with other high performing health systems in Europe (Sentinel Stroke National Audit Programme, 2018).

Although stroke care has been transformed by evidence-based medicine, there are still many areas of stroke care with little evidence to guide practice. One of the reasons for this may be relative underfunding of stroke research: in the United Kingdom for every £10 of health and social care costs attributable to stroke, it received only £0.19 in funding, compared to £1.08 for cancer and £0.65 for coronary heart disease (Luengo-Fernandez, Leal & Gray, 2015). The areas of stroke care with the poorest evidence base are generally the less acute components of care, such as therapy and rehabilitation. Even fundamental questions about rehabilitation, such as when physiotherapy should commence after stroke, and at what intensity, are only now being addressed in randomized controlled trials (AVERT Trial Collaboration Group et al., 2015). Lack of evidence makes it difficult to define what optimal care in these areas should be, contributing to variations in practice. For example, there are wide variations across Europe in the amount of therapy provided to patients after stroke, which are not explained by differences in patient characteristics and likely reflect variation in access and availability (Wolfe et al., 2004; Wellwood et al., 2009).

One of the biggest challenges for stroke medicine in high income countries in the next few years will be in implementing access to thrombectomy. Current provision is largely concentrated in relatively small numbers of specialist hospitals, and even in these hospitals there may not be round-the-clock access. The main barrier to implementation is insufficient numbers of trained neurointerventionists; increasing capacity will take time and there are likely to be resource challenges in maintaining a 24/7 acute thrombectomy service that may only be used relatively infrequently, with only a minority of acute stroke patients being appropriate for this treatment. Another risk is that a focus on developing thrombectomy services will distract attention and resources away from the wider challenge of implementing good quality stroke unit based care and post-stroke rehabilitation.

The future

The challenge for the future involves the twin tasks of implementing an ever-growing evidence base on new interventions and innovations and in improving the availability and quality of the elements of stroke care that we already know to work. As has already been described, wide variations in care quality exist both across and within European countries and these will not be reduced if the focus of clinicians, funders and managers is solely on implementing the "new". Indeed, it is worth emphasizing that from a global perspective most people with stroke do not even receive the most core elements of stroke care such as stroke unit based care. By far the greatest reduction in the future burden of stroke on populations will come about not through new technologies but as a result of public health efforts to reduce stroke incidence through tobacco control, public health programmes to reduce cardiovascular risk factors (such as hypertension, obesity, alcohol and physical inactivity), increasing access to stroke unit based care and rehabilitation, and effective use of secondary prevention.

There are also examples of interventions that are still in use, despite evidence of ineffectiveness or even harm. One of the most prevalent of these is the use of antiplatelet agents in patients with AF. Historically, antiplatelet agents such as aspirin were often used as an alternative to anticoagulants to reduce the risk of stroke in people with AF (particularly in older people), but it is now known that antiplatelets provide much less benefit and are no safer than oral anticoagulants

(Aguilar, Hart & Pearce, 2007). Current guidelines therefore recommend that antiplatelet agents are not used for stroke prophylaxis in AF. However, many patients with AF are still prescribed antiplatelets, and oral anticoagulants remain underused. In England, for example, 31% of eligible patients known to be in AF in primary care were not prescribed an oral anticoagulant in 2013/2014 (NHS Quality and Outcome Framework, 2015), resulting in many thousands of avoidable strokes per year. Newer oral anticoagulants have become available in recent years that offer similar reductions in stroke risk but may have reduced risks of major complications than treatment with warfarin (Gómez-Outes et al., 2013).

As already discussed, the innovation most likely to change stroke care in the next five years in high income countries is thrombectomy for ischaemic stroke. The challenges of implementing this at scale, though, are significant and it is not certain how quickly this will become widely available experience from thrombolysis suggests that it is likely to be slow and highly variable between settings. There are other emerging areas of research that are still at early stages but may lead to significant impacts in the future. One of the most intriguing ideas is of reducing delays in thrombolysis by installing brain CT scanners in ambulances, allowing pre-hospital diagnosis of stroke type and administration of thrombolysis if appropriate. The concept has been demonstrated in a small number of centres (Walter et al., 2012; Parker et al., 2015), and although the real-world feasibility and cost-effectiveness of this model of care remain unproven, using new diagnostic technologies to facilitate pre-hospital stroke diagnosis could transform stroke care pathways. Imaging is an area of fast-moving innovation and development – for example, it is now possible to non-invasively image areas of unstable atherosclerotic plaque that are the source of the majority of strokes, and identify at an early stage the patients at highest risk of new or recurrent stroke (Tarkin, Joshi & Rudd, 2014). Further off, there is the prospect that stem cell technologies may allow the repair of established brain damage occurring as a result of stroke; early-stage clinical trials in stroke patients are already ongoing (Banerjee et al., 2014). Rehabilitation is also increasingly making use of new advances in robotics to provide therapy and augment motor functioning in patients with limb paralysis after stroke (Burgar et al., 2000).

Although exciting, most of these innovations are likely to be applicable only to a minority of stroke patients. The implementation of these new resource-intensive interventions therefore needs to be linked to efforts to develop models of delivery that can provide these in the most clinically and cost-effective way: for many aspects of acute stroke care this is likely to mean further development of networks of care and centralization of specialist services into hub hospitals.

Perhaps of greater medium-term significance to population health will be innovations that are applicable to all patients with stroke: the shift towards increased engagement of patients in managing their own health through shared decision-making and self-management, and in the increasingly sophisticated use of data to support research, quality improvement and new models of care. For example, there is good evidence that helping patients to manage their own blood pressure leads to better blood pressure control than the typical model of clinic-based management (McManus et al., 2014); it is likely that health care services will increasingly take the role of supporting stroke survivors (and their carers) in managing stroke as a long-term condition. Similarly, health care in the future will make much more sophisticated use of real-world data such as electronic health records and clinical registries (Krumholz, 2014). For example, use of such data to generate more accurate predictions of prognosis, or to generate patient-specific estimates of the harms and benefits of interventions, can help in making better decisions about treatment and support patients in shared decision-making (Spertus et al., 2015).

Stroke care in the hospital of the mid-21st century

Stroke care has changed dramatically over recent decades, driven by the development of organized multidisciplinary care and an increasing emphasis on acute intervention. The dependency on advanced medical imaging, resource-intensive multidisciplinary care and acute treatments that can only feasibly be administered in large hospitals means than hospitals are likely to remain the cornerstone of acute stroke care with most patients being admitted for inpatient care. The hospital of the future, if it is to provide comprehensive care for patients with stroke, will therefore need to be organized and designed to deliver:

- round-the-clock access to advanced imaging, diagnostics and neurointervention facilities that are geographically located within the hospital to optimize speed of access;

- stroke units to which patients with acute stroke are admitted without delay and which are the setting for multidisciplinary stroke specialist care;
- the appropriate environment and equipment to enable optimal provision of therapy and to support rehabilitation and recovery; and
- organized pathways of care that reduce treatment delays and support the provision of good quality therapy not just in hospital but also in the community.

In many places this means that some acute hospitals should no longer attempt to treat stroke. Rather, there is a need to find alternative models of care whereby those suffering a stroke will be taken, at least for definitive treatment, to a hospital that can provide a comprehensive care package, including rapid diagnosis and intervention where required. This will often not be the nearest facility. This could have profound implications for the organization of hospitals in a defined area, especially where they have had a high degree of autonomy. It will often be extremely challenging, politically and legally, to tackle this and each solution must be tailored to the particular context.

The critical component of stroke care services will remain not physical assets and medical devices but the MDTs of people that are the core of organized stroke unit care. Maintaining and developing this resource will require long-term investment in the training of the stroke workforce (medical, nursing and allied health professions). Providing ongoing education and training will be of increasing importance in helping clinicians keep up to date with the accelerating pace of new medical knowledge and evidence.

It will be disappointing if the next few decades do not see the development of new, high-impact drugs and devices that improve recovery after stroke, reduce complications, or help survivors manage the long-term consequences of stroke. The development of therapies that facilitate brain repair (for example, through stem cells) could be a real paradigm shift, but the brain is vastly complex and still contains many mysteries; progress in the development of new "brain regeneration" therapies is hard to predict. For patients with permanent impairments after stroke, assistive technologies (such as robotics) are likely to become much more mainstream and sophisticated, and allow more stroke survivors to live independent lives. The challenge for the future will be providing these innovations at scale in a cost-effective way and in speeding up the diffusion of new evidence into widespread clinical practice.

The evidence of current variation in care quality and outcome points to the importance of prioritizing and developing quality improvement in stroke care. This includes supporting and developing current systems of clinical audit (SSNAP, SSCA, Riks-Stroke, Danish Stroke Register) and increasing the capacity of health care systems to deliver continuous quality improvement. As the sophistication and scope of health care data collection increase, this is likely to lead to a growing emphasis on the development of new ways of using data in stroke care as part of clinical care, research and quality improvement. It is hard to foresee in much detail what this new, data-aware world of health care will look like in practice, but it may have a transformative effect on the delivery and organization of stroke care in the next few decades.

References

Aguilar MI, Hart R, Pearce LA (2007). Oral anticoagulants versus antiplatelet therapy for preventing stroke in patients with non-valvular atrial fibrillation and no history of stroke or transient ischemic attacks. *Cochrane Database Syst Rev* 3:CD006186.

American Heart Association/American Stroke Association (2014). Guidelines for the Prevention of Stroke in Patients with Stroke and Transient Ischaemic Attack. *Stroke*, 45(7):2160–236.

Anderson CS et al. (2013). INTERACT2 Investigators. Rapid blood-pressure lowering in patients with acute intracerebral hemorrhage. *N Engl J Med*, 368(25):2355–65.

AVERT Trial Collaboration Group et al. (2015). Efficacy and safety of very early mobilisation within 24 h of stroke onset (AVERT): a randomised controlled trial. *Lancet*, 386(9988):46–55. doi: 10.1016/S0140-6736(15)60690-0. Epub 16 April 2015.

Ayerbe L et al. (2013). Natural history, predictors and outcomes of depression after stroke: systematic review and meta-analysis. *Br J Psychiatry*, 202:14–21.

Ayis SA et al. (2013). Variations in acute stroke care and the impact of organised care on survival from a European perspective: the European Registers of Stroke (EROS) investigators. *J Neurol Neurosurg Psychiatry*, 84(6):604–12.

Banerjee S et al. (2014). Intra-Arterial Immunoselected CD34+ Stem Cells for Acute Ischemic Stroke. *Stem Cells Transl Med*, 3(11):1322–30.

Bottacchi E et al. (2012). The cost of first-ever stroke in Valle d'Aosta, Italy: linking clinical registries and administrative data. *BMC Health Serv Res*, 12:372.

Bray BD et al. (2013a). Associations between the organisation of stroke services, process of care, and mortality in England: prospective cohort study. *BMJ*, 346:f2827.

Bray BD et al. (2013b). Bigger, faster? Associations between hospital thrombolysis volume and speed of thrombolysis administration in acute ischemic stroke. *Stroke*, 44(11):3129–35.

Bray BD et al. (2014). Associations between stroke mortality and weekend working by stroke specialist physicians and registered nurses: prospective multicentre cohort study. PLOS Med, 11(8):e1001705.

Bray BD et al. (2017). The association between delays in screening for and assessing dysphagia after acute stroke, and the risk of stroke-associated pneumonia. *J Neurol Neurosurg Psychiatry*, 88(1):25–30.

Burgar CG et al. (2000). Development of robots for rehabilitation therapy: the Palo Alto VA/Stanford experience. *J Rehabil Res Dev*, 37(6):663–73.

CLOTS (Clots in Legs Or sTockings after Stroke) Trials Collaboration et al. (2013). Effectiveness of intermittent pneumatic compression in reduction of risk of deep vein thrombosis in patients who have had a stroke (CLOTS 3): a multicentre randomised controlled trial. *Lancet*, 382(9891):516–24. doi: 10.1016/S0140-6736(13)61050-8. Epub 31 May 2013.

Cochrane Stroke Group (2013). Organised inpatient (stroke unit) care for stroke. *Cochrane Database Syst Rev*, 9: CD000197.

Cruz-Flores S, Berge E, Whittle IR (2012). Surgical decompression for cerebral oedema in acute ischaemic stroke. *Cochrane Database of Syst Rev*, 1:CD003435.

de Falco FA, Leone MA, Beghi E (2009). Stroke in neurological services in Italy. *Neurol Int*, 1(1):e8.

Di Carlo A et al. (2015). European Implementation Score Collaboration Study Group. Methods of Implementation of Evidence-Based Stroke Care in Europe: European Implementation Score Collaboration. *Stroke*, 46(8):2252–9.

Douw K, Nielsen CP, Pedersen CR (2015). Centralising acute stroke care and moving care to the community in a Danish health region: challenges in implementing a stroke care reform. *Health Policy*, 119(8):1005–10.

Emberson et al. (2014). Effect of treatment delay, age, and stroke severity on the effects of intravenous thrombolysis with alteplase for acute ischaemic stroke: a meta-analysis of individual patient data from randomised trials. *Lancet*, 384(9958):1929–35.

Eriksson M et al. (2010). Dissemination of thrombolysis for acute ischemic stroke across a nation: experiences from the Swedish stroke register, 2003 to 2008. *Stroke*, 41(6):1115–22.

Fassbender K et al. (2013). Streamlining of prehospital stroke management: the golden hour. *Lancet Neurol*, 12(6):585–96.

Feigin VL et al. (2009). Worldwide stroke incidence and early case fatality reported in 56 population-based studies: a systematic review. *Lancet Neurol*, 8(4):355–69.

Feigin VL et al. (2015). Update on the Global Burden of Ischemic and Hemorrhagic Stroke in 1990–2013: The GBD 2013 Study. *Neuroepidemiology*, 45(3):161–76.

Flynn D et al. (2014). A time series evaluation of the FAST National Stroke Awareness Campaign in England. *PLoS One*, 9(8):e104289.

Gache K et al. (2014). Main barriers to effective implementation of stroke care pathways in France: a qualitative study. *BMC Health Serv Res*, 14:95.

Gallacher KI et al. (2014). Stroke, multimorbidity and polypharmacy in a nationally representative sample of 1,424,378 patients in Scotland: implications for treatment burden. *BMC Med*, 12:151.

GBD 2013 Mortality and Causes of Death Collaborators (2015). Global, regional, and national age-sex specific all-cause and cause-specific mortality for 240 causes of death, 1990–2013: a systematic analysis for the Global Burden of Disease Study 2013. *Lancet*, 385(9963):117–71.

Gómez-Outes A et al. (2013). Dabigatran, Rivaroxaban, or Apixaban versus Warfarin in Patients with Nonvalvular Atrial Fibrillation: A Systematic Review and Meta-Analysis of Subgroups. *Thrombosis*, 2013:640723.

Goyal et al. (2016). Endovascular thrombectomy after large-vessel ischaemic stroke: a meta-analysis of individual patient data from five randomised trials. *Lancet*, 387(10029):1723–31.

Guidetti D et al. (2013). Monitoring the implementation of the State-Regional Council agreement 03/02/2005 as to the management of acute stroke events: a comparison of the Italian regional legislations. *Neurol Sci*, 34(9):1651–7.

Hess DC, Audebert HJ (2013). The history and future of telestroke. *Nat Rev Neurol*, 9(6):340–50.

Heuschmann PU et al. (2011). Three-month stroke outcome: the European Registers of Stroke (EROS) investigators. *Neurology*, 76(2):159–65.

Holloway RG et al. (2014). Palliative and end-of-life care in stroke: a statement for healthcare professionals from the American Heart Association/American Stroke Association. *Stroke*, 45(6):1887–916.

Iihara K et al. (2014). Effects of comprehensive stroke care capabilities on in-hospital mortality of patients with ischemic and hemorrhagic stroke: J-ASPECT study. *PLoS One*, 9(5):e96819.

Intercollegiate Stroke Working Party (2016). *National Clinical Guideline for Stroke* (5th edn). London, Royal College of Physicians.

Jennum P et al. (2015). Cost of stroke: a controlled national study evaluating societal effects on patients and their partners. *BMC Health Serv Res*, 15(1):466.

Krumholz HM (2014). Big data and new knowledge in medicine: the thinking, training, and tools needed for a learning health system. *Health Aff (Millwood)*, 33(7):1163–70.

Langhorne P, Baylan S (2017). Early supported discharge services for people with acute stroke. *Cochrane Database Syst Rev* 7:CD000443.

Langhorne P, de Villiers L, Pandian JD (2012). Applicability of stroke-unit care to low-income and middle-income countries. *Lancet Neurol*, 11(4):341–8.

Langhorne P, Pollock A, Stroke Unit Triallists' Collaboration (2002). What are the components of effective stroke unit care? *Age Ageing*, 31(5):365–71.

Lebrun L et al. (2011). Improving stroke care: a French health-care organiser's perspective. *Int J Stroke*, 6(2):123–4.

Leys D et al. (2007). Facilities available in European hospitals treating stroke patients. *Stroke*, 38(11):2985–91.

Leys D et al. (2009). Facilities available in French hospitals treating acute stroke patients: comparison with 24 other European countries. *J Neurol*, 256(6):867–73.

Luengo-Fernandez R, Gray AM, Rothwell PM (2009). Effect of urgent treatment for transient ischaemic attack and minor stroke on disability and hospital costs (EXPRESS study): a prospective population-based sequential comparison. *Lancet Neurol*, 8(3):235–43.

Luengo-Fernandez R, Leal J, Gray A (2015). UK research spend in 2008 and 2012: comparing stroke, cancer, coronary heart disease and dementia. *BMJ Open*, 5(4):e006648.

McKevitt C et al. (2011). Self-reported long-term needs after stroke. *Stroke*, 42(5):1398–403.

McManus RJ et al. (2014). Effect of self-monitoring and medication self-titration on systolic blood pressure in hypertensive patients at high risk of cardiovascular disease: the TASMIN-SR randomized clinical trial. *JAMA*, 312(8):799–808. doi: 10.1001/jama.2014.1005.

McMeekin P et al. (2017). Estimating the number of UK stroke patients eligible for endovascular thrombectomy. *Eur Stroke J*, 2(4):319–326.

Mellon L et al. (2013). Can a media campaign change health service use in a population with stroke symptoms? Examination of the first Irish stroke awareness campaign. *Emerg Med J*, 31(7):536–40. doi: 10.1136/emermed-2012-202280.

Mendelow AD et al. (2013). Early surgery versus initial conservative treatment in patients with spontaneous supratentorial lobar intracerebral haematomas (STICH II): a randomised trial. *Lancet*, 382:397–408. (Erratum appears in *Lancet*, 382(9890):396.)

Meretoja A et al. (2013). Helsinki model cut stroke thrombolysis delays to 25 minutes in Melbourne in only 4 months. *Neurology*, 81(12):1071–6.

Middleton S, Grimley R, Alexandrov AW (2015). Triage, treatment, and transfer: evidence-based clinical practice recommendations and models of nursing care for the first 72 hours of admission to hospital for acute stroke. *Stroke*, 46(2):e18–25.

Middleton S et al. (2011). Implementation of evidence-based treatment protocols to manage fever, hyperglycaemia, and swallowing dysfunction in acute stroke (QASC): a cluster randomised controlled trial. *Lancet*, 378:1699–706.

Morris S et al. (2014). Impact of centralising acute stroke services in English metropolitan areas on mortality and length of hospital stay: difference-in-differences analysis. *BMJ*, 349:g4757.

National Audit Office (2005). Reducing Brain Damage: faster access to better stroke care.

National Institute of Neurological Disorders and Stroke rt-PA Stroke Study Group (1995). Tissue plasminogen activator for acute ischemic stroke. *N Engl J Med*, 333(24):1581–7.

Needleman J et al. (2011). Nurse staffing and inpatient hospital mortality. *N Engl J Med*, 364(11):1037–45.

NHS Quality and Outcome Framework (2015). NHS Digital.

Nor AM (2005). The Recognition of Stroke in the Emergency Room (ROSIER) scale: development and validation of a stroke recognition instrument. *Lancet Neurol*, 4(11):727–34.

North American Symptomatic Carotid Endarterectomy Trial Collaborators (1991). Beneficial effect of carotid endarterectomy in symptomatic patients with high-grade carotid stenosis. *N Engl J Med*, 325(7):445–53.

Parker SA et al. (2015). Establishing the first mobile stroke unit in the United States. *Stroke*, 46(5):1384–91.

Public Health England (2015). *PHE encourages people to act FAST if they experience stroke symptoms* (Online). Available at: https://www.gov.uk/ government/uploads/system/uploads/attachment_data/file/400241/Stroke_ press_release_020215.pdf.

Reeves MJ et al. (2008). Changes in knowledge of stroke risk factors and warning signs among Michigan adults. *Cerebrovasc Dis*, 25(5):385–91.

RiksStroke (2018). URL: www.riksstroke.org/eng/.

Ringelstein et al. (2013). European Stroke Organisation recommendations to establish a stroke unit and stroke center. *Stroke*, 44(3):828–40.

Rizos T et al. (2009). Point-of-care international normalized ratio testing accelerates thrombolysis in patients with acute ischemic stroke using oral anticoagulants. *Stroke*, 40(11):3547–5.

Rothwell PM et al. (2007). Effect of urgent treatment of transient ischaemic attack and minor stroke on early recurrent stroke (EXPRESS study): a prospective population-based sequential comparison. *Lancet*, 370(9596):1432–42.

Saka O et al. (2009). Cost-Effectiveness of Stroke Unit Care Followed by Early Supported Discharge. *Stroke*, 40:24–9.

Sandercock PA et al. (2008). Antiplatelet therapy for acute ischaemic stroke. *Cochrane Database Syst Rev*, 3:CD000029. *Doi: 10.1002/14651858. CD000029.pub2*.

Schmidt A et al. (2015). Acute Ischemic Stroke (AIS) patient management in French stroke units and impact estimation of thrombolysis on care pathways and associated costs. *Cerebrovasc Dis*, 39(2):94–101.

Sentinel Stroke National Audit Programme (2018). *Sentinel Stroke National Audit Programme* (Online). Available at: www.strokeaudit.org.

Sheth KN et al. (2015). Drip and ship thrombolytic therapy for acute ischemic stroke: use, temporal trends, and outcomes. *Stroke*, 46(3):732–9.

Spertus JA et al. (2015). Precision medicine to improve use of bleeding avoidance strategies and reduce bleeding in patients undergoing percutaneous coronary intervention: prospective cohort study before and after implementation of personalized bleeding risks. *BMJ*, 350:h1302.

Stroke Unit Triallists' Collaboration (2007). Organised inpatient (stroke unit) care for stroke. *Cochrane Database Syst Rev*, 4:CD00019.

Tarkin JM, Joshi FR, Rudd JH (2014). PET imaging of inflammation in atherosclerosis. *Nat Rev Cardiol*, 11(8):443–57.

Thrift AG et al. (2014). Global stroke statistics. *Int J Stroke*, 9:6–18.

Turner et al. (2016). Stroke patients admitted within normal working hours are more likely to achieve process standards and to have better outcomes. *J Neurol Neurosurg Psychiatry*, 87:138–43.

Vahedi K et al. (2007). Early decompressive surgery in malignant infarction of the middle cerebral artery: a pooled analysis of three randomised controlled trials. *Lancet Neurol*, 6(3):215–22.

Walter S et al. (2012). Diagnosis and treatment of patients with stroke in a mobile stroke unit versus in hospital: a randomised controlled trial. *Lancet Neurol*, 11(5):397–404.

Wellwood I et al. (2009). An observational study of acute stroke care in four countries: the European registers of stroke study. *Cerebrovasc Dis*, 28(2):171–6.

Wiedmann S et al. (2012). Variations in quality indicators of acute stroke care in 6 European countries: the European Implementation Score (EIS) Collaboration. *Stroke*, 43(2):458–63.

Wiedmann S et al. (2014). The quality of acute stroke care – an analysis of evidence-based indicators in 260 000 patients. *Dtsch Arztebl Int*, 111(45):759–65.

Wolfe CD et al. (2004). Variations in care and outcome in the first year after stroke: a Western and Central European perspective. *J Neurol Neurosurg Psychiatry*, 75(12):1702–6.

Wolfe CD et al. (2011). Estimates of outcomes up to ten years after stroke: analysis from the prospective South London Stroke Register. *PLoS Med*, 8(5):e1001033.

Xian Y et al. (2011). Association between stroke center hospitalization for acute ischemic stroke and mortality. *JAMA*, 305(4):373–80.

4 | Meeting the needs of frail older patients

SHERENA NAIR[1], DAVID OLIVER[2], ALISON
CRACKNELL[3]

[1] Elderly Medicine Registrar, Leeds Teaching Hospitals NHS Trust
[2] Clinical Vice President, Royal College of Physicians, London
[3] Consultant Medicine for Older People and Honorary Clinical
Associate Professor, Leeds Teaching Hospitals NHS Trust

Introduction

The current challenge

All European countries are experiencing rapid demographic transitions, with an increase in the proportion of over 65-year-olds and the most rapid increase in people over 80 years of age (Creighton, 2014). This means that, increasingly, the business of acute hospitals is the care of older people, often with frailty, dementia or multiple long-term conditions complicating their acute illness. Without a radical shift in care models, at scale and surpassing anything we have yet seen, this will continue to be the case for the foreseeable future. There has been a general reduction in hospital beds and increases in ambulatory and community treatment but there remain gaps in services that fail to meet the needs of frail older people, which often result in hospital attendances (NHS Benchmarking, 2013; Cowling et al., 2014; Radvansky, 2014; Melzer et al., 2015). Particular challenges arise for those with frailty, chronic multiple conditions, and those with dementia, adding to the complexity of treatment and care needs of older people (Melzer etv al., 2015).

Some of the key challenges facing hospitals caring for older people with frailty include unmet care needs, health inequalities, and a lack of quality service models and integration between services (European Institute, 2012). There is wide variation in the nature and scope of services addressing the needs of frail older people, with some countries such as Austria having recognized geriatric medicine as a subspecialty of internal medicine only from 2011 (Ekdahl et al., 2012). While countries are acknowledging the need for better integration of services, implementation of more integrated care models has been slow (Curry & Ham, 2010; Shah et al., 2010).

The challenge of frailty

Frailty is defined as a state of increased vulnerability and a disturbance in homoeostasis where a stressor event can lead to dramatic changes to the health status of an individual, which result in increased dependency levels, mobility problems, a change in cognition, such as delirium, and marked levels of functional decline (Clegg et al., 2013) (Figure 4.1; Box 4.1). Frailty is also associated with increased mortality and morbidity, and it is a strong predictor of care home utilization and death (Clegg et al., 2016). There are two common models for defining frailty as a clinical entity and these are increasingly important as ways of segmenting and addressing the needs of hospital patients (Oliver, 2016c). These rest on an identifiable "frailty phenotype" (Fried model) based on the

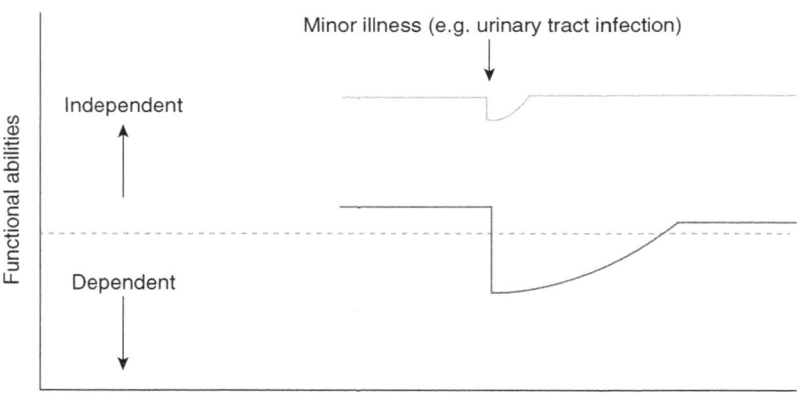

Figure 4.1 Vulnerability of frail older people to a sudden change in health status following a minor illness

Note: The top line represents a fit older person who, following a minor stress such as a urinary tract infection, experiences a relatively small deterioration in function and then returns to homoeostasis. The lower line represents a frail older person who, following a similar stress, experiences a larger deterioration which may manifest as functional dependency and who does not return to baseline homoeostasis.

Source: Clegg et al., 2013

Box 4.1 Common presentations of frail older people

Frailty syndromes (how people with frailty present to services)

- "Non-specific" – e.g. fatigue, weight loss, recurrent infection
- Falls/collapse
- Immobility/worsening mobility
- Delirium ("acute confusion")
- Incontinence (new or worsening)
- Fluctuating disability
- Increased susceptibility to medication side effects – e.g hypotension, delirium

---

presence of three or more characteristics or a "frailty index" (Rockwood & Mitnitski, 2011; Clegg et al., 2016) based on an accumulation of deficits. There is an overlap between frailty, multiple co-morbidity and age-related disability (World Health Organization, 2015; National Institute for Health and Care Excellence, 2016), although it is now possible to identify people with frailty in community settings using existing primary care data (Clegg et al., 2016) (Table 4.1), at the hospital emergency front door or on the inpatient wards, where simple pragmatic case-finding tools are often employed (Royal College of Physicians, 2013; British Geriatrics Society, 2014a; Health Improvement Scotland, 2015).

Adequate assessments and interventions for frailty are important. Survival plots using primary care data in England suggest that those with severe frailty are at higher risk of dying by a factor of five (Bates et al., 2014). A ten-year prospective cohort study involving community-dwelling older people identified frailty to be the leading cause of death, accounting for 28% of deaths compared to organ failure (21%), cancer (19%), dementia (14%) and other causes (15%) (Clegg et al., 2013).

Falls are a common reason for admission to hospital and have come to the attention of policy-makers and payers. Frailty is known to be an independent predictor of falls, and figures over the last five years show that Ireland had spent an estimated €520 million on falls, while in the Netherlands fractures were estimated to have led to 80% of fall-related costs, amounting to approximately €540 million between 2007 and

Table 4.1 *Adjusted 1, 3 and 5 year hazard ratios for outcomes of mortality, unplanned hospitalization and nursing home admission for older people with mild, moderate and severe frailty*

Outcome	Mild frailty (HR, 95% CI)	Moderate frailty (HR, 95% CI)	Severe frailty (HR, 95% CI)
1 year mortality	1.92 (1.81–2.04)	3.10 (2.91–3.31)	4.52 (4.16–4.91)
3 year mortality	1.77 (1.71–1.83)	2.78 (2.68–2.89)	3.99 (3.79–4.20)
5 year mortality	1.72 (1.68–1.77)	2.64 (2.57–2.72)	3.83 (3.68–3.99)
1 year unplanned hospitalization	1.93 (1.86–2.01)	3.04 (2.90–3.19)	4.73 (4.43–5.06)
3 year unplanned hospitalization	1.78 (1.74–1.82)	2.63 (2.55–2.71)	3.76 (3.60–3.94)
5 year unplanned hospitalization	1.71 (1.68–1.74)	2.50 (2.44–2.56)	3.43 (3.31–3.58)
1 year nursing home admission	1.89 (1.63–2.15)	3.19 (2.73–3.73)	4.76 (3.92–5.77)
3 year nursing home admission	1.67 (1.56–1.80)	2.60 (2.40–2.82)	3.55 (3.19–3.96)
5 year nursing home admission	1.59 (1.51–1.67)	2.30 (2.18–2.44)	3.12 (2.88–3.38)

Note: For all outcomes the comparator is fit older people. All data adjusted for age and sex. NB: Hospitalization outcome for external validation cohort includes only those practices (n = 158) with Hospital Episode Statistics (HES) linked data. CI: confidence interval; HR: hazard ratio.

Source: Clegg et al., 2016

2009. In England alone, falls in older people have been estimated to cost the National Health Service £2 billion annually (Fenton, 2014). Across Europe and other high income countries, the estimated costs of falls to health care services are significant.

Minimizing harm in frail older people in hospital

Older people are at significant risk of "harm" often associated with their care and medicalization of their illnesses. Polypharmacy, falls, hospital-acquired infections, malnutrition and immobility are some of the common problems that arise, which can lead to increased morbidity and mortality of older patients admitted to hospital (Barber et al., 2009; Oliver, Foot & Humphries, 2014). Bed rest in itself has also been associated with a range of harms where 10 days of bed rest in healthy older adults can lead to a 14% reduction in leg and hip muscle strength, and a 12% reduction in aerobic capacity (Oliver, Foot & Humphries, 2014). Older people often already have decreased physical function which may be negatively affected by hospitalization. They also have poorer functional outcomes and are less likely to recover from their problems in hospital (Covinsky et al., 2003; Kleinpell, Fletcher & Jennings, 2008; Mudge, O'Rourke & Denaro, 2010).

Models of pre-hospital care

The role of primary care in care coordination and urgent access

Frail older people pose a challenge to primary care although family physicians are ideally posed to incorporate the identification and management of frailty in their practice (Lacas & Rockwood, 2012). Countries are increasingly implementing more proactive personalized care planning, care coordination and case management to enhance primary care services for (frail older) people with one or more long-term conditions (Coulter et al., 2015). These care provisions are often provided by specialist nurses and therapists as well as volunteers in the care sector (Kringos et al., 2013; Bienkowska-Gibbs et al., 2015). At the same time, when the health or independence of older people rapidly deteriorates, it is important to ensure rapid access to urgent care, including effective alternatives to hospital (Oliver, Foot & Humphries, 2014; NHS Benchmarking, 2015). The following sections describe selected models that are being implemented in different settings to meet this need in particular.

Rapid community response teams

Older people with frailty are at a higher risk of unplanned hospital admissions (Boutsioli, 2012; Sona et al., 2012; Wittenberg et al., 2014). In England alone, up to 42% of emergency admissions in 2011 came from care homes with older people who were within the last six months of their life; these patients also often had multiple admissions in the year leading up to death (Smith et al., 2015).

Rapid response teams can offer specialist advice and improve the care for frail older people with long-term conditions (Oliver, Foot & Humphries, 2014; Wittenberg et al., 2014; NHS Benchmarking, 2015). These services may variously include geriatricians, GPs, specialist nurses, physiotherapists, occupational therapists, and sometimes others such as pharmacists, social workers, personal care assistants or generic rehabilitation assistants to address the complex medical needs of frail older people where time is of the essence, and without which the episode may result in hospital admission. These teams can also collaborate with ambulance organizations to divert patients to the community rapid response team and towards the community team. They are most likely to be effective when able to see patients within hours and when they have a range of skills within the team (NHS Benchmarking, 2016; Shepperd et al., 2016).

Ambulatory care clinics

Ambulatory care clinics are defined as units that provide preventative intervention and chronic disease management services for frail older people who may be at risk of future hospital admission (Oliver, Foot & Humphries, 2014). Ambulatory care clinics can be located in hospital outpatient settings or in primary care, and led by GPs or specialist clinicians with a range of multidisciplinary staff that can include pharmacists and social workers to optimize care of the frail older patient. Ambulatory care clinics or "one-stop" frailty clinics are an emerging service in France that provides assessment, management and support for older people with the aim of preventing and minimizing disability among those who are fit enough to attend such services (Tavassoli et al., 2014) and uses a collaborative approach with primary care and other allied professionals (Box 4.2). The overall evidence for impact of such service models remains weak, although a recent randomized controlled trial in Sweden demonstrated improved survival, and reduced length of stay in hospital without increasing cost up to three years after assessment (Ekdahl, Alwin & Eckerblad, 2016). In the United Kingdom, rapid access ambulatory care clinics in community hospitals have shown that frail older patients who are referred from primary care, ambulance services and community teams can be seen more quickly and closer to home,

---

Box 4.2 Gerontopole frailty clinic

A geriatric frailty clinic (structured as a day hospital unit) was established in 2011 in Toulouse, France, for frail people above the age of 65 years, who were referred by their GP, geriatrician or specialist to undergo a multidisciplinary evaluation to assess frailty and underlying risk factors for disability. During a two-year period the clinic assessed over 1000 people and a personalized prevention plan was developed to optimize their care in the community. The unit was led by a physician with ad hoc training in geriatrics at the university hospital outpatient clinic. The physician coordinating the evaluation was supported by other health care professionals (in particular, nurses, nutritionists, neuropsychologists and physical therapists) in the development of a personalized plan of intervention. This was then shared with the person's GP in order to make them aware of the recommendations and promote adherence to the preventive programme. A month after the assessment at the clinic a nurse would make a follow-up call to the patient to ensure that the interventions agreed had been undertaken; if a further deterioration in health was detected at this time, further action/plans were put in place to remedy the situation, where possible through the local GP responsible. This service focuses on secondary prevention for frail older people still completely autonomous in their basic activities of daily living. It was found that almost 94% of patients referred to the service were either frail or pre-frail, according to Fried's definition of frailty.

Source: Tavassoli et al., 2014

---

with a MDT addressing complex care needs effectively, and figures show that only up to 20% of those referred are transferred on to the nearest acute centre, with 56% discharged home or to their previous care setting (Koduah et al., 2014).

Community hospitals and intermediate care units

In Europe, community hospitals are increasingly being (re)considered as a means to address the care needs of older people in particular and are predominantly staffed by GPs and nurses, with some specialist input

(Winpenny et al., 2016). These often provide pre- and post-hospital care and so bridge the gap between care received for an acute illness prior to discharge to home (Oliver, Foot & Humphries, 2014). One recent example is the introduction, in 2012, of municipal acute care beds in Norway, which are organized as part of the municipal health services together with GPs, local emergency services, long-term care services and other parts of social care (Swanson & Hagen, 2016). They are targeted at stable patients who need monitoring or close follow-up from acute illnesses, often exacerbated by chronic medical conditions. Evidence from community hospital-type set-ups are mainly observational in nature, and evaluation of their effectiveness is still lacking (World Health Organization, 2015).

Models of hospital care

Across Europe frail older people account for approximately 20% of total attendance to emergency departments (Sona et al., 2012). The majority of people over 50 years old attending emergency departments have multiple long-term conditions (Quality Watch, 2015). One important response is hospital care based on comprehensive geriatric assessment as the underpinning tenet of assessment and management. The models described in this section can be found in different European countries, although we also consider successful models from other developed health care systems such as the United States.

Comprehensive geriatric assessment for frail older inpatients

Comprehensive geriatric assessment (CGA) is a process of assessing an older person's medical, psychological, physical and social functioning to inform the use of specific interventions and then develop and implement a plan for ongoing treatment and follow-up. There is good evidence from meta-analysis of numerous studies from several European countries that comprehensive interdisciplinary assessment of older people presenting to hospital delivers long-term benefits in terms of survival and the ability to remain in their own homes with less cognitive decline (Ellis et al., 2011). Because this is an iterative process rather than a discrete event, a CGA initiated in hospital can be continued in a person's own home to fully assess the need for support and so enable the frail older person to remain within their own environment (Ellis et al., 2011).

CGA is multidisciplinary, although outcomes are best with a specialist geriatrician leadership or input team on admission of the patient (Ellis et al., 2011; Oliver, Foot & Humphries, 2014). In the United Kingdom standards of care and assessment have been set out by national leadership bodies (British Geriatrics Society, 2014b; Health Improvement Scotland, 2015). Across Europe CGA is gaining momentum and is being used to assess and optimize frailty for a variety of medical and surgical conditions, and as a predictor of adverse outcomes. For examples, see Kristjansson et al. (2010) and Molina-Garrido & Guillén-Ponce (2011).

A recent review of the practice of CGA in high income countries in Europe, North America and Taiwan showed that only 32% of interdisciplinary geriatric consultation teams had used any formal CGA screening aid in intervention decisions. Also, while nurses formed key members of teams, their roles and responsibilities tended not to be clearly identified (Deschodt et al., 2016). There is a need to place implementation barriers of CGA into local contexts and so effectively address its effectiveness, culture change, educational needs of practitioners, research and evolving requirements of service provision (Gladman et al., 2016).

Specialist models of acute hospital care for people with frailty

Acute frailty services are specialist units that focus on specialized and tailored care for complex frail older people at, or close to, the hospital front door and with a focus on older people in the first phase of hospital admission. Where possible, they aim to assess and stabilize patients with a view to early discharge before they move to "deeper" wards within the hospital (Acute Frailty Clinical Network, 2015; Royal College of Physicians, 2015; Oliver, 2016c). There are different models in various acute settings but the most common models include: emergency department-based models and acute frailty units (Van Craen et al., 2010; Deschodt et al., 2013; Conroy et al., 2014).

Emergency department-based geriatrics and frailty services provide specialist geriatric input in decision-making for frail older people who attend the emergency department; other objectives include providing a multidisciplinary assessment using CGA and initiatives to reduce admission rates (Blakemore, 2012). Specialized nurses, who are experienced in falls, dementia, mental health and continence, are often available within these teams to provide support in hospital and coordinate better specialist care in the community at discharge. The overall evidence for emergency frailty units remains weak, with the majority of care models being trials of transitional care, which is a relatively novel concept of providing care for older people (Conroy & Chikura, 2015). Implementation of such care models in the emergency department remains challenging because of the complexity involved in identifying frailty, including the lack of standardized frailty instruments and poor understanding of frailty and the absence of clinical guidelines of frailty management in the emergency setting (Dent et al., 2016).

Acute frailty units, also referred to as "acute geriatric evaluation and management units", are inpatient wards at or close to the hospital "front door" that admit frail older people for assessments, treatment, review and rehabilitation through the use of CGA (Van Craen et al., 2010). A meta-analysis by Van Craen et al. (2010) of American, Austrian, German and Norwegian studies found that acute frailty units showed a significant positive impact on functional decline at discharge and institutionalization at one year. It also demonstrated that multidisciplinary CGA added value to those who were admitted to hospital by meeting the specific needs of frail older people and resulting in higher satisfaction of care provided to the patient.

European countries are at different stages in the development of acute frailty or acute geriatric units, which tend to be concentrated in larger cities, mainly because of the uneven distribution of geriatricians (Kolb, Topinkova & Michel, 2011; Ekdahl et al., 2012) and poor availability outside major centres. Whereas geriatric medicine is the largest internal medical speciality in the United Kingdom (Royal College of Physicians of London, 2015) and acute frailty units are found in small and medium-sized hospitals (Acute Frailty Clinical Network, 2015; NHS Benchmarking, 2016), it is not as well established in many European countries (EUGMS Survey, in press). For example, in Denmark and Sweden specialist geriatric units tend to be based at tertiary hospitals where frail older people undergo assessments that aid further planning of care. In smaller hospitals, geriatric care is embedded within general internal medicine departments on the whole (Kolb, Topinkova & Michel, 2011; Ekdahl et al., 2012).

Delirium units and teams

Delirium units often coexist with dementia wards because of the common coexistence of the two conditions and similar management strategies that are employed to support patients (Lam et al., 2014). Delirium is so widely prevalent among older hospital inpatients that it is unlikely that specialist delirium units could ever look after all patients or that it is possible or desirable to cohort them all in one clinical area (National Institute for Health and Care Excellence, 2010; Oliver, 2016a). And so, it is equally important to ensure that all staff caring for frail older people are able to recognize, prevent and manage delirium and that specialist teams are able to provide support and training of other staff.

One example is the Hospital Elder Life Programme (HELP), which was developed in the USA in 1993; it involves the use of a "multicomponent strategy" with multidisciplinary specialist teams who provide structured support to older people with delirium (Young & Inouye, 2007). HELP has been implemented in more than 11 countries across more than 100 sites (Steelfisher et al., 2013). It has been shown to be cost- and clinically effective, with reduced rates of delirium and functional decline, including the prevention and exacerbation of chronic medical conditions, with improved satisfaction among providers, patients and family (National Institute for Health and Care Excellence, 2010). Health Improvement Scotland is driving a national programme to prevent, recognize and improve outcomes in people with delirium and to share best practice (Health Improvement Scotland, 2016). The European Delirium Association now also has a network to share best practice and research across Europe.

Geriatric–surgical collaboration and liaison for frail older people

Not all frail older people are admitted under geriatric medicine and therefore it is crucial to provide CGAs where possible to optimize the care and health of older people admitted under different specialties. The more familiar and most widely developed liaison service across Europe is orthogeriatric collaboration with available evidence demonstrating cost-effectiveness and significant associations with reduced mortality rates in frail older people with fragility fractures (Sabharwal & Wilson, 2015; Knobe & Pape, 2016; Ozalp & Aspray, 2016). In Germany and Austria the explicit implementation of geriatric trauma centres has been developed where hip fracture patients are co-managed with common ward rounds between geriatricians, orthopaedic surgeons and specialized nurses (Kammerlander et al., 2011; Pape et al., 2014). In the United Kingdom the development of a fracture liaison service has been promoted as a "model of best practice" to provide optimum care to frail older people with hip fractures; a recent analysis of data from 11 hospitals in England points to significant improvements in mortality post surgery (British Orthopaedic Association, 2007; Hawley et al., 2016).

General surgical liaison is now a growing field in the United Kingdom, after its initial liaison model was developed specifically to address the needs of older people undergoing surgery, known as the proactive geriatric liaison with older people undergoing surgery (POPS) model (Harari et al., 2007). A survey of 161 hospitals in the United Kingdom showed that there are varying levels of geriatric-led perioperative services being provided across the country, with a combination of preoperative and postoperative services being offered that covers both acute and elective surgery, although barriers include funding, workforce issues, and a lack of inter-specialty collaboration (Partridge et al., 2014).

Other European countries are at different stages of developing medical liaison services as there is clear recognition of the value of geriatric input into the management of complex medical issues. Belgium introduced the "Geriatric Health Care Programme" in 2007 by adopting the development of a geriatric unit that also provides internal and external liaison services to frail older people on non-geriatric wards through similar tenets of CGA and MDT working (Van Den Noortgate & Petrovic, 2009; Baitar et al., 2015). In Ireland the older person assessment and liaison service (OPAL) showed that the service model provided timely CGA, and facilitated effective discharges from hospital, which may be further enhanced by efficient referrals and assessment processes through the use of clinical nurse managers (Hayes et al., 2016).

The role of outpatient clinics

Outpatient clinics in secondary care serve to bridge the gap between hospital care and the community once a patient has been discharged from hospital. They may also assume the role of "specialist" clinics that assess and treat specific conditions such as Parkinson's disease, respiratory or cardiology conditions, as well as falls and syncope clinics. Falls (prevention) clinics have been shown to reduce the incidence of injurious falls among older people by providing specific interventions around falls prevention with the support of physiotherapists and occupational therapists (Moore et al., 2010; Palvanen et al., 2014). Outpatient falls and syncope clinics are sometimes defined as day clinics, where assessments involve addressing underlying medical conditions to be treated, which are followed by further assessments by the physiotherapist and occupational therapists before an intervention is put into place (Lamb, Gates & Fisher, 2007). Outpatient clinics may also provide day services such as blood transfusion and chemotherapy where appropriate to enable patients to return home without needing inpatient admissions for such procedures. However, the provision of such assessment and follow-up does not necessarily have to happen on hospital sites, especially when travel and repeat attendances could be disruptive and distressing to older people with frailty. In some cases, hospital specialists and skilled MDTs can provide outpatient services in community and primary care settings closer to patients' homes, often in collaboration with primary care teams (British Geriatrics Society et al., 2012; King's Fund, 2014; Gordon, 2015).

End of life care

A study examining the place of death in older people with dementia-related diseases across 14 countries showed that in Europe the proportion of deaths in hospital ranged from 1.6% in the Netherlands to 62.3% in Hungary (31.7% in England, 35.9% in France, 32% in Italy, 33.6% in Spain, 21.6% in Belgium) (Reyniers et al., 2015). A qualitative systematic review of integrated palliative care in Europe found that a palliative care framework is necessary to improve symptom control, lessen care-giver burden, improve continuity and coordination of care, reduce admissions, increase cost-effectiveness and enable patients to die in their preferred place of care (Siouta et al., 2016). In 2010 the National Gold Standards Framework in End of Life Care Centre, a volunteer sector organization in the United Kingdom, was formed to provide support, training, and innovation in delivering better end of life care through advance care planning, with the goal of improving the quality and coordination of care, reducing hospitalization, and enabling more people to live and die at home (Gold Standards Framework, 2012). A 2015 audit on death and dying by the Royal College of Physicians of London (2016) found that of the 93% of patients whose death was predictable and documented, only 54% of case records showed that the needs of the person were asked about, with only 24% of patients having clinically assisted (artificial) hydration; 34% of cases had documented evidence about the need for clinically assisted (artificial) nutrition. Only 67% of hospitals reported that they implemented change to their service by taking into account bereaved family and friends' requests about patient care in their final days (Royal College of Physicians of London, 2016). Between 2005 and 2012 improvements in coverage of palliative care services had been made mostly in western European countries compared to central and eastern European countries, with still significant gaps across services (Centeno-Cortes et al., 2016). There is only one chance to get end of life care right and often this is unfortunately not the case. With a limited number of hospice beds and palliative care specialists available, advance care planning and addressing end of life issues earlier is pivotal, and if the patient does end up in hospital in their final days, then every effort should be made to get it right from the start (Oliver, 2016d; Royal College of Physicians of London, 2016).

Care of older patients with dementia and mental health problems in general hospitals

Dementia encompasses a group of organic brain diseases and the most common forms are Alzheimer's dementia, vascular dementia, mixed dementia (having Alzheimer's and vascular components), Lewy bodies and fronto-temporal dementia (Hackman et al., 2013). The personal, social, and economic costs of dementia are substantial, often complicated by multiple co-morbidities or frailty. The global estimate of older people living with dementia is expected to increase to 81 million by 2040, of whom 30% will be living in Europe (Kaplan & Berkman, 2011). Hospital patients with dementia are typically more frail, and at risk of significant complications of hospital-acquired infections, delirium, loss of function and unplanned readmissions (Hermann, Muck & Nehen, 2015). They can find hospital admission confusing, which can have a negative impact on their health and well-being both physically and mentally. Many who present with delirium are subsequently found to have dementia after discharge from hospital, with the two often coexisting (Jackson et al., 2016).

Countries across Europe have developed national strategies towards the diagnosis and management of dementia in hospitals and the community (Royal College of Psychiatrists et al., 2013). Specialized and appropriate care in hospital is vital for diagnosis and for supporting frail older people with dementia and their families towards a life that is disability-free and productive as far as possible. The main models of care delivered in acute hospital settings include specialist dementia wards, liaison psychiatry teams who provide diagnosis and support to patients, and dementia specialist nurses who work both in the hospital and in the community setting. The following discusses each approach in turn.

Specialist dementia wards

Specialist dementia wards have been in development across European hospitals to cater for the needs of older people with dementia (Wilkinson & Hendriks, 2015; O'Connor et al., 2016). Although such specialist units have not demonstrated measurable impact on hospital and primary care utilization, mainly because patients tend to be at the end of life, the experience of patients and their carers were reported to be significantly better compared to care received on general wards (Goldberg et al., 2013). Goldberg et al. (2013) also demonstrated, in a randomized controlled trial of specialist and mental health units, that patients had more positive interactions and engagement with the staff, families perceived the management of confused patients to be more empathetic, and discharge planning was seen to be more efficient. There is variability in terms of the number of beds available in these facilities and length of stay. Components of care include therapy involvement, spaces for patient interaction, a routine that meets the needs of patients with cognitive deficits, volunteer workers, and specialist staff who provide care and tailored plans for individual patients that take into account their social and cultural backgrounds (Hermann, Muck & Nehen, 2015).

Liaison psychiatry for older people

With so many older hospital patients having dementia or mental problems accompanying their other complaints, there is no prospect of all patients being admitted to specialist units, so other models of specialist input matter. Liaison psychiatry or liaison psychological medicine is defined as a specialty that manages people who present with mental and physical symptoms concerned with the interplay between physiological, psychological and social determinants that cause ill health. Liaison psychiatry teams often consist of a MDT which includes psychiatrists, nurses, support workers and therapists (Royal College of Psychiatrists et al., 2013), and liaison psychiatry for older adults is provided either by psychiatrists with an interest in old age psychiatry or by specialist nurses. Liaison psychiatry for older adults (LPOA) has become embedded in many European hospital settings as part of the routine assessment to improve the quality of life of older people (Mukaetova-Ladinska, 2006). For example, an LPOA service in a tertiary hospital in Portugal found that delirium and dementia accounted for more than 60% of the diagnoses and although the referring complaint was mostly "mood disturbances", it was found that only 24% of these patients had depression, highlighting the poor diagnostic experience of referring clinicians (Nogueira et al., 2013).

Evidence on liaison mental health services points to some benefits for people with dementia, for example increased referral rates for cognitive assessment, better detection and diagnosis, and greater staff confidence in caring for patients with dementia. However, a literature review of dementia care in general hospitals showed that, despite individual case studies demonstrating local benefit, trial evidence around mental health liaison is lacking. Quality of inpatient care improves as a result of these services, but the impact on cost-effectiveness and length of stay remains uncertain (Dewing & Dijk, 2014).

Specialist dementia nurses

The care delivered by specialist nurses has been identified to be of key importance in supporting people with dementia. There has been increasing interest in many settings in developing specialist nurse roles as one approach to improving the care of people with dementia in hospital (Griffiths, Bridges & Sheldon, 2013), and across European countries specialist nurses are being widely used to support frail older people with dementia in acute hospitals and the community (Hermann, Muck & Nehen, 2015). A scoping review of the role of the dementia specialist nurse in acute care working directly with people with dementia and their families for a significant period of time found this model to benefit older people with dementia in hospital and their families (Griffiths, Bridges & Sheldon, 2013).

Models of post-hospital care

Transitional care arrangements that constitute post-hospital care can put pressures on frail older people, and need to be timely and safe to ensure effective and efficient transfers (Allen et al., 2014). Across high income countries various models of post-hospital care are emerging to bridge the gap between hospital and people's homes, with core elements including anticipatory care targeting older people, MDTs, and enhanced interagency working to promote improved outcomes (Philp et al., 2013). These services aim to allow people to leave hospital sooner, reduce the chance of readmission and improve their short- and medium-term health outcomes. This section focuses on a range of models that have been implemented across European countries and describes discharge-to-assess and early discharge approaches, while also considering the role of community geriatricians and of primary care in promoting and supporting post-hospital care in the community. It is sometimes the same teams or referral hubs providing pre-hospital or "step up" care and admission prevention (see Section 2) that are able to provide this transitional or "step down" care and such an arrangement allows for simplicity and continuity of care.

Discharge-to-assess models and early supported discharge

In a discharge-to-assess model, a patient whose acute health needs have been stabilized is subsequently discharged home for rapid assessment of their needs in their own home environment and follow-up of ongoing care by community-based clinicians (Andrew & Rockwood, 2014). An older person who is deemed medically stable for discharge from the emergency department or acute medical unit ward but still requires ongoing support is discharged home with a team of multidisciplinary therapy staff for assessment. A plan of support is put in place immediately; should the patient fail the assessment at home, they would then return to hospital (Silvester et al., 2014). In the United Kingdom a number of local quality improvement studies have shown the benefits of early senior review linked to these models in terms of reduced admission rates, reduced bed occupancy, and higher rates of discharge home within 24 hours of presentation (Fox et al., 2013; Health Foundation, 2013). However, the majority of studies are single case based and there is little robust evidence from controlled trials. Data from such quality studies suggest that effective discharge-to-assess models require timely expert assessment on initial acute presentation to hospital and adequate capacity for medical and nursing care, therapy support, and social care for providing assessment and support at home (Silvester et al., 2014).

Early supported discharge (ESD) enables patients to return home earlier and receive rehabilitation within their own homes. Unlike discharge-to-assess, it tends to rely on more traditional assessment of needs in the hospital setting as the basis for defining ongoing clinical and care needs after discharge. This service is more commonly provided for people who have physical disabilities such as post-acute stroke (Fearon & Langhorne, 2012). In contrast to discharge-to-assess models of care, ESD follows after completion of assessments in the hospital and the patient is found to have met the minimum criteria for transfer back to their own home (Kirk, 2013). EDS is comparatively widely implemented across European countries, with much of the evidence originating from northern Europe and a 2012 Cochrane review concluded that among older patients following stroke, those who were discharged with an ESD service had improved physical outcomes, reduced lengths of stay in hospital, lower dependency rates and reported higher satisfaction with services compared to those receiving conventional services (Fearon & Langhorne, 2012; Mas & Inzitari, 2015).

Hospital at home schemes

A number of countries in Europe have developed innovative models of care in the community to bridge the gap between hospital and home, or to provide extra support at home without hospital admission (Jones & Carroll, 2014; Vilà et al., 2015). Examples include the "hospital at home" model and the "virtual community ward", which enable frail older people to continue to be treated within their familiar environments.

In a hospital at home setting, care is provided within a patient's home, with services similar to those provided in hospital but delivered by a community-based team or hospital-resourced outreach staff through domiciliary visits (Shepperd et al., 2010). There is mixed evidence about the effectiveness of hospital at home services. Systematic reviews of single chronic disease management, such as COPD and heart failure, suggest that patients seem to benefit from the service as the readmission rate is reduced and the system is proving to be more cost-effective. In contrast, frail older people with multiple co-morbidities seem to have an increased rate of readmission (Shepperd et al., 2010; Jeppesen & Jae, 2012; Qaddoura et al., 2015).

End life care seems to be better managed using hospital at home type models. For example, a programme in Barcelona, Spain, found such a service to improve end of life care in patients with terminal illnesses, with up to 72% choosing to remain at home in their final days with support from the community teams (Vilà et al., 2015). A recent systematic review of home-based end of life care found this to significantly increase the likelihood of dying at home compared with usual care, with some evidence of improved patient satisfaction at one-month follow-up (Shepperd et al., 2016).

Virtual and community wards

Virtual wards also replicate a hospital ward. However, contrary to the hospital at home model, which provides acute clinical care, the virtual ward places emphasis on the integration of medical teams, nursing, therapists and social care to provide a proactive approach of care to people at risk of hospital admission (Jones & Carroll, 2014). They can be used to support discharge ("step down") as well as preventing admission. The evidence of the effectiveness of virtual wards in frail older people with complex multimorbidity remains mixed (Bardsley et al., 2013; National Institute for Health and Care Excellence, 2016). Recent evaluations of virtual wards in four parts of England were unable to demonstrate reductions in cost or hospital bed utilization, although there were some reductions in elective activity (Lewis et al., 2013). Similarly, a randomized controlled trial of a virtual ward for high-risk adult hospital discharge patients in Toronto, Canada, did not find a statistically significant effect of a virtual ward model of care on readmissions or death at different points of time after hospital discharge (Dhalla et al., 2014). Lewis et al. (2013) commented, based on the English experience, that where virtual or community wards are developed locally, this should be motivated by patients' needs and the need to provide care closer to home for those at highest risk, rather than because they will deliver savings (Box 4.3).

The role of community geriatricians

We have discussed the role of geriatricians in hospital care but their role in the community is just as important in providing support to community services for frail older people. In some European countries this is the major part of their work, with acute hospital care being more the province of internal medicine physicians (Kolb, Topinkova & Michel, 2011; Ekdahl et al., 2012; Gordon, 2015). The role of community

---

Box 4.3 "virtual ward hub" services for older patients in Bradford, England

In order to improve integration of services, and because of the need to reduce readmission rates, a virtual ward hub was developed by Bradford Teaching Hospitals NHS Trust in 2012 to provide support to frail older patients who were discharged from the elderly admissions unit and general geriatric wards. The service is geriatrician-led, with typical support involving daily nurse visits and therapy staff depending on the needs of the patient and a shared electronic health records system enabling cross-boundary sharing of information and skills to manage a patient within their home. The team consists of 3 advanced nurse practitioners, 4 physiotherapists, 6 nursing sisters, 19 nurses, 18 rehabilitation support workers, and 2 geriatricians. A typical monthly caseload is approximately 40 patients, with multidisciplinary discussions held three times a week. Bed occupancy across geriatric medicine has reduced by 6% (compared to 1.5% across the rest of the hospital), and there has been a perceived reduction of pressure on the acute hospital. This service is continuing to expand with further development of the hub to take on more patients, co-location with social services, and embedding CGA in all their assessments of frail older patients.

Source: Ryland, 2015

---

geriatricians includes support for people in nursing and residential facilities, support for community case management teams or virtual wards or discharge teams, and close work with primary care teams to support high-risk patients with frailty (Oliver & Burns, 2016). For example, in the Netherlands and Norway community geriatricians provide specialist care to frail older people residing in nursing homes through CGA with a network of multidisciplinary professionals to optimize care (Verenso, 2015). Community geriatrician involvement in care homes has been linked to a reduction in medications prescribed and optimizing drug treatment, thereby reducing risks of readmission associated with adverse drug reactions (Burns & McQuillan, 2011). Evidence suggests that adverse drug reactions are common in the post-hospitalization period and this needs to be addressed effectively across transitions of care in order to prevent harm and inconvenience.

Intermediate care rehabilitation services

There are several definitions of intermediate care but the common thread underlying them is the provision of health care services to those who require support in the transitions between acute care, primary care and social care. They vary in their provision of support depending on the needs of the patient to optimize and achieve their baseline function where possible or to provide an environment for further assessments such as CGA to take place (Woodford & George, 2010). The following section discusses each category in turn.

Crisis response teams can take the shape of rapid response teams (see above) that provide step up or step down services. Step up services are targeted at older people who require support in their home or in an intermediate care facility, with the aim of avoiding hospital admission where possible and appropriate. Step down services provide a bridge service for transitions from the emergency department or post discharge from hospital (NHS Benchmarking, 2015).

Home-based intermediate care services are provided within a person's home by a multidisciplinary professional team. In Finland such services are provided by a nurse and home-care aid worker, depending on individualized plans devised by the case manager for a period of time until independence has been restored or regular home care has been put in place (Hammar, Rissanen & Perälä, 2009).

Bed-based intermediate care services overlap with other community-based facilities that are situated within nursing homes or local community hospitals and more commonly accommodate frail older people who have been admitted to hospital and require a period of convalescence and rehabilitation prior to discharge to their home.

Rehabilitation services outside hospital focus on providing a suitable environment to promote functional recovery. Delivered by a MDT, these services aim to meet the rehabilitative goals of service users by concentrating on activities that are important to the individual but which may have been missed in a clinical environment (Pearson et al., 2015). Rehabilitation primarily includes physical therapy and occupational therapy to prevent admission to an acute hospital or facilitate a stepped pathway out of hospital.

Workforce planning in caring for frail older adults

One of the key workforce challenges in the care of frail older adults is a shortage of medical and nursing staff within geriatric care (Kolb, Topinkova & Michel, 2011; Heinen et al., 2013). In the United Kingdom geriatrics is the largest internal medicine speciality with the highest number of training posts. But demand for both geriatric medicine posts and acute internal medicine posts is so high that not all posts are filled currently (Royal College of Physicians of London, 2015). Guidance from the Royal College of Physicians recommends a minimum of one consultant geriatrician per 50 000 population for effective facilitation of geriatric care (Fisher et al., 2014). France, Spain and Ireland have a lower number of geriatricians per capita compared to Belgium, Germany and Switzerland, with vast differences in recruitment and structured training programmes (Kolb, Topinkova & Michel, 2011).

With shortages of geriatrics specialist doctors, nurses and allied health professionals, those in other adult clinical areas all commonly encounter older patients with complex co-morbidities, dementia and frailty as a big part of their core role (British Geriatrics Society, 2014a; Oliver, Foot & Humphries, 2014; Quality Watch, 2015). Non-geriatric trained health care professionals do not always have the competence or confidence to manage frail older people (Alzheimer's Society, 2009). Unfortunately, ageist attitudes persist in parts of the workforce, leading to age discriminatory treatment and service models (Centre for Policy on Ageing, 2009; Economist Intelligence Unit, 2012; British Geriatrics Society, 2014b; World Health Organization, 2015; National Institute for Health and Care Excellence, 2016).

Surveys from North America and Europe have shown that there are shortcomings in the undergraduate curriculum of geriatric medicine for doctors in training, and as a result there are initiatives in place to ensure that resources are allocated towards specialist teaching around geriatric medicine, focusing on attitudes towards older patients, and trying to engage these patients in teaching to enable a broader view of managing frail older patients in practice (Oakley et al., 2014). There are now toolkits available that define core requirements for postgraduate training across Europe in geriatric medicine that can help inform a structured curriculum at the European Union level (Singler et al., 2016).

Nursing staff shortages and issues such as attitudes to older people and the lack of training to work with them are also significant problems

(Capezuti et al., 2012; Heinen et al., 2013). Capezuti et al. (2012) found that geriatric-specific nurse training can contribute to successful recruitment of nurses and provide the high level nursing input required for geriatric patients. Staff development in specialist areas such as dementia is needed to improve their knowledge and competence (Page & Hope, 2013; Hermann, Muck & Nehen, 2015). NHS Education for Scotland in partnership with the Scottish Social Services Council developed a framework for all health and social services staff working with people with dementia, their families and carers in 2011, with four levels of training depending on the amount of contact staff had with the patients (Banks et al., 2014).

Advanced nurse practitioners (ANPs) may carry out CGAs and provide advice about acute care, including managing mental health illnesses, as well as playing a part in rehabilitative medicine and supporting clinical governance, education and innovation (Goldberg et al., 2016). A systematic review of the role of ANPs in long-term residential care concluded that they play a positive role in reducing mental health illnesses, improving urinary continence and pressure ulcer care, improving residents' abilities to meet personal goals and in family satisfaction with medical services (Donald et al., 2013).

Geriatricians are unable to look after all patients with frailty and, with an ageing population, frail older people are seen in all specialties such as surgery, general medicine, and mental health (Bagnall et al., 2013; Oliver, Foot & Humphries, 2014). European countries clearly need an increase in the specialist geriatric medicine workforce as increasingly the core business of acute internal medicine, emergency medicine and general internal medicine is geriatric medicine (Cesari et al., 2016). At the same time, there will never be enough geriatricians or specialist nurses and allied health professionals to look after all older people with frailty and so other specialists will need greater competencies (Oliver & Burns, 2016). This has been recognized in plans for European training curriculums by the European Federation of Internal Medicine (2016 and ongoing).

The challenges facing geriatric medicine call for a new way of collaborative and integrated working across disciplines, and key elements to inform this should include: definition of roles of those managing the patient, goal setting with the patient, team communication between geriatricians and the treating team, care planning with relevant guidelines in place, and leadership to oversee that the overall care is safe, effective and deliverable (Tsakitzidis et al., 2016). The National Institute for Health and Care Excellence guidelines on managing patients with multimorbidity has set out similar messages (Farmer et al., 2016).

Barriers to delivering optimal and integrated hospital and acute care

The quality of geriatric care depends on available resources, structures and a specialized workforce to deliver acute care, rehabilitation, long-term care and palliative care services; however, countries across Europe vary in terms of how well established their geriatric systems are, with some countries having more developed services compared to others (Kolb, Topinkova & Michel, 2011; EUGMS, 2016). But all doctors, nurses and allied health professionals working in acute internal medical and surgical specialties will care for older people with frailty (Oliver, Foot & Humphries, 2014; Oliver & Burns, 2016). Geriatric training curriculums need to change and evolve to reflect the complexities that surround frail older people and the European Union Geriatric Medicine Society (EUGMS) has now set plans in place to develop a curriculum for "geriatric emergency medicine" for this specific purpose (Bellou & Conroy, 2016).

Care for older people is still very much divided into primary care, secondary care and social care, often with a lack of continuity throughout the process of an older person's journey as they transition through any of these systems (Oliver, Foot & Humphries, 2014). One restructuring process that distributed funding and developed an integrated model of health care provision in New Zealand transformed the way older people were cared for, which subsequently improved waiting times, reduced unplanned readmissions and increased the availability of social care to the older population through their "one budget, one system" philosophy (Timmins & Ham, 2013). The province of Quebec in Canada has also been successful in integrating health and social care through structural organizations, contractual agreements, and the sharing of informatics between these systems of care (Vedel et al., 2011).

Improved information systems will be increasingly important but a systematic review (Lluch, 2011) demonstrated that health information technologies are difficult to implement even though evidence suggests that this does improve exchange of data, and subsequently improves the safety and quality of care provided to older people and those with multiple co-morbidities.

System-level changes are required to deliver quality, coordinated and economically viable care to an ageing population that have co-morbidities as the norm rather than the exception (Jeste, 2011). Some authors have suggested that evidence-based practices need to change from traditional randomized controlled trials that are costly and time-consuming to a more pragmatic approach; with quality improvement gaining momentum, implementation research can add great value to innovation and transferability across systems (Balasubramanian et al., 2015; McGrath et al., 2016; Thompson & Jones, 2016). Some countries in Europe are more advanced on their journey to integrated care than others, with governments prioritizing it on national agendas over the last 20 years, and others are less worried and more confident about future challenges (Economist Intelligence Unit, 2012). Finland, for example, has spent the last 30 years developing centralized integrated care approaches aimed at optimizing care for older people, as well as those with issues with mental health or substance misuse and younger children (Mur-Veeman, van Raak & Paulus, 2008). Integration of long-term care to meet the needs of ageing populations will remain challenging but will be an important area for organizational development, training and research in the future (Leichsenring, 2012).

Geriatricians and other staff groups specializing in coordinated care for older people need to lead the way by using their expertise to enter leadership positions and work in partnership with physicians, researchers, and other health care professionals, which is crucial to achieving a critical mass. Together, they can lead a comprehensive national health agenda for frail older people and advocate ground-breaking policy changes (Nikolich-Zugich et al., 2015).

Conclusion

Older people are increasingly the main focus of much of hospital care. Older people with frailty are at high risk of hospital admissions, increased mortality, and care home utilization, and there is much that the design of hospital services and their associated community and primary care services can do to reduce these issues. There are opportunities from a number of new approaches to the management of care for older people and from changes in how professionals work and how they come together in teams more effectively. The acute hospital remains a centre of care provision to the frail and the vulnerable, but it sits within the wider context of the community and social care arrangement, where integration of care is vital to the provision of holistic care to people with frailty. There are major challenges from workforce shortages and a need to equip a wide range of professionals with the skills to help them care for older people more effectively. A shift in focus is needed in managing the complex pathway of patients through the health care system and, in many parts of Europe, reducing their dependence on the hospital.

References

Acute Frailty Clinical Network (2015). *Improving services for frail older people*. Updated 2015. Available at https://www.acutefrailtynetwork.org .uk/about-us

Allen J et al. (2014). Quality care outcomes following transitional care interventions for older people from hospital to home: A systematic review. *BMC Health Services Research*, 14(1):346.

Alzheimer's Society (2009). *Counting the Cost. Caring for people with Dementia on Hospital Wards*. Available at: https://www.alzheimers.org .uk/sites/default/files/2018-05/Counting_the_cost_report.pdf

Andrew MK, Rockwood K (2014). Making our health and care systems fit for an ageing population: considerations for Canada. *Can Geriatr J* 17(4):133–5.

Bagnall NM et al. (2013). What is the utility of preoperative frailty assessment for risk stratification in cardiac surgery? *Interact Cardiovasc Thorac Surg*, 17(2):398–402.

Baitar A et al. (2015). Implementation of geriatric assessment-based recommendations in older patients with cancer: A multicentre prospective study. *J Geriatr Oncol*, 6(5):401–10.

Balasubramanian, BA et al. (2015). Learning Evaluation: blending quality improvement and implementation research methods to study healthcare innovations. *Implementation Science*, 10(1):1.

Banks P et al. (2014). Enriching the care of patients with dementia in acute settings? The Dementia Champions Programme in Scotland. *Dementia (London, England)*, 13(6):717–36.

Barber ND et al. (2009). Care homes' use of medicines study: prevalence, causes and potential harm of medication errors in care homes for older people. *Qual Saf Health Care*, 18(5):341–6.

Bardsley M et al. (2013). *Evaluating integrated and community based care*. London, The Nuffield Trust.

Bates C et al. (2014). *First National Frailty Workshop: White Paper*, 1–13.

Bellou A, Conroy S (2016). European Curriculum of Geriatric Emergency Medicine (ECGEM), 1–12.

Bienkowska-Gibbs T et al. (2015). *New organisational models of primary care to meet the future needs of the NHS: a brief overview of recent reports*. RAND Europe. Available at: https://www.rand.org/pubs/research_reports/ RR1181.html.

Blakemore S (2012). Emergency frailty unit helps get patients home quicker. *Nursing Older People*, 24(2):6–7.

Boutsioli Z (2012). A simple descriptive analysis of hospital admissions' progress: a case study of the Greatest Public General Hospital, Athens, Greece. *Journal of Hospital Administration*, 1(1):36–41.

British Geriatrics Society (2014a). *Fit for Frailty Part 1. Consensus Practice Guidelines for the Care of People with Frailty*. Available at: https://www .bgs.org.uk/sites/default/files/content/resources/files/2018-05-23/fff_full.pdf

British Geriatrics Society (2014b). *Fit for Frailty Part 2. Developing, commissioning and managing services for older people with frailty in community settings* . Available at: http://www.bgs.org.uk/campaigns/fff/fff2_full.pdf

British Geriatrics Society et al. (2012). *"Silver book": quality care for older people with urgent and emergency care needs*. Available at: www.bgs.org .uk/campaigns/silverb/silver_book_complete.pdf.

British Orthopaedic Association (2007). *The care of patients with fragility fracture*. Available at: https://www.bgs.org.uk/sites/default/files/content/ attachment/2018-05-02/Blue%20Book%20on%20fragility%20 fracture%20care.pdf

Burns E, McQuillan N (2011). Prescribing in care homes: the role of the geriatrician. *Ther Adv Chronic Dis*, 2(6):353–8.

Capezuti E et al. (2012). Nurses Improving Care for Healthsystem Elders – a model for optimising the geriatric nursing practice environment. *J Clin Nurs*, 21(21–22):3117–25.

Centeno-Cortes C et al. (2016). Coverage and development of specialist palliative care services across the World Health Organization European Region (2005–2012): Results from a European Association for Palliative Care Task Force survey of 53 countries. *Palliat Med*, 30(4):351–62.

Centre for Policy on Ageing (2009). *Ageism and Age-Discrimination in health and social care in the UK*. Available at: http://www.cpa.org.uk/ agediscrimination/age_discrimination.html.

Cesari M et al. (2016). The geriatric management of frailty as paradigm of "The end of the disease era". *Eur J Intern Med*, 31:11–14.

Clegg A et al. (2013). Frailty in elderly people. *Lancet*, 381(9868):752–62.

Clegg A et al. (2016). Development and validation of an electronic frailty index using routine primary care electronic health record data. *Age and Ageing*, 45(3):353–60.

Conroy S, Chikura G (2015). Emergency care for frail older people — urgent AND important — but what works?, *Age and Ageing*, 44(5):724–5.

Conroy SP et al. (2014). A controlled evaluation of comprehensive geriatric assessment in the emergency department: the "Emergency Frailty Unit". *Age and Ageing*, 43(1):109–14.

Coulter A et al. (2015). Personalised care planning for adults with chronic or long term health conditions. *Cochrane Database Syst Rev*, 3:CD010523

Covinsky KE et al. (2003). Loss of independence in activities of daily living in older adults hospitalized with medical illnesses: Increased vulnerability with age. *J Am Geriatr Soc*, 51(4):451–8.

Cowling TE et al. (2014). Emergency Hospital Admissions via Accident and Emergency Departments in England: Time Trend, Conceptual Framework and Policy Implications. *J R Soc Med*, 107(11):432–8.

Creighton H (2014). *Europe's Ageing Demography*. Available at: https://ilcuk.org.uk/wp-content/uploads/2019/11/Europes-Ageing-Demography.pdf

Curry N, Ham C (2010). *Clinical and service integration: the route to improved outcomes*. London, The King's Fund, 1–64.

Dent E et al. (2016). Frailty in emergency departments. *Lancet*, 387(10017).

Deschodt M et al. (2013). Impact of geriatric consultation teams on clinical outcome in acute hospitals: a systematic review and meta-analysis. *BMC Med*, 11:48.

Deschodt M et al. (2016). Structure and processes of interdisciplinary geriatric consultation teams in acute care hospitals: A scoping review. *Int J Nurs Stud*, 55:98–114.

Dewing J, Dijk S (2014). What is the current state of care for older people with dementia in general hospitals? A literature review. *Dementia (London)*, 15(1):106–24.

Dhalla IA et al. (2014). Effect of a Postdischarge Virtual Ward on Readmission or Death for High-Risk Patients. *JAMA*, 312(13):1305.

Donald F et al. (2013). A systematic review of the effectiveness of advanced practice nurses in long-term care. *JoJ Adv Nurs* 69(10):2148–61.

Economist Intelligence Unit (2012). *A new vision for old age. Rethinking health policy for Europe's ageing society*. Available at: https://www.learneurope.eu/files/5613/7525/7796/Repensando_la_poltica_de_salud_sociedad_europea_envejecida.pdf

Ekdahl A, Alwin J, Eckerblad J (2016). Long-Term Evaluation of the Ambulatory Geriatric Assessment: A Frailty Intervention Trial (AGe-FIT): Clinical Outcomes and Total Costs After 36 Months. *J Am Med Dir Assoc*, 17(3):263–8.

Ekdahl A et al. (2012). Geriatric care in Europe – the EUGMS survey part II: Malta, Sweden and Austria. *European Geriatric Med*, 3(6):388–91.

Ellis G et al. (2011). Comprehensive geriatric assessment for older adults admitted to hospital. *Cochrane Database Syst Rev*, 7:CD006211.

EUGMS (2016). 12th International EUGMS Congress. Lisbon, Portugal.

EUGMS Survey (in press). EUGMS National Societies Profile – questionnaire 2016. Contact: Anne Ekdahl.

European Federation of Internal Medicine (2016 and ongoing). *Internal medicine curriculum project.* Available at: http://www.efim.org/about/ebim-curriculum-project (accessed 6 February 2020).

European Institute (2012). *The future of healthcare in Europe.* Available at: https://www.medischcentrumhuisartsen.be/documents/focus/future-health-care-challenges-in-europe.pdf

Farmer C et al. (2016). Clinical assessment and management of multimorbidity: summary of NICE guidance. *BMJ*, 354:i4843.

Fearon P, Langhorne P (2012). Services for reducing duration of hospital care for acute stroke patients. *Cochrane Database Syst Rev*, 9:CD000443.

Fenton K (2014). The *human cost of falls*. Publisher? Available at: https://publichealthmatters.blog.gov.uk/2014/07/17/the-human-cost-of-falls/ (accessed 25 July 2016).

Fisher JM et al. (2014). Geriatric medicine workforce planning: a giant geriatric problem or has the tide turned? *Clin Med* 14(2):102–6.

Fox G et al. (2013). Introducing interface geriatricians in Leeds. *British Geriatrics Society Newsletter.*

Gladman JRF et al. (2016). New horizons in the implementation and research of comprehensive geriatric assessment: Knowing, doing and the "know-do" gap. *Age Ageing*, 45(2):194–200.

Gold Standards Framework (2012). *NHS National End of Life Care Programme.* Available at: www.goldstandardsframework.org.uk.

Goldberg SE et al. (2013). Care in specialist medical and mental health unit compared with standard care for older people with cognitive impairment admitted to general hospital: randomised controlled trial (NIHR TEAM trial). *BMJ*, 347(1):f4132.

Goldberg SE et al. (2016). Development of a curriculum for advanced nurse practitioners working with older people with frailty in the acute hospital through a modified Delphi process. *Age Ageing*, 45(1):48–53.

Gordon A (2015). Editorial Comment. Specialist services in the community: A qualitative study of consultants holding novel types of employment contracts in England. *Future Hos J*, 2:180–1.

Griffiths P, Bridges J, Sheldon H (2013). *Scoping the role of the dementia nurse specialist in acute care.* University of Southampton, 1–37. Available at: https://eprints.soton.ac.uk/349714/1/dementia%2520specialist%2520nurses%2520appendices.pdf

Hackman E et al. (2013). Reducing patient distress: a model for dementia care. *Br J Nurs*, 22(4):2–6.

Hammar T, Rissanen P, Perälä ML (2009). The cost-effectiveness of integrated home care and discharge practice for home care patients. *Health Policy*, 92(1):10–20.

Harari D et al. (2007). Proactive care of older people undergoing surgery ('POPS'): Designing, embedding, evaluating and funding a comprehensive geriatric assessment service for older elective surgical patients. *Age Ageing*, 36(2):190–6.

Hawley S et al. (2016). Clinical effectiveness of orthogeriatric and fracture liaison service models of care for hip fracture patients: population-based longitudinal study. *Age Ageing*, 45(2):236–42.

Hayes M et al. (2016). An older person assessment and liaison service in an Irish university teaching hospital: a mixed methods critical analysis. *Age Ageing*, 45(s2):ii13–ii56.

Health Foundation (2013). *Improving patient flow: how two trusts focused on flow to improve the quality of care and use available capacity effectively.* London, The Health Foundation.

Health Improvement Scotland (2015). *Older people in acute care (OPAC) standards.* Available at: http://www.healthcareimprovementscotland.org/our_work/person-centred_care/resources/opah_standards.aspx.

Health Improvement Scotland (2016). *Delirium toolkit.* Available at: https://ihub.scot/project-toolkits/delirium-toolkit/delirium-toolkit/ (accessed 6 February 2020)

Heinen MM et al. (2013). Nurses' intention to leave their profession: a cross sectional observational study in 10 European countries. *Int J Nurs Stud*, 50(2):174–84.

Hermann DM, Muck S, Nehen H-G (2015). Supporting dementia patients in hospital environments: health-related risks, needs and dedicated structures for patient care. *Eur J Neurol*, 22(2):239–e18.

Jackson T et al. (2016). Undiagnosed long-term cognitive impairment in acute hospitalised older patients with delirium. A prospective cohort study. *Age Ageing*, 45(4):505–11.

Jeppesen WE, Jae W (2012). Hospital at home for acute exacerbations of chronic obstructive pulmonary disease (Review). *Cochrane Database Syst Rev*, 5: CD003573

Jeste DV (2011). Promoting successful ageing through integrated care. *BMJ (Clinical research ed.)*, 343:d6808.

Jones J, Carroll A (2014). Hospital admission avoidance through the introduction of a virtual ward. *Br J Community Nurs* 19(7):330–4.

Kammerlander C et al. (2011). The Tyrolean Geriatric Fracture Center: an orthogeriatric co-management model. *Zeitschrift für Gerontologie und Geriatrie*, 44(6):363–7.

Kaplan DB, Berkman B (2011). Dementia care: a global concern and social work challenge. *International Social Work*, 54(3):361–73.

King's Fund (2014). *Specialists in out-of-hospital settings.* Available at: https://www.kingsfund.org.uk/publications/specialists-out-hospital-settings (accessed 6 February 2020)

Kirk H (2013). *Early Supported Discharge.* National University Hospital. Available at: http://www.nuh.com.sg/patients-and-visitors/patients-and-visitors-guide/admissions/nuh-2-home/early-supported-discharge.html.

Kleinpell RM, Fletcher K, Jennings BM (2008). Reducing functional decline in hospitalized elderly. In: *Patient Safety and Quality: An Evidence Based Handbook for Nurses.* Agency for Healthcare Research and Quality: Available at: http://www.ncbi.nlm.nih.gov/bookshelf/br.fcgi?book=nursehb&part=ch11.

Knobe M, Pape HC (2016). Focus on co-management in geriatric fracture care. *Eur J Trauma Emerg Surg*, 42(5):533–5.

Koduah DY et al. (2014). Reducing inappropriate admissions of older people into acute hospitals: the role of a rapid access clinic in a community hospital. *Age Ageing*, 43(s1):i3.

Kolb G, Topinkova E, Michel JP (2011). Geriatric care in Europe – the EUGMS Survey part I : Belgium, Czech Republic, Denmark, Germany, Ireland, Spain, Switzerland, United Kingdom. *European Geriatric Med*, 2(5):290–5.

Kringos D et al. (2013). The strength of primary care in Europe: An international comparative study. *Br J Gen Pract*, 63(616):742–50.

Kristjansson SR et al. (2010). Comprehensive geriatric assessment can predict complications in elderly patients after elective surgery for colorectal cancer: a prospective observational cohort study. *Crit Rev Oncol Hematol*, 76(3):208–17.

Lacas A, Rockwood K (2012). Frailty in primary care: a review of its conceptualization and implications for practice. *BMC Med*, 10(1):1.

Lam CY et al. (2014). Prospective observational study of delirium recovery trajectories and associated short-term outcomes in older adults admitted to a specialized delirium unit. *J Am Geriatr Soc*, 62(9):1649–57.

Lamb S, Gates S, Fisher J (2007). *Scoping exercise on fallers' clinics: Report to the National Co-ordinating Centre for NHS Service Delivery and Organisation R & D (NCCSDO).* London Publisher?. Available at: https://njl-admin-test.nihr.ac.uk/document/download/2089827

Leichsenring K (2012). Integrated care for older people in Europe – latest trends and perceptions. *International Journal of Integrated Care*, 12(Jan):1–4.

Lewis G et al. (2013). Integrated Care Case virtual ward model: lessons in the process of care integration from 3 case sites. *Int J Integr Care*, 13(Nov):1–11.

Lluch M (2011). Healthcare professionals' organisational barriers to health information technologies – A literature review. *Int J Med Inform*, 80(12):849–62.

Mas MA, Inzitari M (2015). A critical review of early supported discharge for stroke patients. From evidence to implementation into practice. *Stroke*, 10:7–12.

McGrath K et al. (2016). Rehabilitating the revolving door: reducing readmissions – a multi-disciplinary quality improvement project. *Age Ageing*, 45(s2):ii1–ii12.

Melzer D et al. (2015). *The Age UK almanac of disease profiles in later life*. Age UK.

Molina-Garrido MJ, Guillén-Ponce C (2011). Development of a cancer-specific Comprehensive Geriatric Assessment in a University Hospital in Spain. *Crit Rev Oncol Hematol*, 77(2):148–61.

Moore M et al. (2010). Translating a multifactorial fall prevention intervention into practice: a controlled evaluation of a fall prevention clinic. *J Am Geriatr Soc*, 58(2):357–63.

Mudge AM, O'Rourke P, Denaro CP (2010). Timing and risk factors for functional changes associated with medical hospitalization in older patients. *J Gerontol A Biol Sci Med Sci*, 65 A(8):866–72.

Mukaetova-Ladinska EB (2006). Towards living long and being healthy – the challenge for liaison psychiatric services for older adults. *Age Ageing*, 35(2):103–5.

Mur-Veeman I, van Raak A, Paulus A (2008). Comparing integrated care policy in Europe: Does policy matter? *Health Policy*, 85:172–83.

National Institute for Health and Care Excellence (2010). *Clinical guideline 103. Delirium: prevention, diagnosis and management*. Available at: https://www.nice.org.uk/guidance/CG103/chapter/Introduction.

National Institute for Health and Care Excellence (2016). *Multimorbidity: clinical assessment and management*. Available at: https://www.nice.org.uk/guidance/ng56

NHS Benchmarking (2013). *National Audit of Intermediate Care Report, p.110*. Available at: www.nhsbenchmarking.nhs.uk/National-Audit-of-Intermediate-Care/year-two.php.

NHS Benchmarking (2015). *National Audit of Intermediate Care*. Available at: http://www.nhsbenchmarking.nhs.uk/CubeCore/.uploads/NAIC/Reports/NAICReport2015FINALA4printableversion.pdf.

NHS Benchmarking (2016). *Older people's care in acute care settings*. Available at: http://www.bgs.org.uk/pdfs/1216_op_benchmarking_report.pdf.

Nikolich-Zugich J et al. (2015). Preparing for an Aging World: Engaging Biogerontologists, Geriatricians, and Society. *JJ Gerontol A Biol Sci Med Sci*, 71(4):435–44.

Nogueira V et al. (2013). Improving quality of care: focus on liaison old age psychiatry. *Ment Health Fam Med*, 10(3):153–8.

Oakley R et al. (2014). Equipping tomorrow's doctors for the patients of today. *Age Ageing*, 43(4):442–7.

O'Connor EO et al. (2016). Making a medicine for the elderly ward dementia friendly-phase 1. *Age Ageing*, 45(s2):ii13–ii56.

Oliver D (2016a). Delirium Matters. *BMJ*, 353:i2886.

Oliver D (2016b). *End-of-life care: getting it right for more people, more of the time*. London, The King's Fund Available at: https://www.kingsfund .org.uk/blog/2016/07/end-life-care-getting-it-right.

Oliver D (2016c). Frailty in Acute Care. *BMJ*, 354:i5195.

Oliver D (2016d). *What if there were community services for older people 24/7?* London, The King's Fund Available at: http://www.kingsfund.org .uk/reports/thenhsif/what-if-community-services-older-people/.

Oliver D, Burns E (2016). Geriatric medicine and geriatricians in the UK. How they relate to acute and general internal medicine and what the future might hold? *Future Hosp J*, 3(1):49–54.

Oliver D, Foot C, Humphries R (2014). *Making our health and care systems fit for an ageing population*. London, The King's Fund.

Ozalp B, Aspray TJ (2016). Orthogeriatric medicine and fracture liaison going from strength to strength. *Age Ageing*, 45(2):180–1.

Page S, Hope K (2013). Towards new ways of working in dementia: perceptions of specialist dementia care nurses about their own level of knowledge, competence and unmet educational needs.J Psychiatr Ment Health Nurs, 20(6):549–56.

Palvanen M et al. (2014). Effectiveness of the Chaos Falls Clinic in preventing falls and injuries of home-dwelling older adults: a randomised controlled trial. *Injury*, 45(1):265–71.

Pape H-C et al. (2014). Development of geriatric trauma centers – an effort by the German Society for Trauma and Orthopaedics. *Injury*, 45:1513–15.

Partridge JSL et al. (2014). Where are we in perioperative medicine for older surgical patients? A UK survey of geriatric medicine delivered services in surgery. *Age Ageing*, 43(5):721–4.

Pearson M et al. (2015). Providing effective and preferred care closer to home: a realist review of intermediate care. *Health Soc Care Community*, 23(6):577–93.

Philp I et al. (2013). Reducing hospital bed use by frail older people: results from a systematic review of the literature. *Int J Integr Care*, 13(Dec):e048.

Qaddoura A et al. (2015). Efficacy of hospital at home in patients with heart failure: a systematic review and meta-analysis. *PloS One*, 10(6):1–15.

Quality Watch (2015). *Focus on A&E attendances. Nuffield Trust*. Available at: https://www.nuffieldtrust.org.uk/files/2018-10/qualitywatch-a-and-e-attendances.pdf

Radvansky M (2014). *Effects of demographic changes on hospital workforce in European countries*. Bratislava.

Reyniers T et al. (2015). International variation in place of death of older people who died from dementia in 14 European and non-European countries. *J Am Med Dir Assoc*, 16(2):165–71.

Rockwood K, Mitnitski A (2011). Frailty Defined by Deficit Accumulation and Geriatric Medicine Defined by Frailty. *Clin Geriatr Med*, 27(1):17–26.

Royal College of Physicians of London (2013). *Acute care toolkit 3: Acute medical care for frail older people*. London, Royal College of Physicians Available at: https://www.rcplondon.ac.uk/guidelines-policy/acute-care-toolkit-3-acute-medical-care-frail-older-people.

Royal College of Physicians of London (2015). *2014–15 Census of consultants and registrars*. Available at: https://www.rcplondon.ac.uk/projects/ outputs/2014-15-census-uk-consultants-and-higher-specialty-trainees

Royal College of Physicians of London (2016). *End of Life Care Audit – Dying in Hospital. Healthcare Quality Improvement Partnership*. Available at: https://www.rcplondon.ac.uk/projects/outputs/end-life-care-audit-dying-hospital-national-report-england-2016.

Royal College of Psychiatrists et al. (2013). *National Audit of Dementia Care in General Hospitals 2012–13: Second Round Audit Report and Update*, 2–77.

Ryland E (2015). *Effect of a "discharge to assess" Geriatrician-led Virtual ward promoting integration of services on rates of discharge*. Yorkshire & Humber AHSN.

Sabharwal S, Wilson H (2015). Orthogeriatrics in the management of frail older patients with a fragility fracture. *Osteoporosis International*, 26(10):2387–99.

Shah SM et al. (2010). Identifying the clinical characteristics of older people living in care homes using a novel approach in a primary care database. *Age Ageing*, 39(5):617–23.

Shepperd S et al. (2010). Discharge planning from hospital to home. *Cochrane Database Syst Rev*, 1:CD000313.

Shepperd S et al. (2016). Hospital at home: home-based end-of-life care. Update in *Cochrane Database Syst Rev*, 2:CD009231.

Silvester KM et al. (2014). Timely care for frail older people referred to hospital improves efficiency and reduces mortality without the need for extra resources. *Age and Ageing*, 43(4):472–7.

Singler K et al. (2016). The development of a geriatric postgraduate education assessment instrument using a modified Delphi procedure. *Age Ageing*, 45(5):718–22.

Siouta N et al. (2016). Integrated palliative care in Europe: a qualitative systematic literature review of empirically-tested models in cancer and chronic disease. *BMC Palliative Care*, 15(1):56.

Smith P et al. (2015). *Focus on: Hospital admissions from care homes*. QualityWatch.

Sona A et al. (2012). Determinants of recourse to hospital treatment in the elderly. *Eur J Public Health*, 22(1):76–80.

Steelfisher GK et al. (2013). Learning from the closure of clinical programs: a case series from the Hospital Elder Life Program. *J Amer Geriatr Soc*, 61(6):999–1004.

Swanson JO, Hagen TP (2016). Reinventing the community hospital: a retrospective population-based cohort study of a natural experiment using register data. *BMJ Open*, e012892.

Tavassoli N et al. (2014). Description of 1,108 older patients referred by their physician to the "Geriatric Frailty Clinic (GFC) for assessment of frailty and prevention of disability" at the gerontopole., 18(5):457–64.

Thompson S, Jones R (2016). A Quality Improvement Project to Assess Timing of Initial Investigations in Stroke Medicine. *BMJ Quality Improvement Reports*, 5(1):u209241–w3796.

Timmins N, Ham C (2013). *The quest for integrated health social care – A case study in Canterbury, New Zealand*. London, The King's Fund.

Tsakitzidis G et al. (2016). Outcome Indicators on Interprofessional Collaboration Interventions for Elderly. *Int J Integr Care*, 16(2):1–17.

Van Craen K et al. (2010). The effectiveness of inpatient geriatric evaluation and management units: A systematic review and meta-analysis. *J Amer Geriatr Soc*, 58(1):83–92.

Van Den Noortgate N, Petrovic M (2009). The importance of a geriatric approach in medicine. *Acta Clinica Belgica*, 64(1):7–10.

Vedel I et al. (2011). Ten years of integrated care: backwards and forwards. The case of the province of Québec, Canada. *Int J Integr Care*, 11 Spec Ed(Mar):p.e004.

Verenso (2015). Elderly care physicians in the Netherlands: professional profile and competencies.

Vilà A et al. (2015). Cost-Effectiveness of a Barcelona Home Care Program for Individuals with Multimorbidity. *J Amer Geriatr Soc*, 63(5):1017–24.

Wilkinson A, Hendriks N (2015). Getting to know you the best we can; embedding design in a dementia ward. In: *Proceedings of the Third European Conference on Design4Health*.

Winpenny E et al. (2016). Community hospitals in selected high-income countries: a scoping review of approaches and models. *Int J Integr Care, 16(4):13*

Wittenberg R et al. (2014). *Understanding emergency hospital admissions of older people*. Report no. 6. Oxford, Centre for Health Service Economics & Organisation.

Woodford HJ, George J (2010). Intermediate care for older people in the UK. *Clinical Medicine, Journal of the Royal College of Physicians of London*, 10(2):119–23.

World Health Organization (2015). *World report on Ageing and Health*. Available at: http://www.who.int/ageing/events/world-report-2015-launch/en/.

Young J, Inouye SK (2007). Delirium in older people. *BMJ (Clinical research ed.)*, 334(7598):842–6.

5 | *Oncological hospital care*

ANKE WIND, WIM VAN HARTEN, SIGBJØRN SMELAND,
LUCIA DA PIEVE, WIM GROEN

Introduction

With an estimated 1.75 million deaths from cancer in Europe in 2012 (Ferlay et al., 2013), cancer is the second leading cause of death in Europe (World Health Organization, 2012). Diagnosis, treatment, continuing care, and in many cases palliation account for a substantial volume of the work of the acute general hospital. Yet while the word "cancer" is widely used in popular discourse, it is important to recognize that it is not a single disease but rather a pathological process that can affect almost all organs of the body. This process involves uncontrolled tissue growth, based on changes related to genetic or acquired abnormalities of the DNA, or related processes in the cell. Genetic changes that cause cancer can be inherited or, more commonly, they arise during a person's lifetime as a result of errors that occur by chance as cells divide or because of damage to genes caused by environmental exposures such as chemicals in tobacco smoke or ultraviolet radiation. The clinical management of cancer thus depends on both the nature of the pathological processes involved, increasingly being characterized at the molecular level, and the organs affected. An individual's cancer is thus characterized by a unique combination of genetic changes, which can change over time, for instance as a result of developing resistance by selecting clones of therapy-resistant cells. As a consequence, there has been an important paradigm shift from organ-based interventions to a patient-centred and targeted treatment for which increasingly innovative biological therapies are being discovered. In addition, cancer shares certain risk factors with other diseases. Thus, patients with cancer may be at greater risk of those other conditions. For example, tobacco use, which is the leading preventable cause of cancer in Europe, is associated not only with cancers of the lung but also with many other cancers, while also contributing to other conditions, such as coronary heart disease (Peto et al., 2012).

Cancer diagnosis and treatment have changed substantially in the past decades, with, for example, the advent of new chemotherapeutic agents transforming many cancers from short-lasting fatal illnesses into long-term chronic disorders. With increased understanding of the underlying disease processes, there have been considerable advances in early detection and diagnostic imaging, genetic profiling, and increased treatment options, including the introduction of targeted drugs and multidisciplinary care in many settings. In addition, and related to improved survival rates, cancer care takes account of psychosocial aspects, quality of life, patients' rights, and empowerment and survivorship. In this chapter we explore these shifts in cancer treatment and care, with a focus on oncological hospital care in Europe.

The burden of cancer in Europe

In 2008 one-quarter of the global cancer burden was observed in Europe, which is striking given that the total European population comprises only one-ninth of the world's population (Ferlay et al., 2013). For 2012 the Globocan project predicted an incidence of 3 715 000 cases with a five-year prevalence of 9 701 000 cases. There were an estimated 3.45 million new cases of cancer (excluding non-melanoma skin cancer) and 1.75 million deaths from cancer in Europe in 2012 (Ferlay et al., 2013).

Female breast cancer (464 000 cases), colorectal cancer (447 000), prostate cancer (417 000) and lung cancer (410 000) were the most frequent cancers, together representing half of the overall cancer burden in Europe in 2012 (Ferlay et al., 2013). The most common cancer modalities leading to death in 2012 were lung cancer (353 000 deaths), colorectal cancer (215 000), breast cancer (131 000) and stomach cancer (107 000). Incidence varies across the region, however, with cancers resulting from external carcinogens and bacteria (e.g. stomach cancer) tending to be higher in eastern Europe and Portugal, while breast and prostate cancer are more common in western Europe. Data from the International Agency for Research on Cancer (IARC), an agency within the World Health Organization, found the incidence in western European countries to be over 244 per 100 000 in 2012, compared to between 177.3 and 244.2 per 100 000 in eastern Europe.

Overall, cancer incidence continues to rise, with growth rates of up to 2% or 3% per year across Europe. As survival is also gradually

Table 5.1 *Summary indicators of cancer burden in selected high income regions, 2012*

	North America	EU-28	Western Europe	Northern Europe	Southern Europe	Australia and New Zealand
New cancer cases						
Age-standardized rate (per 100 000)	315.6	273.5	298.7	277.4	253.6	318.5
Risk of getting cancer before age 75 (%)	30.9	27.3	29.6	27.5	25.3	30.7
Cancer deaths						
Age-standardized rate (per 100 000)	105.5	109.4	105.0	108.0	105.2	97.6
Risk of dying from cancer before age 75 (%)	11.2	11.5	11.0	11.2	10.9	9.9
Five-year prevalent cases, adults (per 100 000)	1 888.2	1 690.4	2 018.6	1 658.6	1 585.3	1 901.8
Five most frequent cancers (defined by total number of cases)	Prostate Breast Lung Colorectal Bladder	Breast Prostate Colorectal Lung Bladder	Prostate Breast Colorectal Lung Bladder	Prostate Breast Colorectal Lung Melanoma of skin	Colorectal Breast Lung Prostate Bladder	Prostate Colorectal Breast Melanoma of skin Lung

Note: Estimates of worldwide age-standardized incidence and mortality as provided by GLOBOCAN use the World standard population, while EUCAN uses the European standard population. The World standard population presents a young population compared to the European standard population; EUCAN estimates for individual European countries or regions (such as those reported by Ferlay et al., 2013) are therefore higher than those provided by GLOBOCAN.

Source: adapted from GLOBOCAN, 2014

improving, prevalence is growing at an even quicker pace, leading to increased numbers of cancer patients (those still alive but in various stages of disease after primary treatment) and cancer survivors (those who have ended therapy and are in follow-up schedules).

Cancer survival rates are typically used as an indicator of the quality of cancer care, from prevention and screening to treatment. In Europe the EUROCARE study has systematically collected survival data from national cancer registries to monitor trends in cancer survival in children and adults (Berrino et al., 2007; De Angelis et al., 2014). EUROCARE data show large differences in survival, with some analyses linking differences in survival to differences in spending on cancer care, with the Nordic countries and Switzerland scoring favourably compared to the rest of Europe (Luengo-Fernandez et al., 2013). However, interpretation of the data is challenging because of persisting variations in the quality of data available, and the challenges of adjusting for case mix-when interpreting observational studies (Lyman, 2013), as well as how best to respond to this evidence (Whalen, 2010). What is clear is that greater resources will be needed to respond to the combination of a projected rise in the number of cancer cases and technological innovations that could potentially improve outcomes (Aggarwal, Ginsburg & Fojo, 2014).

The development of contemporary cancer care

Cancer diagnosis and treatment have progressed rapidly since the discovery of the cellular origins of cancer in the 1860s, but mainly in incremental steps. Important developments came about from the 1950s onwards, with advances in radiation technology and, in particular, cancer chemotherapy such as the treatment of childhood leukaemia and, in adults, Hodgkin's disease from the mid-1960s, with success of adjuvant treatment of breast cancer since the 1970s (DeVita & Rosenberg, 2012). At the same time, a greater understanding of the causes of cancer has increased scope for primary prevention, reducing the risk of developing disease. The most prominent example is perhaps the discovery of tobacco smoking as a cause of cancers of the lung and various other organs, with declines in the occurrence of lung cancer and subsequently mortality as a consequence of antismoking measures (Jha & Peto, 2014). The discovery of certain viral infections as a cause of cancer has also led to the development of vaccines against, for example, certain types of human papilloma virus (HPV) for the prevention of cervical cancer or hepatitis B virus for liver cancer.

Recent advances in the understanding of biological functioning of the cell have increased our understanding of cellular mechanisms, enabling the development of targeted drugs that have been very successful in certain subgroups of patients. Among the most recent developments is immunotherapy, which provides for progression-free survival in tumours that were previously considered to be uniformly fatal, such as metastatic melanoma and lung cancer.

While advances in screening have enabled early detection of certain cancers, albeit at a risk of over diagnosis for some (Viguier, 2015), these changes have had considerable implications for the management of cancer, which increasingly involves a complex array of interventions that require different professionals working together in a coordinated fashion to enhance outcomes for people with cancer. As it can involve many disciplines, sequential and parallel process steps, different handovers and frequent patient contacts by different disciplines, cancer care is increasingly organized through MDTs and along cancer care pathways.

The cancer care pathway

The cancer care pathway describes the patient's journey from the initial suspicion of cancer and symptom-based investigations, or through screening and early detection, to the various diagnostic procedures leading to a diagnosis of cancer, followed by treatment, which typically involves a selection of one or more interventions, such as surgery, radiotherapy, or chemotherapy. Depending on the outcome of the primary treatment, the patient will receive follow-up care and rehabilitation or, where the tumour remains active or is advanced, undergo further treatment or receive palliative and end life care when the tumour proves incurable (Figure 5.1).

The precise nature and scope of the cancer care pathway differs between cancer types and countries. Detailing cancer care pathways provides patients and professionals with a better understanding of the complex processes that are involved in treatment, while also contributing to enhancing the patient journey to strengthen high quality cancer care. Each pathway identifies the different steps and recommended care processes at each stage of the journey (Cancer Council Australia, 2016).

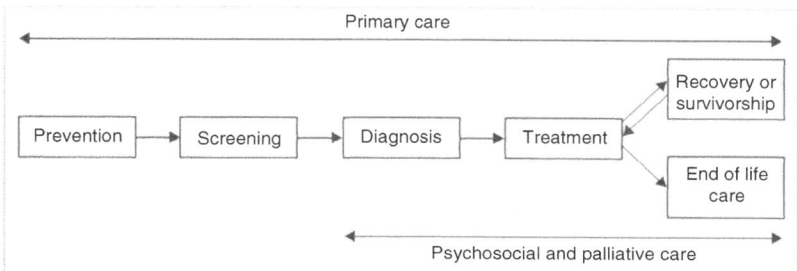

Figure 5.1 The cancer journey

Source: © Cancer Care Ontario

In countries where the general practitioner (GP) acts as gatekeeper to specialist care, such as the United Kingdom and the Netherlands, most cancers are diagnosed by a specialist after presentation of complaints or symptoms to the patient's GP, while others are diagnosed upon emergency presentation (Rubin et al., 2015). A proportion of cancers is detected through screening programmes such as for breast cancer, colorectal and cervical cancer, although percentages differ across cancer sites and coverage of related programmes in different health systems. Countries where patients can directly access specialist care enable direct and extensive diagnostics; this can lead to overuse of diagnostic procedures. On the other hand, there are some concerns that overly stringent primary care gatekeeping may introduce inappropriate delays. Clearly, it is difficult to get the right balance.

As we shall see below, the diagnosis and treatment of common tumour types is commonly provided by medical specialists within a hospital setting. Many countries have also established designated cancer centres for the delivery of specialized care for a large portfolio of common and rare tumours, serving also as tertiary referral centres for patients with rare tumours, late-stage disease or other difficult cases. Comprehensive cancer centres usually undertake a wide range of activities in translational cancer research, from basic scientific discovery, to the delivery of novel approaches, to care of patients with cancer, such as targeted therapies.

The precise nature of the cancer patient journey differs for different types of cancer. Figure 5.2 illustrates a typical pathway for a patient with breast cancer in a cancer centre in the Netherlands. In this example, the

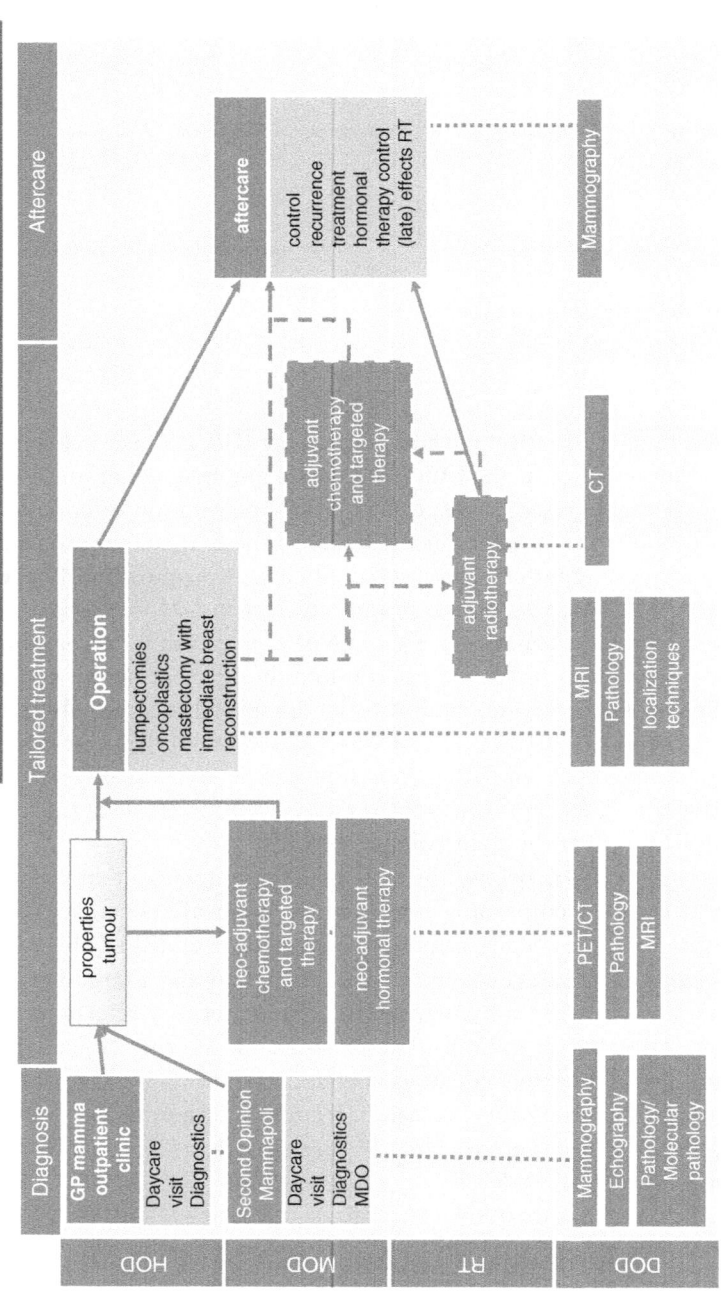

Figure 5.2 Breast cancer patient pathway, the Netherlands

Source: Undisclosed hospital in the Netherlands

patient would typically consult with a range of specialists within the cancer centre, which would also be responsible for aftercare. In some countries therapy is provided in "shared care" arrangements involving office-based physicians or local hospitals, for instance in order to provide chemotherapy closer to the patient's home.

Although most types of cancer care require specialized equipment and staff, there is an increasing trend to move more parts of the cancer care pathway into the community. Care in the community takes several forms, including chemotherapy delivered in people's own homes (Corbett et al., 2015), rehabilitation in community settings, blood and other monitoring tests in general practices or local settings, and increased access to local services and support groups (Macmillan, 2014).

Patient-focused, integrated care initiatives can provide greater quality, efficiency and patient satisfaction (Leutz, 1999; Burns & Pauly, 2002; Kodner & Spreeuwenberg, 2002). Evidence emerging over the past 20 years suggests that the transition of cancer care from oncologist-led models to nurse-led models in cancer centres or primary care-led models in the community may improve cancer outcomes (Grunfeld et al., 1999; Wattchow et al., 2006; Lewis et al., 2009; Grunfeld & Earle, 2010; Sussman et al., 2011). Primary care providers are often willing to assume follow-up care with appropriate guidance and a clear path for transition of care for their patients, and they are more likely than oncologists to provide preventive interventions directed at non-cancer conditions (Del Giudice et al., 2009; Grunfeld & Earle, 2010).

Multidisciplinary teams

We have noted above that the management of cancer increasingly involves a complex array of interventions that require different professionals working together in a coordinated fashion to enhance outcomes for people with cancer. Figure 5.3 provides an illustration of the range of staff involved in the breast cancer care pathway introduced in Figure 5.2. Optimizing delivery of the care pathway and patient outcomes will require close coordination and communication among the different professionals involved. Health providers are increasingly drawing on MDT working to enhance decision-making between health care team members and patients (Fleissig et al., 2006; Borras et al., 2014). MDTs usually address one type of cancer or a group of cancers.

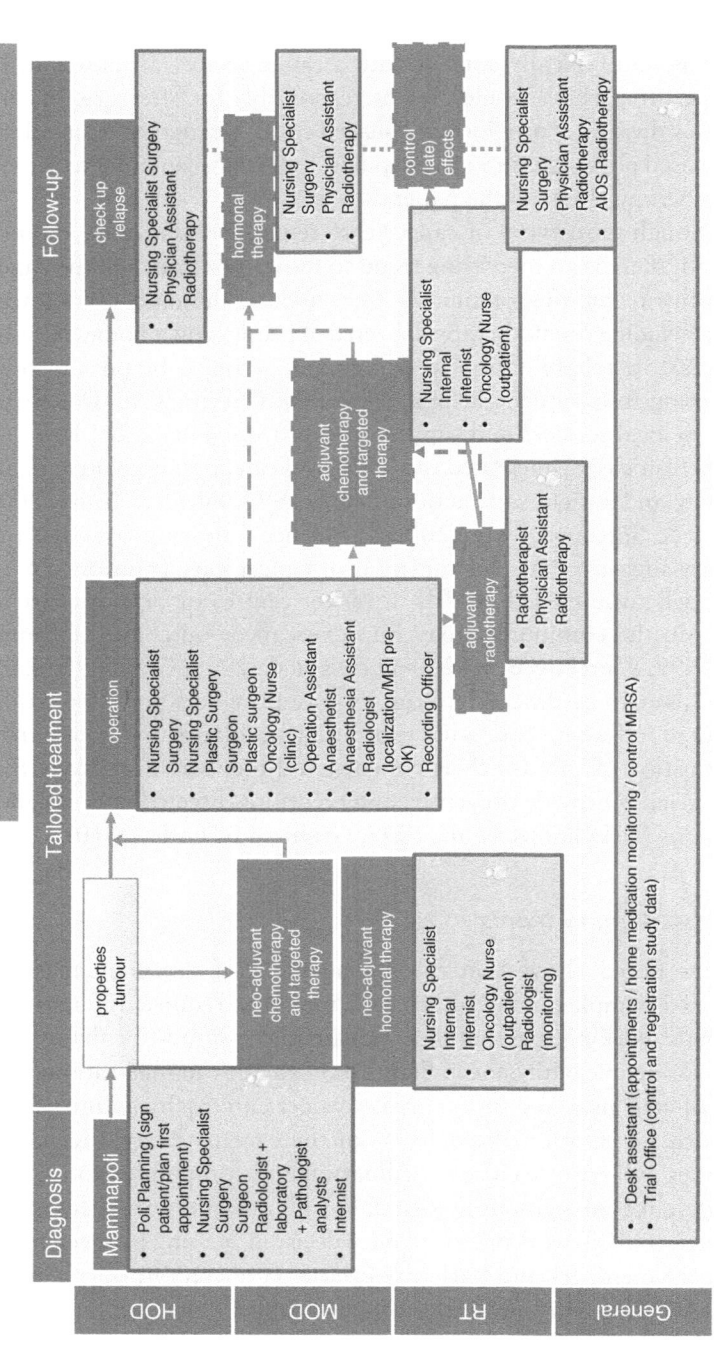

Figure 5.3 Breast cancer pathway for staff, the Netherlands

Source: Undisclosed hospital in the Netherlands

Oncology MDTs can include surgeons, diagnostic and therapeutic radiologists, pathologists, medical and clinical oncologists, nurse specialists, and palliative-care physicians, among others. Such a team will often collaborate closely with other supportive professionals, such as psychologists and psychiatrists (Fleissig et al., 2006).

The move towards MDT working in oncology has been supported by several expert groups and it is now considered the standard in cancer care in most countries in Europe and elsewhere (Borras et al., 2014). Some countries require that the management of all patients with cancer within MDT conferences should be the norm, although some cases that are uncomplicated will be dealt with according to standard guidelines without being discussed by all involved.

Overall, the adoption of MDTs in cancer care has been rapid. For example, in England in the mid-1990s fewer than 20% of cancer patients were managed by an MDT compared with more than 80% in 2004 (Griffith & Turner, 2004). In the Netherlands the peer review system for hospital cancer services, which was introduced in 1994, provided a strong stimulus for the adoption of MDT working (Kilsdonk et al., 2015a, 2015b). Although it is difficult to evaluate the exact mechanism through which an MDT exerts its effect and little direct evidence exists, MDT working has been linked to improved patient outcomes, increased recruitment into clinical trials, and better job satisfaction and psychological well-being among health professionals (Fleissig et al., 2006; Pillay et al., 2016). For example, Pillay et al. (2016) found, based on a systematic review, that MDT meetings impact positively upon the ways cancer patients are assessed and managed. This is consistent with a review by Taplin et al. (2015), which suggests that using team-based approaches across the care continuum can improve access to and the quality of care processes and structures. However, robust evidence on the impact of MDTs on patient outcomes such as survival remains weak. Overall, while they appear intuitively to be beneficial, the current evidence base provides only a limited degree of support for their widespread use (Pillay et al., 2016) and, at least for now, it may be more cost-effective to limit MDT meetings to the discussion of particularly complex or controversial patients.

Barriers to delivering optimal care and the sustainability of the oncological service system

Workforce

The hospital workforce more broadly, and the oncology workforce specifically, face several barriers regarding the delivery of optimal and sustainable cancer care. Key challenges include demographic changes in the composition of the workforce, including an ageing health workforce, leading to shortages due to retirement (European Commission, 2008), along with fewer younger generations entering the workforce due to the limited attractiveness of employment in the health sector (European Commission, 2008). Further challenges are related to the mobility of the workforce across the EU, in particular the movement of some health professionals from poorer to richer countries within the EU, as well as the health brain drain from third countries (European Commission, 2008).

Expensive biological drugs

A review of market access to cancer drugs in Europe found that reimbursement mechanisms, the use of cost-effectiveness analysis in decision-making, and the extent of pharmaceutical price regulation schemes vary considerably across countries (Pauwels et al., 2014; van Harten et al., 2016). Most countries have some form of risk-sharing agreement for high value drugs, be it financial agreements where rebates are offered to third-party payers for the cost of increased expenditure over an annual subsidization cap, or performance or outcome-based agreements (Cheema et al., 2012).

Overall, there are marked differences in the availability and reimbursement of new and often expensive cancer drugs. For example, in Italy innovative new cancer drugs are classified as Class H, qualifying their use in the hospital setting. Class H drugs are bought directly by hospitals from the manufacturers, enabling them to benefit directly from cost sharing agreements and minimum discounts of 50%. This has enabled expansion of patient access to pharmaceuticals (Folino-Gallo et al., 2008). In the United Kingdom the National Institute of Health and Care Excellence (NICE) provides advice on whether or not to reimburse innovative drugs; in other countries there are comparable agencies although the implications of their decisions vary. Differences in the availability of cancer medicines across countries, and the cost of cancer treatment, have prompted considerable public debate in a number of countries. However, the impacts of variation in access to innovative medicines on cancer outcomes at population level are difficult to ascertain.

Radiotherapy and radiology

Unlike cancer drugs, the evaluation of radiation technologies has attracted less attention although it is an area that has undergone significant development over the past 5 to 10 years. Radiotherapy is considered a necessary component of treatment in about half of all newly diagnosed cancers (Delaney et al., 2005). However, European countries are in the paradoxical situation where delivering affordable radiotherapy over the next 20 years is being compromised by both current under-capacity and under-investment in "standard" radiotherapy and also over-penetration of newer radiotherapy technologies that have far greater associated costs (Van Loon et al., 2012). A recent analysis of the Directory of Radiotherapy Centres (DIRAC) database demonstrated variation in radiotherapy capacity and quality across the EU (Rosenblatt et al., 2013).

Imaging techniques and radiology play a major role in the management of many patients, including cancer patients (see Chapter 9). The quality of imaging has improved significantly over recent decades and the use of these new devices has increased, although often because of a belief – not always justified – that "newer is better" (Deyo, 2002). However, the greater use of these techniques has created a larger problem. They often lead to diagnosis of lesions of dubious clinical significance (Lumbreras et al., 2010).

An unexpected finding can trigger additional medical care, including unnecessary tests and other diagnostic procedures and treatments which, in some cases, may pose an additional risk to the patient. This process has been called the "cascade effect" (Whiting et al., 2003). A review by Lumbreras et al. (2010) found that a considerable percentage of patients in whom incidental findings were observed underwent further evaluation with additional expensive and often uncomfortable or risky imaging tests or other diagnostic tests and procedures. Radiologists and clinicians have to balance the diagnostic potential against unnecessary testing and treatment (Lumbreras et al., 2010). Some measures have been recommended to clarify the situation (Whiting et al., 2003), including explicit assessment of the potential risk of the incidental finding for the patient or the availability of a beneficial treatment that justifies follow-up, although the optimum strategy will depend greatly on the particular circumstances.

General trends in oncology care

Looking ahead, there are some trends in cancer care that will have especially profound consequences for the hospital. These include precision medicine, targeted treatment, and immunotherapy; image guided interventions; and improved survivorship and survivorship care.

Precision medicine, targeted treatments, and immunotherapy

Greater understanding of the mechanisms by which cancers develop has provided important insights into interventions targeting underlying mechanisms and treating the condition (Sager, 1997). The primary treatment option is removing the tumour through surgical or radiotherapeutic intervention (often accompanied), which remains by far the most common treatment by which patients are cured (World Health Organization, 2016). However, a considerable percentage of patients are not cured or experience relapse or metastatic disease. Here, chemotherapy and the more recently developed targeted treatments provide important therapeutic options.

Until recently, chemotherapy was given to a large number of patients on the understanding that only a certain percentage would benefit. A better understanding of the underlying pathways has helped to develop treatments that target mechanisms acting at cellular, subcellular or molecular levels. These targeted treatments rely on molecular diagnostics of underlying cell abnormalities, and expertise in genetic aberrations of tumours (Gingeras et al., 2005). Targeted therapies have shown promising results in a number of tumours, especially in advanced stages where so far very few therapeutic options were otherwise available, requiring genome sequencing and analytical techniques along with professional expertise to interpret and weigh findings. It is expected that this trend towards precision medicine, which includes health care innovations involving molecular diagnostics and pharmacogenomics, will continue to bring promising results. This is expected to generate a rapidly growing industry in which genetic markers of disease and treatment responses are searched on a larger scale (Dzau et al., 2015), but which could come at a price that can threaten the financial sustainability of health systems.

In recent years immunotherapy (also referred to as biological therapy) has been shown to be promising in treating certain cancers (and other diseases). This was informed by the observation of "spontaneous" cures in some patients, stimulating research into immune reactions around and inside tumours (as, for instance, observed by white blood cell activity). Immunotherapeutic drug options are available for (metastasized) lung and renal cancer and melanoma, with further experimentation under way with other tumour types. DNA vaccination, stimulating antitumour cell reaction, is also being tested (Stockwell, 2015; Blank et al., 2016) . It is estimated that up to 20% of tumours may benefit from some form of immunotherapy in future. This method has the potential to provide treatment for patients who until recently have had no curative options. However, the costs involved have meant that there is considerable variation in access to new immunotherapeutic drugs and treatments across countries, generating debate on pricing levels and sustainability of the financing of cancer treatment. Recent studies have shown marked differences in list prices and actual prices in a number of European countries; overall access to innovative drug treatment in cancer seems especially difficult in the less developed economies in Europe (Johnsson et al., 2016; Van Harten et al., 2016; Vogler, Vitry & Babar, 2016).

Image guided interventions

Surgical and radiotherapeutic removal of the tumour (bulk) tissue are the primary treatment options if curative treatment is considered. Complete removal is essential but is not always successful. For example, a study on prostatectomy showed that 38% of patients had not had the tumour tissue completely removed (Retel et al., 2014). Here, imaging guidance, a technique available in fields such as cardiology and neurosurgery, has become an important aide to distinguish normal from malignant tissue, or where the tumour is hard to delineate from the surrounding environment. These include perioperative CT scanning, smart needles with optical features and navigation technology combined with image integration. These methods require expertise and infrastructure in imaging modalities as well as biomedical technology expertise within the operating theatre (see Chapter 9). The investments related to these developments can lead to the gradual concentration of diagnostic and intervention infrastructure and expertise. Most technologies are in "proof of principle" or early phased clinical studies and in oncology in innovator locations, such as the Netherlands Cancer Institute in Amsterdam and the Institut Gustaphe Roussy in Paris.

Improved survivorship and survivorship care

Improved survival rates (Stockwell, 2015) have led to a continuously growing number of cancer patients who have survived primary treatment but require ongoing treatment, including cancer survivors treated with curative intent, and who require follow-up and symptom-related aftercare (Van Harten et al., 2013).

Improved cancer survivorship poses challenges for health services, requiring a rethink of how services should be reconfigured to enhance care for cancer survivors (Stovall et al., 2006). The increasingly chronic nature of cancer means that survivors require ongoing support and care in specialist settings and the community. Guidelines for follow-up and survivorship care are being developed in many countries, and research and development into interventions and service development are ongoing. Cancer and cancer treatments are associated with a wide range of physical and psychological challenges, some of which may even appear only years after the initial treatment. Person-centred and stepped care approaches are considered to be the most appropriate way forward, but evidence remains weak on the best ways of providing care that optimizes symptom treatment and problem solving for different cancer sites. For example, Tsianakas et al. (2012), in a study of patient experience of cancer services, found that while those with breast and lung cancer reported broadly similar experiences, they differed in the nature of information they required and the priorities they attached to service improvement activities. New care models are emerging that emphasize the importance of supporting patients to engage in self-management activities and to enable them to make informed choices about the type of support they need. It is apparent that cancer survivors must become more effective coproducers in their own care, with Tsianakas et al. (2012) proposing experience-based codesign as an approach to ensure that patients will be involved as active partners in the care process.

Patient empowerment will be at the core of new approaches to cancer care in hospitals, with Groen et al. (2015) identifying five key attributes: (1) being autonomous and respected; (2) having knowledge; (3) having psychosocial and behavioural skills; (4) perceiving support from community, family, and friends; and (5) perceiving oneself to be useful. The latter two are essential in the cancer setting. Information and communication technology (ICT) and eHealth initiatives are playing an increasing role in supporting cancer patients (McAlpine et al., 2015). Technology ranges from electronic patient portals to electronic decision aids or online cognitive behavioural therapy programmes. The majority of eHealth initiatives in cancer care tends to focus on providing patients with information about their disease and treatments to enable shared decision-making, with only a minority aimed at patients to build the skills necessary to cope with the symptoms they experience (Groen et al., 2015).

The fragmentation of ICT services poses a major challenge to realizing their potential benefits. In the Netherlands, for example, many hospitals have their own patient portal system and do not easily connect to other systems in the cancer care trajectory. If they are to increase patient-centredness and shared care, IT services need to be linked in a way that makes information available for every health care provider in the chain ("shared care"). This most probably will lead to a medical record that is owned by the patient and has connections to multiple health care providers.

Organizational trends in cancer care and hospital-based oncology across the EU

Networks

The development of advanced diagnostics in nuclear medicine, MRI, molecular pathology, and genetic sequencing requires specialist staff and investments in infrastructure and equipment (see Chapter 9). In combination with a growing awareness that in some areas hospitals with a greater volume of patients with certain conditions achieve better outcomes, we see a gradual trend towards cooperation between hospitals in networks, with centralization, especially of complex low volume interventions. This requires providers to formalize agreements on cooperation, division of labour and handovers, and to discuss pathways across organizational boundaries. In 2018 the Organisation of European Cancer Institutes (OECI) started the development of Patient-centred

Quality Standards for Cancer Networks (Organisation of European Cancer Institutes, 2018). We here use the examples of the Netherlands (Box 5.1) and Italy (Box 5.2) to illustrate these trends.

Box 5.1 The emergence of cancer networks in the Netherlands

In the Netherlands most hospitals provide cancer care, although there has been a steady trend towards the centralization of, in particular, low volume and complex treatments. University centres specialize in rare cancers and large hospitals have a leading role in the treatment of high volume tumours such as breast, lung, colorectal and prostate cancer. This trend was initially stimulated by the setting of minimum volume standards for various procedures by government and health insurance companies. This role has now been taken on by professional associations, which are defining norms and quality criteria; they have also introduced quality registries.

The Netherlands Comprehensive Cancer Organization (IKNL) is the quality institute for oncological and palliative research and practice in the Netherlands. It collaborates with health care professionals and managers and patients on the continuous improvement of oncological and palliative care, encourages knowledge exchange and organizes consultation service between centres of expertise and regional hospitals. IKNL also coordinates the issuing and maintenance of care guidelines (Volksgezondheid en zorg, 2016).

In response to the centralization of cancer services, and to clarify the role of various types of hospital and university medical centres (UMCs), regional cancer centre networks (CCNs) are being established. The CCNs will focus on improving treatment, care and clinical research in oncology across the network. It remains challenging to implement CCNs, however, as not all UMCs cover all relevant high volume tumours. Importantly, so far the Netherlands has only one comprehensive cancer centre – the Netherlands Cancer Institute – that has received formal accreditation by the OECI. Also, it was only recently that it was decided to concentrate all paediatric oncology in one national centre (construction started in 2016). As the total number of new cases amounts to around 500 per year, this guarantees state-of-the-art expertise for every individual case (Prinses Maxima Centrum, 2016).

Box 5.2 The emergence of cancer networks in Italy

The Italian National Cancer Plan is increasingly focusing on the concept of regional oncology networks, according to a federal model, of which the Lombard Oncology Network (Regione Lombardia, 2006) is the most representative example in the national network Alleanza Contro il Cancro. Locally, the network provides significant benefits in terms of resources and information optimization; at a national and international level it helps to maximize the collaboration and the sharing of best practices.

The EU has established European reference networks (ERNs) for rare diseases, with networks for paediatric, haematological, and solid tumours approved in December 2016. These are intended to improve the quality of care, to coordinate knowledge dissemination and to facilitate cross-border care. By early 2017 the first European reference networks became operational (European Commission, 2018). Palm et al. (2013) highlighted various challenges in the implementation of European reference networks. For example, for Denmark it was shown to be challenging to identify the right national balance in terms of geographical coverage and capacity of "good clinics", and for monitoring and evaluating the system. There remain questions about how the concept of reference centres and networks should be defined, the management of the process of identifying centres, and the implications of the establishment of such networks for funding of services and coverage of the population.

Organization

There is an increasing trend to centralize cancer services through the formation of cancer centres (outside or within the hospital structure), with a growing number of hospitals and cancer centres in a range of EU countries entering the Accreditation and Designation (A&D) programme of the OECI (Organisation of European Cancer Institutes, 2018).

There remains debate about the optimal model of organizing cancer care; the added value of different forms is difficult to establish, with little robust evidence on the best way of delivering cancer services.

Germany provides an example of a distinct organizational model, which involves a three-tier approach (DKG German Cancer Society, 2014). The first tier comprises comprehensive cancer centres (*Onkologische Spitzenzentren*), which are the leading oncology centres holding a major research portfolio. The cancer centres focus primarily on rare cancers and specialized aspects of care, with a specific programme by the Deutsche Krebshilfe periodically designating 14 centres as comprehensive cancer centres, which will receive considerable additional funding for their translational research. The second tier includes oncology centres, which cover several cancer sites or specialties, particularly rare cancers. The designation as an oncology centre is led by the German Cancer Society (GCS) and aims to guarantee high quality of services for payers, the public and government. The third tier includes organ cancer centres, which specialize in one organ or specialty (e.g. breast, bowel, lung, prostate, skin, and gynaecological tumours). The organ cancer centres are also covered by the GCS programme (DKG German Cancer Society, 2014).

At the European level there are various professional and institutional oncology societies. Professional societies include the European Society of Medical Oncologists (ESMO) and the European Society for Radiotherapy and Oncology (ESTRO). An example is the European Cancer Organization (ECCO), a multidisciplinary organization that connects all stakeholders in oncology across Europe. ECCO is a not-for-profit federation that aims to uphold the right of all European cancer patients to the best possible treatment and care, promoting interaction between all organizations involved in cancer at European level (ECCO, 2016). Another is the Organization of European Cancer Institutes (OECI). The OECI is a non-governmental, non-profit organization with the primary objective to improve communication and bringing together cancer research and care institutions across the European Union, in order to create a critical mass of expertise and competence (Organisation of European Cancer Institutes, 2016).

Patient registries

Patient registries (to be distinguished from the more traditional cancer registries) that collect and enable the monitoring of data on treatments and tumour characteristics have been established in Norway, Sweden and, more recently, the Netherlands. The population-based cancer registries in the Nordic countries include more comprehensive disease-specific quality registries covering treatment data and detailed outcomes data (Møller et al., 2002).

In Italy the Italian Association of Cancer Registries (AIRTUM) established a network of registries which gained international importance in contributing to European survival studies (De Angelis et al., 2014), international prevalence comparisons (Crocetti et al., 2013) and the consolidation of partnerships within the network of cancer registries in the Mediterranean area, including the southern coast (Hamdi Cherif et al., 2015), through the Euromed (EEAS, 2016) project.

Cancer Care in the hospital of the mid-21st century

Cancer will account for a growing volume of hospital activity in coming years. Not only does this mean that more patients will be offered innovative and promising treatments, but the sustainability of the health system, in terms of human and financial resources, will remain under continuous strain.

Perhaps the most important message from this chapter is that the care of cancer in hospitals has become vastly more complex than in the past, in terms of both the technical ability to characterize and understand tumours and to individualize their treatment, and the organizational responses that bring together staff with differing types of expertise. This will require close coordination between clinicians and managers. Further concentration and specialization of services will be inevitable, and this will require continuing networking, increasingly using innovative information technology, telehealth, and telemedicine to ensure that concentration of services does not undermine geographical access to services. It is very likely that regional networks of hospitals will organize cancer care among themselves, concentrate and share expensive diagnostics and intervention capacity, and establish liaisons with referral centres of expertise for rare tumours. Networks of reference centres are established in the EU and offer considerable potential for promoting research and innovative treatments for patients with some very rare tumours, or tumour subtypes.

References

Aggarwal A, Ginsburg O, Fojo T (2014). Cancer economics, policy and politics: what informs the debate? Perspectives from the EU, Canada and US. *Journal of Cancer Policy*, 2(1):1–11.

Berrino et al. (2007). Survival for eight major cancers and all cancers combined for European adults diagnosed in 1995–99: results of the EUROCARE-4 study. *Lancet Oncol*, 8(9):773–83.

Blank CU et al. (2016). The "cancer immunogram". *Science*, 352:658–60.

Borras JM et al. (2014). Policy statement on multidisciplinary cancer care. *Eur J Cancer*, 50(3):475–80.

Burns LR, Pauly MV (2002). Integrated delivery networks: a detour on the road to integrated health care? *Health Aff (Millwood)*, 21(4):128–43.

Cancer Council Australia (2016). Optimal cancer care pathways. Health Professionals (Online). Available at: http://www.cancer.org.au/health-professionals/optimal-cancer-care-pathways.html (accessed 22 January 2016).

Cheema P et al. (2012). International variability in the reimbursement of cancer drugs by publicly funded drug programs. *Curr Oncol*, 19:e165.

Corbett M et al. (2015). The delivery of chemotherapy at home: an evidence synthesis. *Health Services and Delivery Research*, 3.14.

Crocetti E et al. (2013). Cancer prevalence in the United States, Nordic Countries, Italy, Australia, and France: an analysis of geographic variability. *Br J Cancer*, 109(1):219–28.

De Angelis et al. (2014). Cancer survival in Europe 1999–2007 by country and age: results of EUROCARE-5 – a population-based study. *Lancet Oncol*, 15(1):23–34.

Del Giudice et al. (2009). Primary care physicians' views of routine follow-up care of cancer survivors. *J Clin Oncol*, 27(20):3338–45.

Delaney G et al. (2005). The role of radiotherapy in cancer treatment. *Cancer*, 104(6):1129–37.

DeVita VT Jr, Rosenberg SA (2012). Two hundred years of cancer research. *N Engl J Med*, 366(23):2207–14.

Deyo RA (2002). Cascade effects of medical technology. *Annual review of public health*, 23(1):23–44.

DKG German Cancer Society (2014). Certification of health-care structures in oncology – development and effects. Available at: https://www.krebsgesellschaft.de/gcs/german-cancer-society/certification.html (accessed 17 December 2015).

Dzau VJ et al. (2015). Aligning incentives to fulfil the promise of personalised medicine. *Lancet*, 385(9982):2118–19. doi: 10.1016/S0140-6736(15)60722-X. Epub 6 May 2015.

ECCO (2016). European CanCer Organisation web site. Available at: https://www.ecco-org.eu/.(accessed 2 February 2020).

EEAS (2016). Euro-Mediterranean Partnership (EUROMED). Available at: http://eeas.europa.eu/euromed/index_en.htm (accessed 1 February 2016).

European Commision (2008). GREEN PAPER On the European Workforce for Health. Available at: https://ec.europa.eu/health/ph_systems/docs/workforce_gp_en.pdf (accessed 2 February 2020).

European Commission (2018). *European reference networks.* (Online) Directorate-General for Health and Food Safety. https://ec.europa.eu/health/ern/overview_en (accessed 2 February 2020).

Ferlay J et al. (2013). Cancer incidence and mortality patterns in Europe: estimates for 40 countries in 2012. *Eur J Cancer*, 49(6):1374–403.

Fleissig A et al. (2006). Multidisciplinary teams in cancer care: are they effective in the UK? *Lancet Oncol*, 7(11):935–43.

Folino-Gallo P et al. (2008). Pricing and reimbursement of pharmaceuticals in Italy. *Eur J Health Econ*, 9:305–10.

Gingeras TR et al. (2005). Fifty years of molecular (DNA/RNA) diagnostics. *Clin Chem*, 51(3):661–71.

Griffith C, Turner J (2004). United Kingdom National Health Service. Cancer Services Collaborative "Improvement Partnership". *Eur J Surg Oncol*, 30 suppl:1–86.

Groen WG et al. (2015). Empowerment of Cancer Survivors Through Information Technology: An Integrative Review. *J Med Internet Res* 17(11):e270.

Grunfeld E, Earle CC (2010). The interface between primary and oncology specialty care: treatment through survivorship. *J Natl Cancer Inst Monogr*, 2010(40):25–30. doi: 10.1093/jncimonographs/lgq002.

Grunfeld E et al. (1999). Comparison of breast cancer patient satisfaction with follow-up in primary care versus specialist care: results from a randomized controlled trial. *Br J Gen Pract*, 49(446):705–10.

Hamdi Cherif M et al. (2015). Cancer estimation of incidence and survival in Algeria 2014. *J Cancer Res Ther*, 3(9):100–4.

Jha P, Peto R (2014). Global effects of smoking, of quitting, and of taxing tobacco. *N Engl J Med*, 370:60–8.

Johnsson B et al. (2016). The cost and burden of cancer in the European Union 1995–2014. *Eur J Cancer*, 66:162–70. doi: 10.1016/j.ejca.2016.06.022. Epub 31 Aug 2016.

Kilsdonk M et al. (2015a). Evaluating the impact of accreditation and external peer review. *Int J Health Care Qual Assur*, 28(8):757–77.

Kilsdonk MJ et al. (2015b). Two decades of external peer review of cancer care in general hospitals; the Dutch experience. *Cancer Med*, 5(3):478–85.

Kodner DL, Spreeuwenberg C (2002). Integrated care: meaning, logic, applications, and implications – a discussion paper. *Int J Integr Care*, 2:e12.

Leutz WN (1999). Five laws for integrating medical and social services: lessons from the United States and the United Kingdom. *Milbank Q*, 77(1):77–110, iv–v.

Lewis RA et al. (2009). Patients' and healthcare professionals' views of cancer follow-up: systematic review. *Br J Gen Pract*, 59(564):e248–e259. doi: 10.3399/bjgp09X453576.

Luengo-Fernandez R et al. (2013). Economic burden of cancer across the European Union: a population-based cost analysis. *Lancet Oncol*, 14(12):1165–74.

Lumbreras B et al. (2010). Incidental findings in imaging diagnostic tests: a systematic review. *Br J Radiol*, 83(988):276–89.

Lyman GH (2013). Counting the costs of cancer care. *Lancet Oncol*, 14(12):1142–3.

McAlpine H et al. (2015). A systematic review of types and efficacy of online interventions for cancer patients. *Patient Educ Couns*, 98(3):283–95.

Macmillan (2014). Working Together. Challenges, opportunities and priorities for the UK's cancer workforce. Available at: https://www.macmillan .org.uk/documents/getinvolved/campaigns/weareaforeceforchange/ workforcediscussiondoc.pdf

Møller B et al. (2002). Prediction of cancer incidence in the Nordic countries up to the year 2020. *Eur J Cancer Prev*, 11(s1):S1–96.

Organisation of European Cancer Institutes (2016). Member List. Available at: https://www.oeci.eu/MemberList.aspx (accessed 20 February 2020).

Organisation of European Cancer Institutes (2018). How to establish patient-centred quality standards for various types of cancer networks. *OECI Invitational meeting*, 19 April 2018. Available at: http://www.oeci.eu/ Attachments/OECI_Paris_Meeting_19042018.pdf (accessed 1 May 2018).

Organisation of European Cancer Institutes (web site). Available at: http:// www.oeci.eu (accessed 6 March 2018).

Palm W et al. (2013). Building European Reference Networks in Health Care: Exploring concepts and national practices in the European Union., WHO Regional Office for Europe, on behalf of the European Observatory on Health Systems and Policies.

Pauwels K et al. (2014). Market access of cancer drugs in European countries: improving resource allocation. *Target Oncol*, 9(2):95–110.

Peto R et al. (2012). Mortality from smoking in developed countries 1950–2000 or later, updated March 2012. Oxford, Oxford University Press. Available at: https://www.deathsfromsmoking.net/download%20

files/Original%20research/Mortality%20from%20smoking%20in%20 developed%20countries%201950-2000%20(2nd%20ed.).pdf

Pillay B et al. (2016). The impact of multidisciplinary team meetings on patient assessment, management and outcomes in oncology settings: a systematic review of the literature. *Cancer Treat Rev*, 42:56–72.

Prinses Maxima Centrum (2016). Prinses Maxima Centrum voor kinderoncologie. Available at: http://www.prinsesmaximacentrum.nl/ (accessed 2 February 2020).

Regione Lombardia (2006). *Rete Oncologica Lombardo*. Available at: http:// www.progettorol.it/ (accessed 1 February 2016).

Retel VP et al. (2014). Determinants and effects of positive surgical margins after prostatectomy on prostate cancer mortality: a population-based study. *BMC Urol*, 14:86.

Rosenblatt E et al. (2013). Radiotherapy capacity in European countries: an analysis of the Directory of Radiotherapy Centres (DIRAC) database. *Lancet Oncol*, 14(2):e79–e86.

Rubin G et al. (2015). The expanding role of primary care in cancer control. *Lancet Oncol*, 16:1231–72.

Sager R (1997). Expression genetics in cancer: shifting the focus from DNA to RNA. *Proc Natl Acad Sci USA* 94(3):952–5.

Stockwell, S. (2015). Online First: ASCO Names "Cancer Advance of the Year": Transformation of Treatment for CLL. *Oncology Times*, 20 January.

Stovall E et al. (2006). From Cancer Patient to Cancer Survivor: Lost in Transition. Washington, DC, National Academies Press.

Sussman J et al. (2011). The impact of specialized oncology nursing on patient supportive care outcomes. *J Psychosoc Oncol*, 29(3):286–307. doi: 10.1080/07347332.2011.563342.

Taplin SH et al. (2015). Reviewing cancer care team effectiveness. *J Oncol Pract*. 11(3):239–46. doi: 10.1200/JOP.2014.003350. Epub 14 Apr 2015.l

Tsianakas V et al. (2012). Implementing patient-centred cancer care: using experience-based co-design to improve patient experience in breast and lung cancer services. *Support Care Cancer*, 20(11):2639–2647.

Van Harten WH et al. (2013). The role of comprehensive cancer centers in survivorship care. *Cancer*, 119(s11):2200–1.

Van Harten et al. (2016). Actual costs of cancer drugs in 15 European countries. *Lancet Oncol*, 17(1):18–20. doi: 10.1016/S1470-2045(15)00486-6. Epub 4 Dec 2015.

Van Loon J et al. (2012). Evaluation of novel radiotherapy technologies: what evidence is needed to assess their clinical and cost effectiveness, and how should we get it? *Lancet Oncol*, 13(4):e169–e177.

Viguier J (2015). Future perspectives for cancer screening. *Eur J Cancer Prev*, suppl:S87–9.

Vogler S, Vitry A, Babar Z (2016). Cancer drugs in 16 European countries, Australia, and New Zealand: a cross-country price comparison study. *Lancet Oncol*, 17(1):39–47.

Volksgezondheid en zorg (2016). [Integral cancer centres play an important role in care provision]. Available at: https://www .volksgezondheidenzorg.info/onderwerp/kanker/preventie-zorg/organisatie-van-zorg.

Wattchow DA et al. (2006). General practice vs surgical-based follow-up for patients with colon cancer: randomised controlled trial. *Br J Cancer* 94(8):1116–21.

Whalen J (2010). Europe targets drug price cuts. *Wall Street Journal*. New York, Dow Jones & Company, Inc.

Whiting P et al. (2003). The development of QUADAS: a tool for the quality assessment of studies of diagnostic accuracy included in systematic reviews. *BMC Med Res Methodol*, 3(1):1.

World Health Organization (2012). Leading causes of death in Europe: fact sheet. Copenhagen, WHO Regional Office for Europe.

World Health Organization (2016). Treatment of cancer. Cancer (Online). Available at: http://www.who.int/cancer/treatment/en/ (accessed 22 January 2016).

6 COPD *as an exemplar of a chronic health condition*

C MICHAEL ROBERTS[1], JOSE LUIS LÓPEZ-CAMPOS[2], ROBAB BREYER-KOHANSAL[3]

[1] UCLPartners Academic Health Sciences Network; Queen Mary University of London; Royal College of Physicians; Princess Alexandra NHS Trust, United Kingdom.
[2] Unidad Médico-Quirúrgica de Enfermedades Respiratorias; Instituto de Biomedicina de Sevilla (IBiS); Hospital Universitario Virgen del Rocío/Universidad de Sevilla, Spain; CIBER de Enfermedades Respiratorias (CIBERES); Instituto de Salud Carlos III, Madrid Spain.
[3] Department of Respiratory and Critical Care Medicine and Ludwig Boltzmann Institute for COPD and Respiratory Epidemiology, Otto Wagner Hospital, Vienna, Austria.

Introduction

Studies suggest that around 25% of the European population receive treatment for a chronic condition. As the population ages, the prevalence of chronic diseases increases, with an average of two per person in their mid-60s and three for those surviving to their mid-70s (Barnett et al., 2012). People with chronic diseases now form a sizeable proportion of all hospital admissions both elective and emergency. Once admitted to hospital, people with multiple complex conditions may require a long length of stay and place a significant demand on acute hospital services.

Chronic obstructive pulmonary disease (COPD) is such a condition which affects between 3% and 10% of Europe's adult population and accounts for 1.1 million hospital admissions per year (Gibson et al., 2013). While it is a preventable condition, once contracted it is not curable and management strategies aim to reduce the burden of disease both on the individual and on society, which is currently estimated to cost the EU €200 billion per year (Gibson et al., 2013). Managing COPD and other long-term conditions effectively is critical not only for patients and carers but for the effective functioning of the health system itself.

In this chapter we use COPD as an exemplar of a chronic condition whose management depends on the work of the acute general hospital. As noted in Chapter 1, while the care of patients with COPD involves many specific features, it also raises issues of more general relevance to many common chronic disorders. Here we describe the burden of the disease in detail, the current management of the condition within the hospital system, and options for future care pathways illustrated by innovations that have already been implemented across a range of European health systems.

What is COPD?

Chronic obstructive pulmonary disease is an overarching term for the clinical and patho-physiological manifestations of the inflammatory response of the lungs to the repeated inhalation of noxious particles and fumes. This inflammation over time results in damage to both the airways, causing narrowing, and to the alveoli, manifesting as emphysema. People with COPD will characteristically exhibit the symptoms of cough, often with sputum production and usually worse over the winter months, with breathlessness being the most prevalent symptom (Aitsi-Selmi & Hopkinson, 2015) that tends to be progressive over time and may be accompanied by wheeze. The condition results in airflow limitation in both the small and large airways that is detected by lung function tests, notably spirometry, which are used to confirm the diagnosis (Barnes et al., 2015). People who develop COPD probably have a genetic predisposition so that when exposed to noxious inhaled substances, most commonly cigarette smoke but also occupational dusts and, especially in low income countries, biomass fumes in poorly ventilated housing, they react with an increased inflammatory response that causes intrinsic lung damage.

The clinical course once COPD develops is variable but overall is progressive and may lead to death from respiratory failure or as a result of respiratory infection, which may cause intermittent acute exacerbations of the condition. There are a number of identifiable phenotypical expressions of the condition that provide an opportunity for delivering more personalized interventions to individuals. The one intervention that would make most difference to all those with COPD, however, is to remove the exposure to the noxious substances provoking the lung inflammation (Vestbo et al., 2013).

Additionally, co-morbidities may have a significant impact on clinical presentation and prognosis (Laforest et al., 2016) and reduced physical activity is a well recognized consequence of the condition (Hopkinson & Polkey, 2010). Accordingly, there is a need for early intervention to prevent later more severe and expensive disease.

The burden of COPD

It is difficult to provide reliable estimates about the population health burden that can be associated with COPD. This is in part because the disease is often under-diagnosed as it is not usually recognized until it is clinically apparent and moderately advanced (Lamprecht et al., 2015). Furthermore, where estimates are available, these frequently draw on varying definitions and diagnostic criteria. For example, studies of COPD prevalence have variously used self-reported respiratory symptoms, physician diagnosis of COPD, or the presence of airflow limitation with or without spirometric tests as criteria. As a consequence, available estimates vary by study design.

The recent 2010 update of the Global Burden of Disease (GBD) study revisited previous estimates on respiratory diseases and estimated the number of people to have COPD at 328 million globally (Vos et al., 2012). Worldwide the prevalence of COPD is rising, with the highest rise in the eastern Mediterranean region (119% between 1990 and 2010) and the lowest rise in Europe (22.5%), both, however, being substantial. Overall prevalence among men is around twice that of women but there are significant national variations (Adeloye et al., 2015). More recently there is evidence of falls in COPD prevalence within some western European countries, for example in Spain (Soriano et al., 2010) and Finland (Pelkonen et al., 2014), thought to be as a result of tighter tobacco controls.

COPD is one of the major causes of mortality worldwide (Figure 6.1). There has been a steady increase in mortality over time (Jemal et al., 2005) and it was estimated that COPD would become the fourth leading cause of death globally by the year 2030 (Mathers & Loncar, 2006), a projection that was confirmed by the 2010 GBD study, when COPD became the third leading cause of death globally (Lozano et al., 2012). Within Europe it is estimated to have caused 150 000 deaths in 2010, potentially rising to 338 000 a year by 2030 (Gibson et al., 2013).

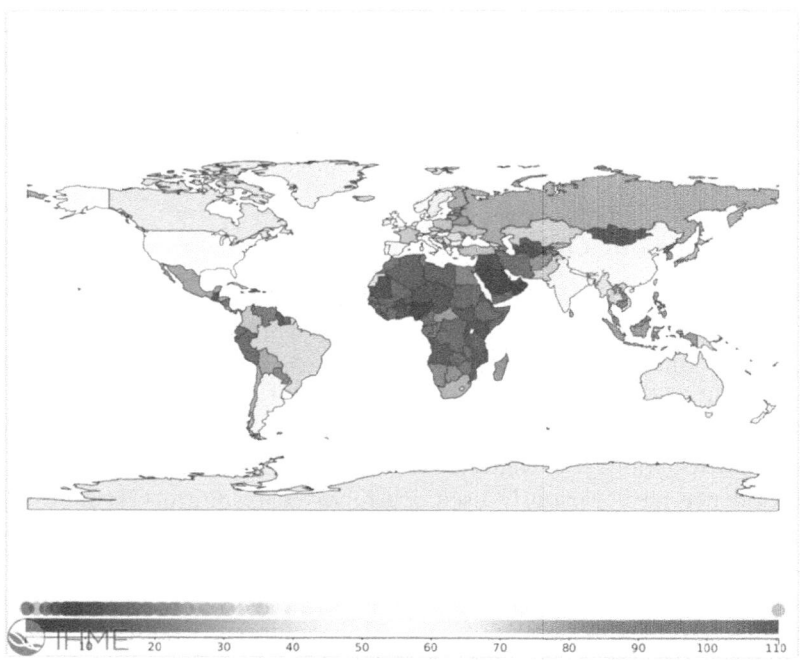

Figure 6.1 Age-standardized death rate from COPD per 100 000, both sexes, 2016

Source: Institute for Health Metrics and Evaluation, 2014

Economic costs that can be associated with the burden of COPD

As noted, COPD has been associated with considerable economic costs to the health system (Khakban et al., 2015) and projections suggest a significant further increase in direct costs by the year 2030 because of population ageing (Herse, Kilijander & Lehtimaki, 2015). COPD also poses a substantial burden at individual level in terms of activity limitation and disability and to society more broadly because of lost productivity and associated costs (Patel, Nagar & Dalal, 2014).

The predominant health care cost item is hospital utilization for exacerbations, which, in the United States in the early 2000s, was estimated to account for $18 billion (€14 billion) annually (Anzueto, Sethi & Martinez, 2007). In southern Spain the annual cost of hospital admissions for COPD exacerbation was estimated to be €27 million in 2000 (López-Campos Bodineau et al., 2002), with admissions to intensive care accounting for one-fifth of the total costs for COPD management (Dalal et al., 2011). Estimates of the mean actual cost per severe exacerbation range from €1711 in Greece (2006–07) (Geitona et al., 2011) to €3985 in Italy (2006) (Blasi et al., 2014). Co-morbidities such as cardiovascular disease, diabetes, asthma and anaemia (Mannino et al., 2015) were shown to further increase the economic burden that can be associated with COPD (Huber et al., 2015), as they drive increased service utilization among people with COPD (Simon-Tuval et al., 2011). With the advent of new pharmacological treatments for COPD (Barjaktarevic, Arredondo & Cooper, 2015), it is reasonable to expect that health care costs that can be associated with COPD will rise further, despite the evidence that pharmacotherapy for COPD in ambulatory care is cost-effective (Simoens, 2013). In summary, available data highlight the need to prioritize interventions aimed at delaying the progression of COPD, preventing exacerbations and reducing the risk of co-morbidities, in order to alleviate the clinical and economic burden of COPD (Wouters, 2003; Foster et al., 2006; Anzueto, Sethi & Martinez, 2007; Mannino et al., 2015).

The COPD care pathway

It is suggested that a high proportion of people with COPD remain undiagnosed either because they have few if any symptoms in the milder stages of the disease or because clinicians are slow to associate common symptoms of cough or breathlessness with the need to screen for COPD (Llordes et al., 2015). People with diagnosed COPD present usually with symptoms on the background of an exposure history, most commonly to cigarette smoke, but in around 5–15% of cases to occupational fumes, with exposure to biomass fuels a particular challenge in low and middle income countries (Smith, Mehta & Maeusezehal-Fauz, 2004). The diagnosis is made clinically but by definition it must be confirmed by spirometry lung function testing.

Once a diagnosis is made, the underlying lung damage is largely permanent and the prognosis is of a slow decline in lung function and symptoms related to the continuing exposure to the causative agent. Thus in a cigarette smoker, stopping smoking will halt further decline but not resolve any existing disease (Box 6.1).

Box 6.1 Evidence-based interventions for the management of COPD: smoking cessation

Smoking is a major risk factor for the development of COPD and current smoking is also higher among people with COPD compared to the general population, up to 47% and 20%, respectively (Schauer et al., 2014). Anthonisen et al. (1994) demonstrated that among people with early-stage COPD annual lung function decline was reduced following a smoking intervention compared to people with COPD who did not receive the intervention. There is also evidence of improvements in the presence of respiratory symptoms and quality of life over time. Against this background, smoking cessation has been proposed as an intervention with the highest impact on the natural history of COPD (Vestbo et al., 2013).

Evidence further suggests that even brief advice provided by physicians to quit smoking can significantly increase the likelihood of successfully quitting smoking (Bao, Duan & Fox, 2006; Stead et al., 2013). At the same time, while behavioural interventions (including simple advice) have modest efficacy in improving smoking quit rates among people with COPD, the combination of counselling and pharmacotherapy tends to be more effective and more cost-effective than either on its own (Hoogendoorn et al., 2010; Tashkin, 2015). International guidance recommends a five-step programme, involving brief strategies to help patients willing to quit smoking (Vestbo et al., 2013), while recognizing that more complex interventions will increase quit rates. Smoking cessation has been identified to be a cost-effective intervention for patients with COPD independently of stage of disease and should therefore be offered to every single smoking COPD patient (Buck, Richmond & Mendelsohn, 2000; Wouters, 2003).

There are no interventions other than smoking cessation that impact the natural history of the disease and arrest the decline in COPD. Management outside of smoking cessation is therefore largely designed to improve symptoms and functional status, and interventions outside smoking cessation tend to be matched to the stage of the disease and the severity of symptoms. This is further illustrated in Figure 6.2, which provides an example of a care pathway to improve outcomes in COPD.

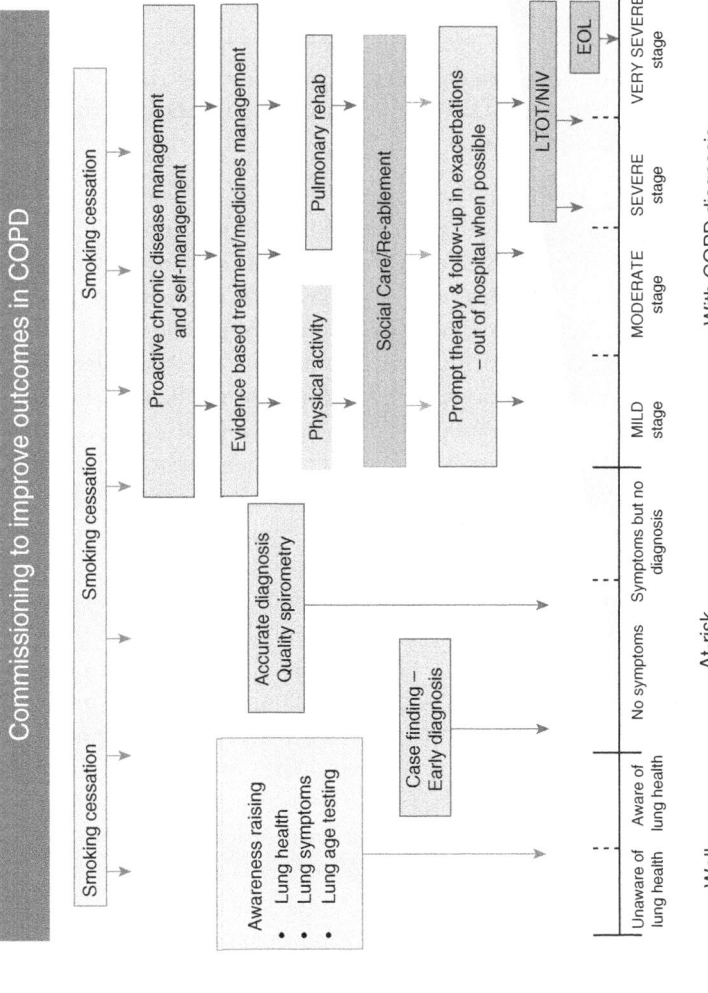

Figure 6.2 Example of a care pathway to improve outcomes in COPD

Source: Matt Kearney. Available at: https://www.networks.nhs.uk/nhs-networks/east-of-england-respiratory-programme/key-documents/documents/Commissioning%20for%20Better%20Outcomes%20in%20COPD.pdf (accessed 20 February 2020)

In the late stages of the disease, long-term oxygen therapy (LTOT) and non-invasive ventilatory (NIV) support may prolong life (Box 6.2) and optimizing palliative care interventions may also improve both quality and length of life. Lung transplantation in selected patients is an ultimate option in very severe COPDs, although this tends to be available to a small minority of end-stage patients only (Lane & Tonelli, 2015).

Box 6.2 Evidence-based interventions for the management of COPD: long-term oxygen therapy and non-invasive ventilatory support

Long-term oxygen therapy has been shown to prolong life in patients with COPD and chronic respiratory failure (hypoxia; deficiency of oxygen in the tissues) (Stoller et al., 2010). Effects on survival are only achieved if LTOT is given for at least 15 hours per day. LTOT is usually provided in the home environment of people with COPD. Ambulatory devices can increase the mobility of the patient and provide longer oxygen usage with resultant patient benefit (Bradley & O'Neill, 2005). Ambulatory oxygen may in some cases also reduce breathlessness on exertion in some patients who do not fulfil the strict criteria for LTOT. Providing LTOT for citizens who wish to spend time across national borders is challenging as there is no established European oxygen prescribing system and using oxygen aboard commercial flights can also be difficult and expensive with each airline following its individual set of rules.

Non-invasive ventilation (NIV) has been shown to be effective in patients with stable but very severe COPD and chronic respiratory failure (hypercapnia; high concentration of carbon dioxide in the blood), with evidence of positive effects on health status and survival (Kohnlein et al., 2014; Struik et al., 2014). NIV in acute respiratory failure in COPD due to exacerbation has been shown to positively impact respiratory acidosis, symptoms, prevalence of ventilator-associated pneumonia, and length of hospital stay (Ram et al., 2004b). Evidence suggests that NIV and invasive mechanical ventilation (IMV) are increasingly used in hospitals, primarily in emergency departments and intensive care units, and access to this therapy has been increased within recent years (López-Campos et al., 2014).

Progressive decline in lung function may lead to significant disability and quality of life impairment where palliative care interventions are most appropriate. For some people COPD leads to death; the condition accounts for around 2.5% of all deaths in Europe (Global Health Observatory, 2008). Death from respiratory causes is, however, not inevitable in COPD and a number of patients will die from linked conditions that share the same aetiology of cigarette smoking, for example heart disease and lung cancer (Zielinski et al., 1997; McGarvey et al., 2007).There is growing recognition that older patients with COPD suffer with multiple morbidities, all of which contribute to the state of frailty, that must be factored into their management. Death will more likely result from one of these diseases than it will from COPD, which in itself will be a major driver in future hospital models of care.

The effect of social factors on the outcome determinants of this complex health picture will further motivate collaboration between social and health care providers. As with many chronic diseases, the care provided to people with COPD tends to be fragmented in most system contexts. Countries are experimenting with new models of care that are designed to better meet the needs of people with long-term conditions (Nolte, Knai & Saltman, 2015), including for COPD, based on the available evidence of the (cost-)effectiveness of structured disease management of COPD (Steuten et al., 2009; Kruis et al., 2013).

The level of interaction between the patient and the hospital will depend very much upon the stage of disease of the patient, the level of support available for out-of-hospital care and the complexity of the individual case. While stable patients with COPD are typically managed outside hospital, there are a number of indications for specialist input that will require hospital care, even in those stable patients. But again these are most often delivered in the outpatient or ambulatory care setting rather than resulting in an admission to hospital. In cases where the diagnosis remains unclear or where, despite optimal treatment in primary care, a patient remains symptomatic, referral for a hospital-based specialist opinion is appropriate. In complex cases at the more severe end of the spectrum some interventions such as endoscopic lung volume reduction and surgical techniques are only available within the hospital setting (Box 6.3).

Box 6.3 Evidence-based interventions for the management of COPD: surgical treatment

Stable COPD patients with severe emphysematous lung damage (hyperinflation) can benefit from surgical treatment such as lung volume reduction surgery (LVRS). This intervention has been shown to lead, in an appropriately selected subgroup of patients with COPD, to better functional outcomes and improved survival compared to standard medical therapy (Naunheim et al., 2006). Similar to other invasive procedures, surgical treatment carries an operative mortality risk compared with medical management. The cost per quality adjusted life year (QALY) in appropriately selected individuals is estimated to be between $40 000 and $55 000 (Ramsey et al., 2007).

Bronchoscopic lung volume reduction (BLVR) is a novel treatment option, with clinical trials showing improvements in symptoms, exercise capacity, and lung function (Davey et al., 2015). Some countries in Europe, notably Germany and Switzerland, have now incorporated this intervention into usual clinical pathways (Pertl et al., 2014). Others are awaiting further evidence. Effective BLVR appears to be associated with a survival benefit in carefully selected patients (Hopkinson et al., 2011; Klooster et al., 2015; Garner et al., 2016; Herth et al., 2016). The cost per QALY for BLVR in that subgroup is around €25 000 (Pietzsch, Garner & Herth, 2014).

The acute exacerbation patient pathway

The main cause for a person with COPD to be admitted to hospital as an emergency will be as a result of an exacerbation of his/her condition. Exacerbations are characterized by increasing breathlessness and accompanied frequently by worsening cough and increased volume or discoloured sputum production. In many cases these acute attacks are caused by infection, while in other cases they represent a deterioration in the underlying condition worsened by atmospheric changes or other environmental factors. Exacerbations can be treated out of hospital but may also result in hospital admission; exacerbations constitute a common cause of hospitalization across Europe (Librero et al., 2016).

People admitted to European hospitals with acute COPD exacerbations have an inpatient mortality of around 4.9% and a 90 day readmission rate of 35% (Hartl et al., 2016). It is against this background that much focus has recently been given to preventing hospital admissions (Vestbo & Lange, 2015). A number of interventions including combination therapy with inhaled corticosteroids and broncho-dilating drugs (Spencer et al., 2011), prophylactic antibiotics (Herath & Poole, 2013) and patient education with self-management (Zwerink et al., 2014) have been shown to effectively reduce exacerbation frequency and hospital admission, with evidence suggesting that these should be implemented for all patients identified to be at risk. There is less evidence that self-management with provision of "rescue packs" of antibiotics and steroid tablets in isolation of a robust education programme is effective at reducing hospital admission (Walters et al., 2010).

While it may have previously been considered that hospitals and their teams should concentrate on hospital care, it is clear that if patients are to receive a more joined-up and consistent level of care, then the influence of the hospital must extend outside of the physical bounds of the buildings themselves. There is some evidence that early self-management and proactive community interventions may reduce hospital admissions for patients with COPD at risk of exacerbation by up to a third (Effing et al., 2007; Suh, Mandal & Hart, 2013). Supporting both clinicians and patients and carers to better manage conditions to avoid unscheduled care and emergency admissions can best be facilitated by collaborative care linking to the education resources now found in abundance on the world wide web provided by national and international patient support groups (European Lung Foundation, 2013).

Which organization takes responsibility for interventions designed to reduce unscheduled care and admission to hospital will depend upon local systems but the skills and resources found in hospitals can enrich such out of hospital services through a variety of models. One example is the Kings Health Partners (London) Integrated Respiratory Team, which involves a partnership between hospital, community and primary care clinicians who form a collaborative team to manage out-of-hospital patients (Box 6.4). In the Spanish Ribera Salud model, a more formal vertically integrated accountable care organization directly employs an integrated community and primary team (Ribera Salud, 2016). Such integrated teams tend to be nurse-led and often include multidisciplinary members such as a physiotherapist and a social care case worker who can address the social aspects and may prevent an otherwise unnecessary admission. MDTs have been shown to be more effective at reducing admissions than nurse mono-professional teams (Wong, Carson & Smith, 2012; Kruis et al., 2013).

Box 6.4 Integrated Respiratory Team (IRT), Kings Health Partners, London, UK

The Integrated Respiratory Team works across King's College Hospital and Guy's and St Thomas' NHS Foundation Trusts and the community in London to deliver care to patients with COPD, including oxygen, pulmonary rehabilitation and supported discharge services. Key components include the IRT working in acute care hospitals to support accurate diagnosis and acute management, communication and post-discharge care, VCs in the community, a single point of referral to IRT from the community and optimizing respiratory prescribing. Respiratory virtual clinics (VCs) run twice a week in primary care. The focus of VCs is joint working between primary care teams and the IRT to systematically review the diagnosis and long-term management of the respiratory patient caseload. Since its launch in 2012 the service has seen a 34% reduction in COPD admissions and a 17% reduction in length of stay.

Source: d'Ancona et al., 2014

Intervention teams may be COPD specific or have a general remit to reduce hospital admissions across a range of patient diagnostic groups. Some are specifically targeted at reducing readmissions to hospital while others provide a prevention service for a broader range of at-risk patients identified through primary care and secondary care ambulatory services. A key enabler for effective team working, particularly across sites and organizations, and to link with the patients across a geography, is technology (see Box 6.5 below). While the evidence for primary technology-based interventions in COPD care is currently weak (Lundell et al., 2015), it seems sensible to suggest that integrated electronic patient care records, web-based self-management programmes (Luckett et al., 2016) and greater use of communication technologies to facilitate coordinated and specialist support to generalist care are to be of increasing importance in the future.

While promising, preventative services such as those described in Box 6.4 are not currently implemented widely across Europe and will therefore be available to only a minority of patients. Most patients will be evaluated by their community-based primary care or specialist doctor and either treated or referred to the hospital. The decision-making process may be supported by (national) guidelines for the diagnosis and management of COPD that have been established in many countries (Effing et al., 2007).

Frequently, however, an acute exacerbation requires assessment in an emergency department (ED) and hospitalization. Across Europe there will be on average 200 hospital admissions for acute COPD per 100 000 population but with a 10-fold difference between countries with high and low admission rates (Gibson et al., 2013). The reasons for such variation are not known but it is hypothesized that this reflects the maturity of primary and community services, prevalence of COPD and the availability of hospital beds (Gibson et al., 2013). While much of the variation may be attributed to "system and population factors", it seems clear that if hospitals are to moderate admissions for long-term conditions, there will be a need to extend their influence outside the physical walls of their estate.

Hospital care for exacerbations of COPD

While efforts are made to prevent admission to hospital, there is a need for severe exacerbation cases to receive the kind of management that currently can only be provided in hospital. The ideal pathway for a COPD admission can be seen to involve early triage to a specialist unit and provision of appropriate care using a MDT, to include ventilatory support where appropriate, and then discharge once safe with entry to a rehabilitation programme at an early stage following discharge (Vestbo et al., 2013). For the minority of end of life patients palliative care services should be provided (Vestbo et al., 2013).

However, hospital services are currently organized very differently across Europe, both within and between countries, which will influence the pathway for the individual COPD patient into the hospital and upon discharge. Data from the 2010–2011 European Respiratory Society audit of hospital care of people with COPD admitted to hospital with exacerbations (European COPD Audit) highlighted this variation (López-Campos et al., 2014). It showed that, for example, triage was operated in only 7% of Belgian hospitals included in the audit compared to 67% in Slovakia and 60% in Croatia. Specialist respiratory wards were available in 93% of UK hospitals but only in 27% of hospitals in

Austria. While all, or the majority, of patients in Belgium and Switzerland (90%) were seen by a nurse or physiotherapy respiratory specialist, this was only the case for 35% of patients in Poland and 20% in Turkey.

Around 5% of admissions will die in hospital, although there are now predictive tools that allow the identification of those with a much higher risk of death who are most likely to benefit from the potentially life-saving interventions of ventilator support. Respiratory acidosis is one such predictor that affects about 20% of COPD admissions and has a mortality of between 20% and 30% without assisted ventilation support. In contrast there is a significant cohort of admissions at very low risk of death who could safely be managed in the community by a MDT as described earlier. The European COPD Audit found that a considerable share of admissions is for people with mild disease (Global initiative for chronic Obstructive Lung Disease (GOLD) stage I or II), ranging from 54% admissions in Romania and 51% in Switzerland to only 35% in the United Kingdom and 30% in Turkey (López-Campos et al., 2014). This suggests that many people with COPD exacerbations currently admitted to hospital could potentially be managed in the community if appropriate services (such as MDTs) were available. In contrast, patients requiring ventilatory support, or who are at risk of developing ventilatory failure requiring such support, should be managed in hospital according to national and international management guidelines. Yet, as data from the European COPD Audit indicate, availability of high dependency units that deliver ventilatory support varies substantially across countries, from 95% of Swiss hospitals to only 22% in Greece and 10% in Romania. Non-invasive ventilation was provided in all hospitals in Switzerland, Ireland and Slovakia but only in 70% of Croatian and 60% of Romanian units. For some patients the key hospital intervention can be palliative and end of life care, yet in the audit this service was available in only 13% of Greek hospitals and 5% in Turkey compared with 91% in Ireland and 92% in the United Kingdom.

Furthermore, the European COPD Audit found that hospital adherence to the 2010 GOLD standards varied considerably both within and across countries (Roberts et al., 2013). Spirometric confirmation of diagnosis was available in just 59% of cases, while even in patients with previous admissions with the same diagnosis 37% had no record of lung function confirmed diagnosis. Further more, of those with a spirometry result recorded, 13% had a result incompatible with the diagnosis of COPD. Taking arterial blood gases on admission, which provides essential information about prognosis and the need for key interventions, was performed in 91.5% cases with an interquartile range (IQR) between hospitals of 78.4% and 98.7% and an IQR between countries of 81.9% and 93.5% (Table 6.2).

As indicated above, diversity of pathways, if not quality of care, for people with COPD admitted to hospital with exacerbations across different health systems is in part the consequence of the different organizational structures that are based on medical models rather than population need. For example, the hospital infrastructure in many countries distinguishes smaller local units and larger regional institutions that are often associated with a university and thus include teaching and research functions. A small number of European countries operate a national respiratory centre of excellence, such as Romania and Slovakia, while elsewhere expertise is spread among several tertiary institutions, including in Spain and the United Kingdom (López-Campos et al., 2014). The resources and organization of care vary widely, with larger hospitals tending to have a higher number of specialist doctors and offering a wider range of specialist services while not necessarily providing better quality care to patients or improving patient outcomes (López-Campos et al., 2014) (Table 6.1).

Care experiences and standards of care that people with COPD in European countries can expect when admitted with a COPD exacerbation will depend very much on the particular hospital they present to. Data from both the European and UK audits of hospital COPD care suggest that the number of specialists per 1000 beds is the single most important resource factor in determining outcomes for patients (Hartl et al., 2016; Price et al., 2006).

Data further suggest that current service delivery often falls short of international guideline standards and that there is major variation in quality of care not just between countries but equally within them (Table 6.2).

Post-acute care

There is growing recognition that the hospital has potential to influence out-of-hospital care not just to prevent admission but also to prevent

Table 6.1 *Selected characteristics of hospital centres participating in the 2010–11 European COPD Audit Variation*

Country	Number of hospital centres participating	Median number of beds per hospital (10th, 90th percentile)	Median catchment population (10 000s) per unit (10th, 90th percentile)	Number of respiratory specialist doctors per unit (10th, 90th percentile)
Austria	47	377 (169–1 098)	10.6 (2.87–25)	7 (3–12)
Belgium	21	450 (240–935)	20 (6–100)	5 (3–12)
Croatia	8	461 (105–1 191)	34 (11–75)	7 (2–13)
Greece	22	575 (200–700)	32.5 (6–15)	5 (2–6)
Republic of Ireland	11	343 (131–851)	25 (12–50.6)	2 (1–6)
Malta	1	850	41.8	5
Poland	38	400 (182–1 002)	25 (5.8–21)	6 (2–16)
Romania	9	185 (118–517)	47.5 (17–77)	11 (7–21)
Slovakia	3	644 (400–887)	106 (12–200)	7 (2–11)
Spain	91	460 (150–1 023)	25 (3.7–99.9)	8 (3–16)
Switzerland	18	245 (161–784)	15 (3.5–40)	3 (1–6)
Turkey	20	610 (133–1 200)	100 (9.6–1 000)	6 (3–14)
United Kingdom	112	527 (290–1 000)	30 (17–55)	4 (2–8)

Source: López-Campos et al., 2014

Table 6.2 *Quality of COPD care across European hospitals against recommendations of the GOLD strategy document*

Audit standard	Compliance at case level (%)	Absolute case numbers	Median by hospital (%)	IQR by hospital (%)	Median by country (%)	IQR by country (%)
Spirometry result available at admission	59.4	9 513/16 018	63.1	43.4–83.3	64.7	49.3–69.9
Arterial blood gas performed at admission	82.4	13 191/16 018	91.5	78.4–98.7	88.1	81.9–93.5
Chest radiograph performed at admission	98.6	15 790/16 018	100	98.6–100	99.0	98.0–99.4
Controlled oxygen therapy used	84.9	13 602/16 018	89.7	76.9–97.9	85.7	79.8–88.5
Short-acting bronchodilator use	91.1	14 594/16 018	95.9	89.1–100	91.4	80.3–94.7
Non-use of intravenous methylxanthines	85.7	13 742/16 018	96.8	83.3–96.	79.9	54.7–97.4
Systemic corticosteroids given	82.3	13 187/16 018	87.9	77.3–95.0	76.9	62.7–88.3
Antibiotics given if sputum purulence or IMV	90.5	8 457/9 347	93.5	85.7–100	89.5	86.3–93.6
NIV given if pH <7.35 and $PaCO_2$ >6 kPa	51.0	1 133/2 222	58.6	40–77.8	47.0	40.9–66.6
IMV given if pH <7.25 and $PaCO_2$ >8 kPa	15.4	73/473	50.0	33.3–100	31.6	22.2–44.4
Fulfilled all 10 recommendations	15.3	2 444/16 018	16.6	9.09–25.0	10.1	5.18–17.8

Source: Roberts et al., 2013

readmission and there are excellent examples of where such influence has major benefits to the patient and to the system. Once a patient has recovered from their acute illness they are usually discharged back to the environment they came from, such as the community or their own home. In some cases, the deterioration in their condition will not have improved enough to allow this to happen and in some health systems a period of convalescence or rehabilitation may be arranged. In other cases this is not an option and a patient may be placed within institutional care, such as residential care or a nursing home. Available evidence supports the use of ESD for selected patients with acute exacerbation of COPD as an effective and safe intervention (Echevarria et al., 2016). Such schemes aim to accelerate discharge from hospital with the provision of continued support in a community setting, typically at the same intensity that would have been provided had the patient remained in hospital, and involving MDTs to prevent (re)admissions. Although countries are increasingly introducing these type of programmes, their availability varies considerably. For example, the European COPD Audit found that 75% of participating UK hospitals offered early discharge support programmes compared to only 37% in Switzerland, the next most frequent user. In many of the participating countries there was no use of such programmes (López-Campos et al., 2014). This suggests that many patients may be receiving suboptimal care.

There are also concerns about the transition from hospital to community, with patient experience varying both within and between countries. This ranges from simple discharge from hospital without coordination of care post discharge to that of an integrated care system where there is seamless continuity of care with a single organization responsible for both secondary and primary care services with a shared electronic health record (Ribera Salud, 2016). Telehealth may offer opportunities to link the hospital to the patient after discharge and to provide monitoring to ensure clinical improvement but also to then provide early warning signs of a deterioration that initiates an early intervention to prevent readmission (Box 6.5), with telemedicine considered more broadly as an aid to the management of long-term conditions (McKinstry, Pinnock & Sheikh, 2009; Hernandez, Mallow & Narsavage, 2014). However, rigorous evaluation is required as in other areas of medicine it has often failed to live up to what has been promised.

Box 6.5 Telehealth teams for monitoring patients with COPD post discharge, Barcelona, Spain

As part of the EU-funded Supporting Healthier and Independent Living for Chronic Patients and Elderly (NEXES), a multidisciplinary telehealth team was established in one of the four health sectors of the city of Barcelona, Spain, to monitor post COPD exacerbation discharge patients. Patients were monitored remotely and had access to regular video conferencing, a dedicated call centre and an online patient management web portal. The call centre was managed by a health coach who might deal with problems directly or refer to the patient's case manager who in turn could access other services as required, including the GP, other health care professionals or a respiratory specialist depending upon the issue identified. The intervention was associated with significantly fewer hospitalizations among patients with chronic respiratory diseases, reduced in-hospital days for patients in a Home Hospitalization/Early Discharge scheme, and increased quality of monitoring of patients receiving additional support.

Source: Hernandez et al., 2015

Where care provision remains fragmented, alternative approaches to providing more joined-up care include a discharge bundle quality improvement tool (Box 6.6), which promotes a standardized set of processes designed to enhance optimal transition back to the community (Turner, 2015) and which has been shown to reduce emergency readmission to hospital post discharge (Hopkinson et al., 2012).

Box 6.6 COPD discharge care bundle project, London, UK

A care bundle is a structured way of improving the processes of care and patient outcomes. It involves a small set of between three and five evidence-based practices that, when performed collectively and reliably, have been shown to improve patient outcomes. The project involved the design and implementation of a COPD discharge care

---

Box 6.6 (cont.)

bundle in northwest London. The bundle includes: (i) smoking cessation advice; (ii) assessment and referral for post-discharge pulmonary rehabilitation; (iii) patient education and self-management plans; (iv) medication review including inhaler technique checks; and (v) assured follow-up post discharge. Evidence from the initial implementation phase suggested that the introduction of the care bundle had reduced readmission rates and improved both staff and patient satisfaction with the discharge process. Further evaluation of the subsequent roll-out of the care bundle to other acute hospitals in London provided further evidence that the introduction of the bundle was associated with a reduction in readmission rates (Laverty et al., 2015).

Source: Hopkinson et al., 2012

Other interventions that can reduce readmission rates and which lie within the influence of the hospital include early pulmonary rehabilitation (Puhan et al., 2011), while for those with end-stage disease, and a high chance of relapse, advanced care planning may result in the avoidance of future admissions. Evidence suggests that in those cases care provided in the patient's own home or in a community setting that is more suited to end of life care can be effective in reducing the symptom burden for patients (Gomes et al., 2013).

Rehabilitation

As noted above, pulmonary rehabilitation has been shown to be a very cost-effective therapy in COPD (Spruit et al., 2013; McCarthy et al., 2015). Reported benefits include improved exercise capacity and quality of life, reduced symptoms, anxiety and depression, and enhanced medications effects. Rehabilitation has further been shown to reduce hospitalizations and length of hospital stay as well as improving the recovery after hospitalization because of COPD exacerbation (Puhan et al., 2016). Components of pulmonary rehabilitation can vary but a comprehensive programme typically includes smoking cessation, exercise training, nutrition therapy, and patient education. Programmes are designed to improve the physical and psychological condition of people with chronic respiratory disease and to promote the long-term adherence to health-enhancing behaviours. The collaborative approach of multiple provider services working across organizational boundaries to provide rehabilitation at its best can have much wider system impacts as exemplified by the Copenhagen SIKS programme (Box 6.7), which has become a model for locality-based integrated care systems in Denmark (Jacobsen et al., 2014).

Box 6.7 Integrated effort for people living with chronic diseases (SIKS) project, Copenhagen, Denmark

Set up as a research project for the period 2005–2007, the SIKS project focused on the implementation of rehabilitation programmes for people with type 2 diabetes, COPD, and heart disease or with balance problems following falls, requiring close collaboration between a local health care centre, a local hospital, and GPs. Standard packages of rehabilitation included disease-specific education and patient self-management sessions, a physical training session, nutritional consultation sessions and smoking cessation programmes. The programmes lasted 7–12 weeks depending on the specific disease. Patients were followed up upon completion of the programme. An evaluation of the impact of rehabilitation on health-care utilization found that compared with their matched controls, patients with COPD participating in the programme in the health care centre showed smaller increases in hospital admissions, bed days and outpatient visits over a two-year period that were statistically significant (at 18%, 34%, and 24%, respectively). The SIKS project is reported to have influenced the way integrated care has been conceptualized in Denmark. For example, after completion of the project, health care centres based on the SIKS model were established across Denmark and the experiences informed wider policy development for coordinated care approaches in Denmark.

Source: Jacobsen et al., 2014

Despite its demonstrable benefits, rehabilitation after an exacerbation is not widely offered in Europe and elsewhere. Data from the European COPD Audit showed that in 2010–11 pulmonary rehabilitation at discharge was available in just half of participating hospitals, ranging from 91% in Ireland and 88% in the United Kingdom to just 18% in Austria and 20% in Romania (López-Campos et al., 2014). Also drawing on the European COPD Audit and additional data, Spruit et al. (2014) reported large differences among pulmonary rehabilitation programmes in mostly high income countries in Europe and North America as they relate to the setting, composition of the pulmonary rehabilitation team, methods of referral and types of reimbursement, among others. For example, in North America the majority of programmes (~70%) were delivered in outpatient settings whereas in European countries this was the case for half of the programmes while another 30% were offered in both inpatient and outpatient settings. There was also substantial heterogeneity in referral practices, in terms of the types of practitioners who refer patients and the types of patients referred, which was attributed, in part, to varying knowledge, attitudes, and perceptions of pulmonary rehabilitation within and across countries, and which may impact on patient outcomes. Importantly, the survey found that only a small number of patients were enrolled in pulmonary rehabilitation across the centres studied, highlighting that a potentially large number of people with potential to benefit from pulmonary rehabilitation are either not referred, not enrolled, lack access, or choose not to participate (Rochester & Spanevello, 2014).

Workforce

The workforce required to staff the future European hospitals will need to meet the challenges posed by advances in medical innovation and technology, the changing population needs as reflected by older people with complex multiple chronic conditions, but most of all by the impending shortages of clinical staff. While there is no European standard for what constitutes an ideal hospital staffing level to make such a judgement, evidence from large-scale studies suggests that higher numbers of doctors and of nurses per hospital bed correlate with better outcomes for patients (Needleman et al., 2011; Hartl et al., 2016). For example, using data from the European COPD Audit, Hartl et al. (2016) found that a higher number of respiratory specialists per 1000 beds reduced the risk of post-discharge mortality for patients with COPD. As we have noted above, the European and UK/England and Wales COPD Audits highlight not only large variations in clinical staff per 1000 beds between countries but also within each country (López-Campos et al.,

2014; Stone et al., 2015). This suggests that workforce distribution is not necessarily based upon workload or patient need but is dependent upon other factors that might include local funding, hospital status or specialty and academic interest, geography and social factors, or simply historical models of care.

The optimal management of patients with COPD faces the same challenges as the health care sector does more widely in deploying an appropriately trained workforce, with shortages in some medical specialties, and especially nurses, alongside demographic changes. Countries are experimenting with extended and new roles for nurses in particular to support nurses and physicians working within the hospital system. Such roles include physician associates with a science-based first degree plus a vocational master's degree who are trained to perform a number of duties, including taking medical histories, performing examinations, diagnosing illnesses, analysing test results, and developing management plans. They are supervised by a senior doctor but take on many of the more routine duties that a physician might otherwise fulfil. Respiratory nurses or physiotherapy specialists are independent practitioners with master's level or equivalent training in respiratory medicine and often specifically in COPD care. They may be deployed as part of a hospital or joint community team bridging the gap between hospital and community care with in-reach or outreach connectivity. They may lead a multiprofessional team with or without medical input. Key roles are within supported discharge, admission prevention teams and pulmonary rehabilitation. The exercise physiologist is a professional role developed in the United States and now adapted in some European systems. They usually hold a biomedical sciences degree with an additional master's qualification in exercise physiology, and specializing further in the management of people with chronic conditions, notably heart and lung disease. Exercise physiologists may prescribe and oversee a personalized exercise programme for patients with COPD and may also supervise a pulmonary rehabilitation programme for a larger number of patients with COPD. The ability to plan and oversee tailored exercise programmes raises the potential to extend rehabilitation to those with co-morbidities with perhaps greater confidence than staff trained purely in COPD or respiratory health care. The result is a blurring of traditional responsibilities in an attempt to provide a wider professional team contributing to a competencies-based workforce. The benefits of this trend include a refocusing of roles around the needs of the patient today rather than to continue a pattern of service delivery configured decades in the past, and to provide multiskilled staff who can meet most of the patient's needs in a single episode of care rather than requiring multiple professionals to input multiple narrow specialized interactions.

COPD teams have been at the forefront of developing new professional roles but there is little consistency of adoption across Europe. The aforementioned European COPD Audit report found that at the time of the study participating hospitals in several countries did not have specialist respiratory trained physiotherapists (Romania, Spain, Turkey), or nurse specialists (Austria, Poland, Switzerland) and while all countries recognized respiratory function technicians as a team member, they were not employed in all hospitals (Roberts et al., 2013). Even where there are roles with similar titles, their competencies and scope are often difficult to compare because of differences in training, and the clinical systems within which they operate.

Specialist resources

There is no equivalence across Europe in terms of function and size or resource level for hospitals that establishes either a minimum or optimum standard, although there are standards described within international COPD recommendations for the interventions that should be available to patients admitted to hospital with exacerbations of COPD (GOLD, 2017). The patient might reasonably expect to receive the same high quality care wherever they present, accepting that this might not be all provided in one location. A range of factors will determine what can be provided, ranging from geography and accessibility to workforce availability and financial pressures on resource allocation. Within any one country, however, systems that share data and promote real-time interaction between clinicians working separately have the potential to reduce the variation in quality of care that is currently the reality. Life-saving treatments can be administered if patients are appropriately diagnosed and triaged in terms of severity using history taking and clinical examination followed by basic blood tests, arterial blood gas measurement and a chest radiograph which should be available at all hospital sites. Severely ill patients with acute respiratory acidosis need to have access to ventilatory support within a period of 1 to 3 hours of presentation according to management guideline recommendations (Celli, MacNee & ATS/ERS Task Force, 2004; Vestbo et al., 2013). This is one key and potentially life-saving intervention outside the basic level of care that can be provided in all locations, i.e. antibiotics, steroids, bronchodilators and oxygen therapy. NIV, while currently often delivered by respiratory specialists, is also managed in some countries by anaesthetists, and some services are led by specialist nurses or physiotherapists who could be supported remotely by specialist doctors if not available on site (Bierer & Soo Hoo, 2009; Pinto et al., 2010; Cabrini et al., 2015; Ambrosino et al., 2016). Invasive ventilation required for those who fail on non-invasive support or where there are other factors making this the more appropriate intervention is more complex and is nearly always delivered by anaesthetic-trained staff in an intensive care unit setting. Ideally such facilities – i.e. the equipment, monitoring facilities, the staff and the specialist unit – should be available in every hospital admitting COPD exacerbations or be accessible by rapid site transfer. This is not the case at present (Roberts et al., 2013; López-Campos et al., 2014).

For the subacute situation all hospitals should also provide diagnostic facilities available to hospital, primary care and community physicians that will ensure accurate diagnosis of COPD. These would include lung function testing and imaging, notably chest radiography and CT scanning. Advice from an expert clinician would be helpful in making the more difficult diagnostic cases where other conditions may exist as co-morbidities or as differential diagnoses.

Stable patients at the advanced stage of the disease will require more complex investigation and interventions that may include LVRS and potentially, in a very small number of cases, lung transplantation. Such patients would be referred to a specialist centre with specific expertise in these techniques and with the expensive equipment and clinical staff available. Once again the implementation of technological solutions would provide opportunities for patients in this situation to be considered regardless of their physical location by the transmission of images, electronic patient records and by video interviews between clinicians and patients. In this manner a hub and spoke model provides an efficient and effective use of resources.

In summary, a technological interconnectivity of hospitals provides an opportunity for all patients to access specialty opinions regardless of their location and situation. Critical to good patient care will be establishing the correct diagnosis at an early stage and, for patients admitted to hospital, early access to assisted ventilation if needed and then prior to discharge a comprehensive care package that will reduce the progression of the disease and risk of further admission. A small number of highly specialized units could provide nationally available expertise to all while networked to a larger number of more local provider units. These in turn, or through the national specialty units, could also provide networked support to both primary care health professionals and to patients and carers facilitated by technological solutions.

Barriers to delivering optimal care

Optimal care can be defined as a composite of evidence-based and consensus-based interventions that promote good outcomes for patients, and guidelines, or in a resource-constrained system might more productively be considered as the appropriate implementation of these interventions within a value-based hierarchy. Unlike for most chronic medical conditions, this value-based approach is well documented for COPD and it provides a useful reminder to clinicians of their responsibilities to the system as well as to the patient (Figure 6.3).

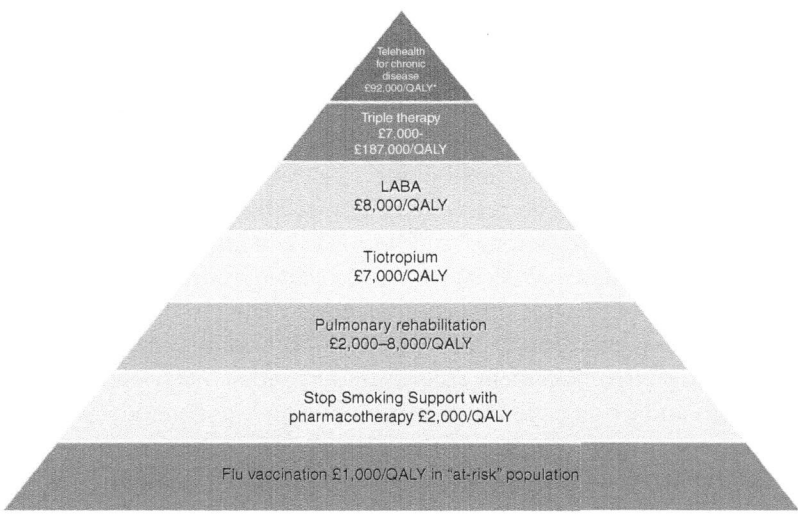

Figure 6.3 The pyramid of value for COPD interventions

Source: IMPRESS Guide to the relative value of COPD interventions (2012). British Thoracic Society Reports, Vol. 4, Issue 2. ISSN 2040-2023.

Implementing optimal care is a multifaceted challenge with the need to modify clinical behaviours and a culture that requires a shift in the balance of control towards patients and away from clinicians. The European evidence relating to the quality of care offered by hospitals confirms that the complex interactions that constitute an organization account for the majority of the variation between units (Ruparel et al., 2016). The principle of value to the system is equally valid when applied to a hospital as it is to the care offered to an individual patient. The evidence that resource-rich organizations perform better in delivering high quality COPD care is relatively weak and although there are some associations between medical staffing levels and better care outcomes (Roberts et al., 2013; Hartl et al., 2016), there is no direct evidence of a link with other inputs. However, it is concerning that European audits reveal that some elements of treatment that have been shown to benefit patients with COPD are unavailable in many of the hospitals that care for these patients.

A useful example of the complex organizational interactions that account for some unwarranted variations in care is the degree to which specialist COPD care is offered to patients within any institution. Much care of patients with COPD in hospitals is delivered by non-respiratory specialists and the evidence is that generalists are less likely to deliver optimum COPD care to their patients with COPD (Hosker et al., 2007; López-Campos et al., 2015). At a population level, most COPD care is delivered out of hospital by generalists, while most of the expertise remains locked within hospital buildings. Providing greater access to that expertise both within and outside the hospital is an important facet of delivering optimal care. Sadly, patients themselves are unlikely to understand what good care looks like and are therefore unlikely to be able to negotiate high quality care with their health teams. Better-informed patients might drive better COPD care.

Until regular measurement of care quality becomes a routine element of clinical care it remains difficult to identify areas of excellence or those where improvement is required. Engaging clinicians in reviewing performance data is a key challenge but if successful promotes the improvement of clinical practice (Flottorp et al., 2010). Leadership is required if Europe is to move forward in redesigning hospital care for patients with COPD. That must come from the health professions and from politicians. At present, there is no functional European health profession voice to provide that leadership and little evidence of a united political will.

COPD and the future hospital – summary

The hospital of the future is likely over time to be admitting sicker and frailer patients with COPD exacerbations. The evidence for ambulatory care as an alternative to admission (Ram et al., 2004a) and early discharge once admitted is compelling (Echevarria et al., 2016) but will not be appropriate for all individuals who require a greater level of support. Particularly in health systems with under-developed primary care, these measures offer huge potential benefits to hospitals in the future. Such a hospital would be a central hub, supported by technology that could provide a learning and education resource supporting patient self-management (Smidth et al., 2013) for a large population, over a geographical area well beyond its historical area of influence. Patients at risk of acute deterioration and admission could be directly linked to a COPD clinical monitoring team to provide the opportunity for early interventions to improve patient well-being (McLean et al., 2011). Patients would be managed at distance, gaining specialist expertise without the need to regularly travel to hospital appointments (D'Ancona et al., 2014). Clinicians too could be connected using digital communication, sharing patient clinical records, laboratory results, and imaging, and holding multidisciplinary discussions with colleagues via video conferencing and email to provide wider access to expertise extending well outside the physical buildings of the hospital itself. The challenge has always been how to provide equality of access to higher standards of care regardless of geography. Providing a technological network of the highest level of expertise available to all provides an opportunity to make progress towards that ideal while managing more people in an out-of-hospital setting.

References

Adeloye D et al. (2015). Global and regional estimates of COPD prevalence: systematic review and meta-analysis. *J Glob Health*, 5:020415.

Aitsi-Selmi A, Hopkinson NS (2015). Breathlessness, physical activity and sustainability of healthcare. *Eur Respir J*, 45:284–5.

Ambrosino N et al. (2016). Tele-monitoring of ventilator-dependent patients: a European Respiratory Society Statement. *Eur Respir J*, 48(3):648–63. doi: 10.1183/13993003.01721-2015. Epub 7 Jul 2016.

Anthonisen NR et al. (1994). Effects of smoking intervention and the use of an inhaled anticholinergic bronchodilator on the rate of decline of FEV1. The Lung Health Study. *JAMA*, 272:1497–505.

Anzueto A, Sethi S, Martinez FJ (2007). Exacerbations of chronic obstructive pulmonary disease. *Proc Am Thorac Soc*, 4:554–64.

Bao Y, Duan N, Fox SA (2006). Is some provider advice on smoking cessation better than no advice? An instrumental variable analysis of the 2001 National Health Interview Survey. *Health Serv Res*, 41:2114–35.

Barjaktarevic IZ, Arredondo AF, Cooper CB (2015). Positioning new pharmacotherapies for COPD. *Int J Chron Obstruct Pulmon Dis*, 10:1427–42.

Barnes PJ et al. (2015). Chronic obstructive pulmonary disease. *Nat Rev Dis Primers*, 1:15076.

Barnett K et al. (2012). Epidemiology of multimorbidity and implications for health care, research, and medical education: a cross-sectional study. *Lancet*, 380:37–43.

Bierer GB, So Hoo GW (2009). Noninvasive ventilation for acute respiratory failure: a national survey of Veterans Affairs hospitals. *Respir Care*, 54(10):1313–20.

Blasi F et al. (2014). The clinical and economic impact of exacerbations of chronic obstructive pulmonary disease: a cohort of hospitalized patients. *PLoS One*, 9:e101228.

Bradley JM, O'Neill B (2005). Short-term ambulatory oxygen for chronic obstructive pulmonary disease. *Cochrane Database Syst Rev*, 4:CD004356.

Buck DJ, Richmond RL, Mendelsohn CP (2000). Cost-effectiveness analysis of a family physician delivered smoking cessation program. *Prev Med*, 31:641–8.

Cabrini L et al. (2015). An international survey on noninvasive ventilation use for acute respiratory failure in general non-monitored wards. *Respir Care*, 60(4):586–92. doi: 10.4187/respcare.03593. Epub 18 Nov 2014.

Celli BR, MacNee W, ATS/ERS Task Force (2004). Standards for the diagnosis and treatment of patients with COPD: a summary of the ATS/ERS position paper. *Eur Respir J*, 23:932–46.

D'Ancona G et al. (2014). P29 Impact of Respiratory Virtual Clinics in Primary Care on Responsible Respiratory Prescribing and Inhaled Corticosteroid Withdrawal on Patients with COPD: a Feasibility Study. *Thorax*, 69:A90.

Dalal AA et al. (2011). Costs of COPD exacerbations in the emergency department and inpatient setting. *Respir Med*, 105:454–60.

Davey C et al. (2015). Bronchoscopic lung volume reduction with endobronchial valves for patients with heterogeneous emphysema and intact interlobar fissures (the BeLieVeR-HIFi study): a randomised controlled trial. *Lancet*, 386:1066–73.

Echevarria C et al. (2016). Early Supported Discharge/Hospital at Home for Acute Exacerbation of Chronic Obstructive Pulmonary Disease: a Review and Meta-Analysis. *COPD*, 13:523–33.

Effing T et al. (2007). Self-management education for patients with chronic obstructive pulmonary disease. *Cochrane Database Syst Rev*, 4:CD002990.

European Lung Foundation (2013). *Lung Health in Europe. Facts and Figures.* United Kingdom, European Lung Foundation.

Flottorp SA et al. (2010). *Using audit and feedback to health professionals to improve the quality and safety of health care*, Copenhagen, WHO Regional Office for Europe.

Foster TS et al. (2006). Assessment of the economic burden of COPD in the U.S.: a review and synthesis of the literature. *COPD*, 3:211–18.

Garner J et al. (2016). Survival after Endobronchial Valve Placement for Emphysema: A 10-Year Follow-up Study. *Am J Respir Crit Care Med*, 194:519–21.

Geitona M et al. (2011). The cost of COPD exacerbations: a university hospital-based study in Greece. *Respir Med*, 105:402–9.

Gibson GJ et al. (2013). Respiratory health and disease in Europe: the new European Lung White Book. *Eur Respir J*, 42:559–63.

Global Health Observatory (2008). *Causes of death in 2008* (Online). World Health Organization. Available at: http://www.who.int/gho/mortality_burden_disease/causes_death_2008/en/ (accessed 9 December 2016).

GOLD (2017). Global Strategy for the Diagnosis, Management and Prevention of COPD, Global Initiative for Chronic Obstructive Lung Disease. Available at: http://goldcopd.org (accessed 2 February 2020).

Gomes B et al. (2013). Effectiveness and cost-effectiveness of home palliative care services for adults with advanced illness and their caregivers. *Cochrane Database Syst Rev*, 6:CD007760.

Hartl S et al. (2016). Risk of death and readmission of hospital-admitted COPD exacerbations: European COPD Audit. *Eur Respir J*, 47:113–21.

Herath SC, Poole P (2013). Prophylactic antibiotic therapy for chronic obstructive pulmonary disease (COPD). *Cochrane Database Syst Rev*, 11:CD009764.

Hernandez C, Mallow J, Narsavage GL (2014). Delivering telemedicine interventions in chronic respiratory disease. *Breathe (Sheff)*, 10:198–212.

Hernandez C et al. (2015). Integrated care services: lessons learned from the deployment of the NEXES project. *Int J Integr Care*, 15:e006.

Herse F, Kiljander T, Lehtimaki L (2015). Annual costs of chronic obstructive pulmonary disease in Finland during 1996–2006 and a prediction model for 2007–2030. *NPJ Prim Care Respir Med*, 25:15015.

Herth FJ et al. (2016). Endoscopic Lung Volume Reduction: An Expert Panel Recommendation. *Respiration*, 91:241–50.

Hoogendoorn M et al. (2010). Long-term effectiveness and cost-effectiveness of smoking cessation interventions in patients with COPD. *Thorax*, 65:711–18.

Hopkinson NS, Polkey MI (2010). Does physical inactivity cause chronic obstructive pulmonary disease? *Clin Sci (Lond)*, 118:565–72.

Hopkinson NS et al. (2011). Atelectasis and survival after bronchoscopic lung volume reduction for COPD. *Eur Respir J*, 37:1346–51.

Hopkinson NS et al. (2012). Designing and implementing a COPD discharge care bundle. *Thorax*, 67:90–2.

Hosker H et al. (2007). Variability in the organisation and management of hospital care for COPD exacerbations in the UK. *Respir Med*, 101(4):754–61. Epub 11 Oct 2006.

Huber MB et al. (2015). Excess costs of comorbidities in chronic obstructive pulmonary disease: a systematic review. *PLoS One*, 10:e0123292.

Institute for Health Metrics and Evaluation (2014). Web site. Available at: http://www.healthdata.org/ (accessed 20 February 2020).

Jacobsen R et al. (2014). The effect of rehabilitation on health-care utilisation in COPD patients in Copenhagen. *Clin Respir J*, 8(3):321–9. doi: 10.1111/crj.12074. Epub 23 Dec 2013.

Jemal A et al. (2005). Trends in the leading causes of death in the United States, 1970–2002. *JAMA*, 294:1255–9.

Khakban A et al. (2015). Ten-Year Trends in Direct Costs of COPD: A Population-Based Study. *Chest*, 148:640–6.

Klooster K et al. (2015). Endobronchial Valves for Emphysema without Interlobar Collateral Ventilation. *N Engl J Med*, 373:2325–35.

Kohnlein T et al. (2014). Non-invasive positive pressure ventilation for the treatment of severe stable chronic obstructive pulmonary disease: a prospective, multicentre, randomised, controlled clinical trial. *Lancet Respir Med*, 2:698–705.

Kruis AL et al. (2013). Integrated disease management interventions for patients with chronic obstructive pulmonary disease. *Cochrane Database Syst Rev*, 10:CD009437.

Laforest L et al. (2016). Frequency of comorbidities in chronic obstructive pulmonary disease, and impact on all-cause mortality: a population-based cohort study. *Respir Med*, 117:33–9.

Lamprecht B et al. (2015). Determinants of underdiagnosis of COPD in national and international surveys. *Chest*, 148:971–85.

Lane CR, Tonelli AR (2015). Lung transplantation in chronic obstructive pulmonary disease: patient selection and special considerations. *Int J Chron Obstruct Pulmon Dis*, 10:2137–46.

Laverty AA et al. (2015). Impact of a COPD discharge care bundle on readmissions following admission with acute exacerbation: interrupted time series analysis. *PLoS One*, 10(2):e0116187. doi: 10.1371/journal.pone.0116187.

Librero J et al. (2016). Trends and area variations in Potentially Preventable Admissions for COPD in Spain (2002–2013): a significant decline and convergence between areas. *BMC Health Serv Res*, 16:367.

Llordes M et al. (2015). Prevalence, Risk Factors and Diagnostic Accuracy of COPD Among Smokers in Primary Care. *COPD*, 12:404–12.

López-Campos JL et al. (2014). Variability of hospital resources for acute care of COPD patients: the European COPD Audit. *Eur Respir J*, 43(3):754–62. doi: 10.1183/09031936.00074413.

López-Campos JL et al. (2015). Antibiotic Prescription for COPD Exacerbations Admitted to Hospital: European COPD Audit. *PLoS One*, 10(4):e0124374. doi: 10.1371/journal.pone.0124374.

López-Campos Bodineau JL et al. (2002). [Analysis of admissions for chronic obstructive pulmonary disease in Andalusia in 2000]. *Arch Bronconeumol*, 38:473–8.

Lozano R et al. (2012). Global and regional mortality from 235 causes of death for 20 age groups in 1990 and 2010: a systematic analysis for the Global Burden of Disease Study 2010. *Lancet*, 380:2095–128.

Luckett T et al. (2016). Content and quality of websites supporting self-management of chronic breathlessness in advanced illness: a systematic review. *NPJ Prim Care Respir Med*, 26:16025.

Lundell S et al. (2015). Telehealthcare in COPD: a systematic review and meta-analysis on physical outcomes and dyspnea. *Respir Med*, 109:11–26.

McCarthy B et al. (2015). Pulmonary rehabilitation for chronic obstructive pulmonary disease. *Cochrane Database Syst Rev*, 2:CD003793.

McGarvey LP et al. (2007). Ascertainment of cause-specific mortality in COPD: operations of the TORCH Clinical Endpoint Committee. *Thorax*, 62:411–15.

McKinstry, B, Pinnock H, Sheikh A (2009). Telemedicine for management of patients with COPD? *Lancet,* 374:672–3.

McLean S et al. (2011). Telehealthcare for chronic obstructive pulmonary disease. *Cochrane Database Syst Rev,* 7:CD007718.

Mannino DM et al. (2015). Economic Burden of COPD in the Presence of Comorbidities. *Chest,* 148:138–50.

Mathers CD, Loncar D (2006). Projections of global mortality and burden of disease from 2002 to 2030. *PLoS Med,* 3:e442.

Naunheim KS et al. (2006). Long-term follow-up of patients receiving lung-volume-reduction surgery versus medical therapy for severe emphysema by the National Emphysema Treatment Trial Research Group. *Ann Thorac Surg,* 82:431–43.

Needleman J et al. (2011). Nurse staffing and inpatient hospital mortality. *N Engl J Med,* 364:1037–45.

Nolte E, Knai C, Saltman RB (2015). *Assessing chronic disease management in European health systems: concepts and approaches.* Copenhagen, WHO Regional Office for Europe on behalf of the European Observatory for Health Systems and Policies

Patel JG, Nagar SP, Dalal AA (2014). Indirect costs in chronic obstructive pulmonary disease: a review of the economic burden on employers and individuals in the United States. *Int J Chron Obstruct Pulmon Dis,* 9:289–300.

Pelkonen MK et al. (2014). Twenty-five year trends in prevalence of chronic bronchitis and the trends in relation to smoking. *Respir Med,* 108:1633–40.

Pertl D et al. (2014). Effectiveness and efficacy of minimally invasive lung volume reduction surgery for emphysema. *GMS Health Technol Assess,* 10:Doc01.

Pietzsch JB, Garner A, Herth FJ (2014). Cost-effectiveness of endobronchial valve therapy for severe emphysema: a model-based projection based on the VENT study. *Respiration,* 88:389–98.

Pinto A et al. (2010). Home telemonitoring of non-invasive ventilation decreases healthcare utilisation in a prospective controlled trial of patients with amyotrophic lateral sclerosis. *J Neurol Neurosurg Psychiatry,* 81(11):1238–42. doi: 10.1136/jnnp.2010.206680.

Price LC et al. (2006). UK National COPD Audit 2003: impact of hospital resources and organisation of care on patient outcome following admission for acute COPD exacerbation. *Thorax,* 61:837–42.

Puhan MA et al. (2011). Pulmonary rehabilitation following exacerbations of chronic obstructive pulmonary disease. *Cochrane Database Syst Rev,* 10:CD005305. doi: 10.1002/14651858.CD005305.pub3.

Puhan MA et al. (2016). Pulmonary rehabilitation following exacerbations of chronic obstructive pulmonary disease. *Cochrane Database Syst Rev,* 12:CD005305. doi: 10.1002/14651858.CD005305.pub4.

Ram FS et al. (2004a). Hospital at home for patients with acute exacerbations of chronic obstructive pulmonary disease: systematic review of evidence. *BMJ,* 329:315.

Ram FS et al. (2004b). Non-invasive positive pressure ventilation for treatment of respiratory failure due to exacerbations of chronic obstructive pulmonary disease. *Cochrane Database Syst Rev,* 1:CD004104.

Ramsey SD et al. (2007). Updated evaluation of the cost-effectiveness of lung volume reduction surgery. *Chest,* 131:823–32.

Ribera Salud (2016). *Ribera Salud's contribution to the public healthcare system in Spain.* Valencia, Ribera Salud Grupo.

Roberts CM et al. (2013). European hospital adherence to GOLD recommendations for chronic obstructive pulmonary disease (COPD) exacerbation admissions. *Thorax,* 68:1169–71.

Rochester CL, Spanevello A (2014). Heterogeneity of pulmonary rehabilitation: like apples and oranges – both healthy fruit. *Eur Respir J,* 43:1223–6.

Ruparel M et al. (2016). Understanding variation in length of hospital stay for COPD exacerbation: European COPD audit. *Eur Respir J Open Res,* 2(1):pii:00034–2015.

Schauer GL et al. (2014). Smoking prevalence and cessation characteristics among U.S. adults with and without COPD: findings from the 2011 Behavioral Risk Factor Surveillance System. *COPD,* 11:697–704.

Simoens S (2013). Cost-effectiveness of pharmacotherapy for COPD in ambulatory care: a review. *J Eval Clin Pract,* 19:1004–11.

Simon-Tuval T et al. (2011). Determinants of elevated healthcare utilization in patients with COPD. *Respir Res,* 12:7.

Smidth M et al. (2013). The effect of an active implementation of a disease management programme for chronic obstructive pulmonary disease on healthcare utilization – a cluster-randomised controlled trial. *BMC Health Serv Res,* 13:385.

Smith KR, Mehta S, Maeusezehal-Fauz M (2004). Indoor air pollution from household solid mass fuel use. In: M Ezzati et al. (eds.) *Comparative quantification of health risks: global and regional health burden of disease attributable to selected major risk factors.* Geneva, World Health Organization.

Soriano JB et al. (2010). Recent trends in COPD prevalence in Spain: a repeated cross-sectional survey 1997–2007. *Eur Respir J,* 36:758–65.

Spencer S et al. (2011). Inhaled corticosteroids versus long-acting beta(2)-agonists for chronic obstructive pulmonary disease. *Cochrane Database Syst Rev*, 10:CD007033.

Spruit MA et al. (2013). An official American Thoracic Society/European Respiratory Society statement: key concepts and advances in pulmonary rehabilitation. *Am J Respir Crit Care Med*, 188:e13–64.

Spruit MA et al. (2014). Differences in content and organisational aspects of pulmonary rehabilitation programmes. *Eur Respir J*, 43:1326–37.

Stead LF et al. (2013). Physician advice for smoking cessation. *Cochrane Database Syst Rev*, 2:CD000165.

Steuten LM et al. (2009). Identifying potentially cost effective chronic care programs for people with COPD. *Int J Chron Obstruct Pulmon Dis*, 4:87–100.

Stoller JK et al. (2010). Oxygen therapy for patients with COPD: current evidence and the long-term oxygen treatment trial. *Chest*, 138:179–87.

Stone RA et al. (2015). *COPD: Who cares matters*. London, Royal College of Physicians.

Struik FM et al. (2014). Nocturnal noninvasive positive pressure ventilation in stable COPD: a systematic review and individual patient data meta-analysis. *Respir Med*, 108:329–37.

Suh ES, Mandal S, Hart N (2013). Admission prevention in COPD: non-pharmacological management. *BMC Med*, 11:247.

Tashkin DP (2015). Smoking Cessation in Chronic Obstructive Pulmonary Disease. *Semin Respir Crit Care Med*, 36:491–507.

Turner C (2015). Mobile working: positively engaging community nurses. *Br J Community Nurs*, 20: 134–8.

Vestbo J, Lange P (2015). Prevention of COPD exacerbations: medications and other controversies. *ERJ Open Res*, 1.

Vestbo J et al. (2013). Global strategy for the diagnosis, management, and prevention of chronic obstructive pulmonary disease: GOLD executive summary. *Am J Respir Crit Care Med*, 187:347–65.

Vos T et al. (2012). Years lived with disability (YLDs) for 1160 sequelae of 289 diseases and injuries 1990–2010: a systematic analysis for the Global Burden of Disease Study 2010. *Lancet*, 380:2163–96.

Walters JA et al. (2010). Action plans with limited patient education only for exacerbations of chronic obstructive pulmonary disease. *Cochrane Database Syst Rev*, 5:CD005074.

Wong CX, Carson KV, Smith BJ (2012). Home care by outreach nursing for chronic obstructive pulmonary disease. *Cochrane Database Syst Rev*, 3:CD000994.

Wouters EF (2003). Economic analysis of the Confronting COPD survey: an overview of results. *Respir Med,* 97 suppl C, S3–14.

Zielinski J et al. (1997). Causes of death in patients with COPD and chronic respiratory failure. *Monaldi Arch Chest Dis,* 52:43–7.

Zwerink, M et al. (2014). Self management for patients with chronic obstructive pulmonary disease. *Cochrane Database Syst Rev,* 3:CD002990.

7 | *Emergency medicine*

MATTHEW COOKE, CLIFFORD MANN, NIGEL
EDWARDS

Introduction

Emergency medicine specializes in acute illness and injury (Edwards, 1996; Tang et al., 2010). It has developed from the realization that these conditions can occur at any time and that dealing with many of these events within more traditional medical specialties led to suboptimal care. Recently the increasing relevance of time-critical interventions such as those associated with complex trauma care, stroke thrombolysis and sepsis therapies have further underlined the importance of a clinically broad but temporally focused specialty. The provision of emergency care is therefore a key function of most major hospitals.

Irrespective of most other health system features, patients with acute severe illness or injury present to or are taken to an emergency department (ED). In the United Kingdom these departments have been officially termed accident and emergency (A&E) departments since the Platt report of 1961 (Anon, 1961). However, accidents and associated injuries have diminished in frequency across western Europe, with a particularly large reduction in injuries associated with road traffic accidents, interpersonal violence and occupational activities (Eurostat, 2017). Consequently, the mix of patients presenting to the ED or A&E has changed significantly over the last 50 years. Case volumes have, however, continued to rise in excess of population growth, especially since 2000; the reasons for this vary but most countries have seen an increased demand for the treatment of acute exacerbations of chronic disease and conditions associated with frailty and ageing (see Chapter 4). Ageing and population growth do not fully explain this growth in demand.

It is increasingly recognized that the presentation of illness is not related solely to aetiology or pathology and it is apparent that we are witnessing a changing utilization of emergency medical systems by patients of all age cohorts.

This chapter looks at the branch of medicine responsible for the initial treatment of many of these emergencies and the emergency departments within the acute general hospitals in which they are usually based.

The development of contemporary emergency medicine

Emergency medicine is a relatively new specialty. First formally recognized in the United Kingdom and the USA in the mid-1960s, it has undergone major changes in many countries since then (Totten & Bellou, 2013). Often starting as a service that provided triage and emergency treatment for victims of injury, modern emergency medicine covers the early management and investigation of a broad range of conditions in addition to trauma, from infectious diseases to psychiatric illness (Box 7.1). Most recently the specialty has evolved in response to pressures to specialize and standardize with demonstrable improvement in outcomes. For conditions such as sepsis, major trauma and stroke it has become increasingly clear that early expert intervention makes a significant difference (Cameron, 2014).

Box 7.1 Defining emergency medicine

Emergency medicine has been defined as "a field of practice based on the knowledge and skills required for the prevention, diagnosis and management of acute and urgent aspects of illness and injury affecting patients of all age groups with a full spectrum of episodic undifferentiated physical and behavioural disorders; it further encompasses an understanding of the development of pre-hospital and in-hospital emergency medical systems and the skills necessary for this development" (International Federation for Emergency Medicine, 2018).

"It is a specialty in which time is critical. The practice of Emergency Medicine encompasses the pre-hospital and in-hospital triage, resuscitation, initial assessment and management of undifferentiated urgent and emergency cases until discharge or transfer to the care of another physician or health care professional." (European Society for Emergency Medicine, 2007)

In some countries it became common for patients admitted as acute emergencies to be dealt with in a single specialist emergency department rather than in different wards, clinics and departments within the hospital. This provided a rationale for the development of a separate specialty. There were also historic factors, including the development of major trauma care first developed in North America, in part in response to experience gained in the Vietnam War, spreading first to the British Isles in the 1980s and adopted more widely in Europe after 1994.

The provision of emergency medical care varies widely between and, at times, within countries. Internationally, two principal models have evolved, the continental European model (sometimes referred to as the "Franco-German" model) and the Anglo-Australasian-American model (Cone et al., 2015). In continental Europe emergency care tends to focus on the critical care end of the spectrum and the management and investigation of emergencies requiring hospital care is undertaken by inpatient specialties. In this model the most seriously injured and ill are typically attended to by anaesthetist-led teams at the scene and often receive extensive treatment before transfer to the operating theatre, intensive treatment unit, or medical or surgical ward. In the Anglo-Australasian-American model treatment at the scene is usually more limited and predominantly paramedic led; the emphasis is on rapid transport to an appropriate hospital where emergency department clinicians are responsible for the investigation and management of the patients and the consequent decision to discharge or admit them.

Proponents of the European model assert that better outcomes are achieved when organ-specific specialists lead the investigation and treatment of patients. The Anglo-Australasian-American model contends that most patients do not arrive with an organ or even a specialty-based diagnosis but have multiple and often interacting conditions. However, the models have in general arisen not as a reflection of deliberate policy choices based on these views but because of circumstance, resource availability and history.

There are no high quality comparative studies of different systems. Moreover, most countries operate some components of each model. Thus, trauma care has evolved to reinforce pre-hospital interventions and direct transfer to major trauma units and centres, whereas patients who meet criteria to consider sepsis are often insufficiently "labelled" to allow triage to particular hospitals or even inpatient teams.

The emergency medicine care pathway

Ideally the emergency care system should commence at the first point of contact between the patient and a clinician or emergency call system. Current systems, though far from mature, aim to coordinate services to provide the most appropriate response to the medical needs of the patient. Where this is achieved, such a system should reduce the inappropriate use of hospitals, ensure that patients who require urgent care receive it promptly, and make best use of limited resources.

Entering the emergency department

In most countries significant numbers of patients self-present to the emergency department. The remainder attend following advice or referral from a general practitioner (GP) or other clinician, by way of a telephone triage service, or following an attendance and subsequent conveyance by an ambulance. In Denmark and Norway patients are required to have sought advice from the GP or ambulance service prior to coming to the emergency department. In the Netherlands this approach is strongly encouraged by the use of insurance deductibles and by providing very accessible general practice services.

Most countries now have a telephone service dedicated to providing urgent health care advice and signposting. The United Kingdom uses lay advisers assisted by computer algorithms; these do not attempt to provide a diagnosis but instead lead to a recommended course of action (disposition). The limitations of this approach and the consequent over-triage to both GP and emergency department care has led to a recent commitment to increase the proportion of calls handled by a clinician, as happens routinely in the systems operated in Sweden and Denmark. All these systems aim to ensure that patients are directed to the right point of care without unreasonable delay or duplication of effort, although the extent to which they achieve this can be unclear (see below).

The Franco-German model has traditionally put doctors in ambulances or cars as a key part of the immediate response. There are some signs of convergence between the United Kingdom model and Franco-German models of pre-hospital care, with initiatives to "front-load" more highly trained clinicians (doctors, paramedics and advanced nurse practitioners), either as staff on an ambulance or dispatched by car from a hospital. The evidence from the United Kingdom for better patient outcomes from pre-hospital deployment of doctors is very limited. The use of medically staffed helicopters for this role has grown significantly but there are major concerns about their cost-effectiveness (Bledsoe et al., 2006; Butler, Anwar & Willett, 2010; Delgado et al., 2013).

The ambition of all systems is to bring triage and immediate treatment to the earliest safe and effective point in the pathway. In consequence it is expected that the development of ambulances staffed with personnel and equipment that allow greater assessment and evaluation skills will enable these same services to either treat and discharge more patients at the scene or convey them to non-hospital providers of health care.

Paramedics can also transport patients to specialist units directly, bypassing non-specialist hospitals and in some cases the emergency department. Hyperacute stroke centres (Ramsay et al., 2015), trauma units and specialist ST elevation myocardial infarction units have evolved across Europe over the last 10 years. Accessing these facilities without intermediate delays has seen an improvement in outcomes that has more than offset the consequential increased journey time, although in many countries only limited progress has been made in achieving change in structures and processes (Albrecht et al., 2017).

These "condition-specific" diversion protocols require either autonomous paramedic practice or make use of telephone/online support from a specialist clinician based at the hospital. In the United Kingdom enhanced paramedic training and autonomy has enabled up to 40% of emergency ambulance calls to be managed without transport to an emergency department (National Audit Office, 2017).

In a number of countries (including the Netherlands, Spain, England, and Norway) primary care centres staffed by GPs or nurses can offer a range of treatment for minor injuries and minor ailments.

Minor injury units were associated with many community hospitals in the United Kingdom even before the creation of the National Health Service (NHS). These units have been variously staffed by GPs and nurse practitioners. The effectiveness and utility of such units, especially in more rural settings, has become increasingly recognized.

In urban areas of the United Kingdom the recognition that at least 20% of patients attending an emergency department can be better dealt with by primary care staff has incentivized the development of co-located primary/urgent care services. Such facilities can decongest the emergency department. These are also an increasing feature of the Dutch system.

The hospital emergency department

The emergency department provides care in the first phase of almost all acute medical episodes that are of a severity sufficient to require hospital resources. Traditionally this was not the case. For most of the 20th century, the majority of acute admissions were seen and assessed by a GP/family doctor who arranged both transfer to hospital and direct admission to an appropriate ward under an inpatient specialty team. In 2017 fewer than 25% of admissions were managed in this way in the United Kingdom; 75% of acute admissions now enter the hospital via the emergency department.

By necessity, emergency departments usually offer care to all types of acute illness and injury, physical and mental health problems, and to all ages. However, the way services are organized varies considerably within and between health systems. For example, obstetric emergencies are usually seen in maternity units, while isolated mental health problems may be seen in a geographically separate mental health facility. Paediatric attendances represent one in four emergency department visits (Tang et al., 2010) and although few in number in the United Kingdom, specialist paediatric emergency departments are common in other parts of Europe, especially in France.

Triage is widely used in emergency departments to prioritize cases so that those with time-critical conditions and greatest symptom severity are treated first. Although formal systems have been evaluated and shown to be reliable they do have significant over and under triage consequences with both resource and risk implications (Parenti et al., 2014).

Ideally triage would not be required because patients could be treated immediately. "See and treat" approaches (Parker, 2004) aim to use triage resources to treat patients rather than risk managing the queue. Such approaches may be difficult to maintain during periods of peak demand.

Senior physician involvement in the initial assessment of all attenders has benefits for ED performance (Abdulwahid et al., 2016) and quality of care (Oredsson et al., 2011). This, however, creates a paradox in resource-constrained services with the least ill or injured being assessed by the most senior clinician.

There is only limited published evidence that streaming of patients into different tracks, performing laboratory analysis in the emergency department, or shifting responsibility for ordering certain radiological investigations to nurses results in shorter waiting time and length of stay (Oredsson et al., 2011), although this is likely to reflect the absence of rigorous research rather than the lack of any effect, as their advantages are intuitive.

The performance of some of these models may also depend on local circumstances – for example, streaming of primary care type patients may be of limited value where most patients see a GP prior to attending, but may be very useful in circumstances where access to local primary care is poor. Data from the United Kingdom indicate that there is considerable variation in the proportion of patients whose needs can be better addressed by primary care clinicians (15% to 40%) (Moulton, Mann & Tempest, 2014). This is an area in which further research and evaluation is required.

Resuscitation is a core component of all emergency medicine systems. In most cases resuscitation of the most seriously ill and injured will be led by an emergency medicine team. They will usually be supported by other specialties – in particular, anaesthesia, intensive care, surgery, and orthopaedics. In some European systems the intensive care team is responsible for resuscitation. Nevertheless, irrespective of the lead clinicians the process of care of seriously ill and injured patients is becoming more standardized with evidence-based guidelines for the management of cardiac arrest, major trauma, paediatric resuscitation and other severe illness such as septic shock.

Improvements in road safety measures, falling levels of interpersonal violence, improving workplace safety, and reductions in suicide (European Association for Injury Prevention and Safety Promotion (EuroSafe), 2013) mean that while major trauma is an important component of emergency medicine, its share of the work of the emergency department is decreasing. In the United Kingdom major trauma accounts for less than 1% of emergency department attendances. It was therefore apparent by the 1990s that it was neither appropriate nor feasible for every emergency department/acute hospital to maintain and deliver high quality trauma care. In consequence trauma services were reorganized into a tiered response with a network of trauma units acting as spokes to the major trauma centre hubs with a demonstrable improvement in outcomes (Celso et al., 2006). In 2013 results from the Trauma Audit and Research Network (TARN) national audit show that one in five patients who would have died before the networks are now surviving severe injuries (McCullough et al., 2014).

The formal designation of trauma centres in Europe has been a slower process than in the USA, which may reflect a lower incidence of severe trauma – in particular the much lower incidence of penetrating trauma associated with gun and knife crime. There are also significant historical, logistical and political difficulties in ensuring that the wide range of specialist services required for an integrated trauma centre are located on the same site. An issue in eastern Europe and the countries of the former Soviet Union is the siting of specialist institutes on different sites that would need to be relocated to create an integrated trauma service.

A significant proportion of patients attending an emergency department will require hospital admission. In the United Kingdom this varies from 15% to 35% depending on case-mix. The proportion is higher in the Netherlands and higher again in Norway. Of those not requiring admission a proportion will require a short period of observation, further investigation or time to establish the efficacy of initial treatment. Historically such patients were admitted to a co-located observation ward. Such units continue to provide appropriate care for many patients attending emergency departments, including those recovering from procedures requiring sedation or anaesthesia, or awaiting specialist interpretation of radiological investigations, such as computerized tomographic pulmonary angiograms. Other patient groups that benefit from such a facility include elderly patients who have fallen and are being assessed by therapists and frailty teams (see Chapter 4).

In many countries people with mental health problems requiring an emergency response are taken directly to mental health units. Patients who have self-harmed and need medical treatment for poisoning or injuries may need to attend the emergency department for assessment and treatment of their physical injury or toxicological emergency. For this reason many health systems have established specialized mental health teams based in the emergency departments.

In the United Kingdom recent systems of "street triage" for mental illness have shown a reduction in ED attendances and the number of compulsory detentions (Dyer, Steer & Biddle, 2015). This system combines police, ambulance and a mental health clinician in a single response vehicle. These initiatives have been shown to lead to improvements in the quality of care of mental health patients, reduced delays and have delivered significant resource savings (Tadros et al., 2018).

Emergency departments have an increasing role in secondary prevention. This may be at an individual patient level, e.g. detection and intervention for high risk alcohol intake, or at system level, e.g. injury surveillance to detect trauma hotspots or emerging causes of trauma.

Admission and post-acute care

In some countries, such as the United Kingdom and the Netherlands, many patients who require further investigation and care are moved to acute medical or surgical assessment units. These units may be run either by internal general medicine specialists or by the emerging specialty of acute medicine. These units have a very active approach to treatment with the aim of further front-loading senior review to optimize care and reduce length of stay.

Patient flow is a major issue for many emergency departments. In particular, inability to move patients who require admission into the right hospital bed or promptly arrange a safe discharge home can substantially delay care and impede efficiency. When patients require admission it is highly desirable that they are admitted to a bed managed by the specialty appropriate to their condition. It is clear that admission to a bed that is available but inappropriate is associated with higher mortality (George & Wilkinson, 2016) and increased lengths of stay.

There are also problems in the emergency department if admission is delayed because of lack of bed capacity; staff become stretched as they have to assess and care for new patients as well as those awaiting admission. There is evidence from Canada, Australia and the United Kingdom that high levels of emergency department crowding are associated with treatment delays (Gaieski et al., 2017) and increased mortality (Sun et al., 2013; Filippatos & Karasi, 2015).

Recognition of the iatrogenic harm caused by delays has encouraged greater scrutiny of patient flows and attendant obstacles to prevent or minimize such risks. While there are many internal hospital processes that can facilitate patient flow, effective discharge is particularly important. Shortages of nursing homes, intermediate care, home care and other support have a significant impact on the effectiveness of the emergency care system.

Discharged patients may be referred for follow-up by other specialties, such as follow-up of patients with fractures by the orthopaedic service. Others will be referred back to their GP and many will be discharged with no requirement for further follow-up. It is increasingly recognized that the ability to discharge a patient with a referral to a specialist clinic within 48 hours is both expedient and usually preferable to admission for many patients.

Workforce

The model and levels of staffing of emergency departments vary considerably depending on a combination of history, primary care provision, and the availability of emergency medicine specialists to provide dedicated staffing.

The Franco-German model has generally used junior medical staff, GPs and nurses with early senior specialist review of most cases before further investigation and treatment. By contrast the Anglo-American-Australian model has supported the development of emergency medicine specialists, with referral of about 25% of patients to specialty teams after assessment, stabilization, investigation and treatment has commenced.

The rising workload has outstripped the ability of the United Kingdom, Ireland and New Zealand to provide sufficient fully trained emergency medicine doctors to manage the service safely and within various process targets. Consequently, various strategies to make better use of other staff groups have been introduced. Such staff include advanced nurse/clinical practitioners, physician associates, paramedics and frailty practitioners. However, the changing nature of the case-mix related to an ageing demographic and the attendant problem of multimorbidity has created real problems for the Franco-German model. Patients presenting with single illness issues represent a minority of patients requiring admission; for this reason reliance upon traditional specialist inpatient teams is increasingly malaligned to patient need.

The role of the senior emergency medicine doctor varies among countries. The main determinant seems to be the number of senior doctors within a department at any one time. Many studies have shown the advantages of early senior intervention in a wide range of conditions improving outcomes and increasing admission avoidance (Purdy, 2010). Senior staff leading and supervising cases in the resuscitation room is almost universal but there are varying approaches to the deployment of senior staff within the remainder of the emergency department. The most common models of this role are:

- Delivery – where the senior staff see and treat patients throughout their care.
- Instigation – where the senior clinician undertakes a rapid assessment and defines a plan which is then implemented by junior staff.
- Attending – where junior staff see the patients initially and then check with senior staff before referral or discharge.
- Consulting – where junior staff see the patient and ask for help when they perceive the need.

Emergency nurse practitioners are now well established in the United Kingdom but their acceptance in other countries is limited. They can provide a safe and effective minor injury service, although in some departments they may be more expensive than a junior doctor model as they are relatively well paid and may take longer to complete their work (Sakr et al., 2003; Wilson et al., 2009). The barriers to implementation are related to emergency department culture, physician reimbursement systems and case-mix. In the United Kingdom advanced clinical practitioner programmes have been established to develop nurses, paramedics and pharmacists to become autonomous practitioners seeing a wide range of cases in the emergency department (Swann et al., 2013). Other somewhat niche roles have also been developed, such as emergency department practitioners (with a background as anaesthetic assistants/ operating department practitioners) who can undertake investigations and invasive procedures in the resuscitation room.

The use of geriatricians in the emergency department has been shown to be effective at reducing admissions and is not associated with a high readmission rate (Jones & Wallis, 2013). This may be better in a dedicated unit rather than in the main emergency department (Sophia & Bashir, 2014) and if supported by a wider MDT to facilitate assessment and discharge.

Every emergency department also needs support from imaging and pathology services, although there is an increasing use of near-patient testing (see Chapter 10). Turnaround times can be reduced but quality control may be more difficult and near-patient testing is often relatively expensive (Asha et al., 2014; Larsson, Greig-Pylypczuk & Huisman, 2015). Certain other specialties are often considered mandatory to support any emergency department that receives undifferentiated emergency cases; these include anaesthetics, intensive care, general medicine, general surgery, orthopaedic trauma, and paediatrics.

It is increasingly recognized that emergency medicine can be highly stressful (Berger, 2013) with consequent challenges for both recruitment and retention. High demand and low job control were found to be common in a systematic review but other factors included insufficient support at work, an imbalance between effort and reward, and organizational injustice (Basu, Qayyum & Mason, 2016).

Barriers to delivering optimal care

The key barriers to delivering optimal care are: rising levels of demand; inefficient use of resources; and downstream delays in the system which lead to queues and consequential overcrowding. These are compounded by problems arising from the physical design of some emergency departments and the workforce challenges discussed above.

Managing demand

It has been clearly demonstrated that difficulty in accessing primary care is related to higher emergency department attendances. Conversely, systems that have easy timely access to primary care have less emergency department usage. Similarly many emergency department attendances are preceded by unsuccessful attempts to obtain a primary care appointment. In some studies interventions to improve primary care access have resulted in reduced emergency department attendances (Whittaker et al., 2016), although extending the hours primary care is available has a limited effect and may not be cost-effective. For those systems where the emergency department receives substantial numbers of primary presentations the provision of co-located primary care facilities has been effective in decongesting the emergency department itself. In England alternative sites, such as urgent treatment centres, have been developed so people can be assessed and treated in a lower acuity setting than an emergency department.

Telephone advice lines that aim to direct the user to the most appropriate location in an appropriate timescale do not seem to reduce the workload to emergency departments and there is some evidence they increase overall demand (Turner et al., 2013; Collins, 2015). This may be improved by involving doctors and other clinicians in the call decision-making (Anderson & Roland, 2015).

Good chronic disease management may be able to reduce the number of acute episodes if better control of the patient's condition can result in fewer episodes of acute need, even if the general trajectory is one of deterioration, although this is rarely easy. Equally important is the early detection of, and intervention for, deterioration. A key part of this is patient education and a good understanding of their disease, together with an agreed plan ranging from self-care (e.g. home-held antibiotics for COPD), to seeking urgent advice before deteriorating further. Support for nursing and residential homes can also avoid attendances at the emergency department, by ensuring optimal ongoing care, good end of life planning, and the use of telehealth advice before calling an ambulance (Nick et al., 2015).

There is no evidence to support the idea that public information campaigns can reduce attendance at emergency departments. For most people it is a rare event for a different condition each time, and the appropriateness of attendance depends not only on medical considerations but also factors such as availability of alternatives and social support. Some disease-specific education campaigns have increased the early recognition of acute episodes but invariably have a high cost of false positives with consequent increase in emergency department attendances. Diverting people away is unlikely to be effective as most people believe the emergency department is the correct location for their care (Atenstaedt et al., 2015) and there are some significant risks.

Although often advocated as a means to reduce demand, there is no evidence that co-payment schemes reduce inappropriate attendances (Reed et al., 2005; Selby, Fireman & Swain, 1996; Siddiqui, Roberts & Pollack, 2015) and they bring many other problems, often costing more to operate than they raise, while deterring necessary care. In Ireland attendances at emergency departments have increased significantly despite a co-payment system designed to encourage primary care use.

Finally social changes are also impacting on emergency departments. In the United Kingdom the "liberalization" of the alcohol licensing laws in 2005 has produced a wholly predictable increase in alcohol-related presentations. The public, media and politicians increasingly expect care seven days a week and 24 hours per day; this in turn has produced a disproportionate increase in demand during "anti-social" hours with major consequences for staffing.

Queues and overcrowding

Demand for emergency care is subject to high levels of variability – both seasonal and at different times of day and days of the week. Although there is some predictability to this, average hourly attendances are subject to wide variation (greater than 50%) (Blunt, 2014). Consequently, systems need to be able to deal with surges in demand and hence there needs to be some redundancy built into staffing and the physical environment. The situation is made worse by the fact that activity in planned care is often even more variable. These variations in demand, both predictable and random, combined with capacity constraints associated with historically high bed occupancy rates, ensure that emergency departments are prone to significant overcrowding during peak periods. This phenomenon is endemic to health systems in many countries, including Ireland, the Netherlands, South Africa, the United Kingdom and the USA – indeed, it is the one almost invariable feature of all current health care systems! Avoiding overcrowding requires better alignment of resources to demands. Within the emergency department this means speedy responses for requests for specialist consultation, access to diagnostics, enhanced bed availability, and prompt discharge when hospital care has been completed.

Within the wider hospital, delays in decision-making, investigation, discharge planning and discharge will mean that beds are not available to admit patients. This can lead to extensive overcrowding. Emergency departments are seldom staffed or designed to deal with a large group of patients awaiting admission. As a result standards of care deteriorate, key interventions are delayed or omitted, and both morbidity and mortality rise (Forster et al., 2003; Guttmann et al., 2011; Boden et al., 2016).

Effective design

The design of emergency departments needs to support effective and efficient function and many national guidelines exist (Department of Health and Social Care, 2013). Good design can also improve user experience and reduce aggression (Design Council, 2011). But because buildings persist longer than any models of care, it is important to include flexibility in design to allow for increases in attendances but also to support new and future models of care. This design also needs to address the specific requirements of a range of groups including children, the elderly, those with cognitive impairment, those with mental health problems, and those with infectious diseases.

The future

Prevention measures have had sustained and large effects. Road safety initiatives – including safety belts, crash helmets, speed control, car design, and alcohol limits – have all contributed to the reduction in deaths and injury from vehicle incidents, especially in developed countries. Other health and safety interventions, especially in building design and the workplace, have also reduced the trauma demand in many emergency departments. Trauma is therefore a decreasing component of the workload in many emergency departments and its nature is also changing with the growth of an older population increasing the importance of injuries from falls (Kehoe et al., 2015; Sivarajasingam et al., 2016).

The increase in population size, the current and projected disproportionate increases in the numbers of patients in the ninth decade of life and the consequent importance of managing frailty, co-morbidities, and cognitive impairment are pressing challenges.

Specialization of health care and the growth of new technologies over the past 40 years have delivered extraordinary improvements in patient care and outcomes but this trend now means that seldom can a single inpatient specialist or team deal with the majority of medical or surgical emergencies. Consequently there is a need for more precise diagnosis by the emergency medicine clinician before referral. This has substantial resource implications both for the emergency medicine workforce and the support services of pathology and diagnostic imaging. The development of time-critical interventions similarly requires sufficient resources to deliver such treatments on a 24/7 basis. New staff roles can be developed to help support this – not just as extensions of the roles of nurses and other professionals. Where emergency medicine grows, it will be important to ensure that other specialisms withdraw from offering more general support for emergency care.

Crucially, the need to maintain minimum caseloads to sustain expertise means that often subspecialty services will be reorganized to fewer centres. In the future it is likely that common non-complex conditions will be treated in most hospitals but for less common/more complex conditions and treatments patients will need to be transferred to larger centres. Inevitably such patients will continue to present to any emergency department. Properly configured and resourced networks (akin to those established for trauma) will need to be established and supported to ensure optimal care and appropriate transfer for all patients.

Approximately 15% of all emergency hospital admissions in England involve the 1% of people in their final year of life. There is more to do to ensure that patients who are at the end of life do not spend their last hours in an emergency department through appropriate advanced planning and ensuring that ambulance and other services have information available about these plans immediately available.

Finally Denmark, the Netherlands and the United Kingdom have all seen significant reductions in the number of emergency departments, with more expected in other countries. In addition, some departments may shut to ambulance attendances overnight. The drivers for these changes include the general trend to hospital regionalization, optimal utilization of the scarce emergency medicine workforce, and the need to ensure on-site provision of many other services to support the delivery of 21st-century care that can deliver optimal outcomes.

References

Abdulwahid MA et al. (2016). The impact of senior doctor assessment at triage on emergency department performance measures: systematic review and meta-analysis of comparative studies. *Emerg Med J*, 33:504–13.

Albrecht V et al. (2017). Practice management of acute trauma haemorrhage and haemostatic disorders across German trauma centres. *Eur J Trauma Emerg Surg*, 43:201–14.

Anderson A, Roland M (2015). Potential for advice from doctors to reduce the number of patients referred to emergency departments by NHS 111 call handlers: observational study. *BMJ Open*, 5:e009444.

Anon (1961). The Platt Report. *BMJ*, 2(5263):1341–1342.

Asha SE et al. (2014). Impact from point-of-care devices on emergency department patient processing times compared with central laboratory testing of blood samples: a randomised controlled trial and cost-effectiveness analysis. *Emerg Med J*, 31:714–19.

Atenstaedt R et al. (2015). Why do patients with non-urgent conditions present to the Emergency Department despite the availability of alternative services? *Eur J Emerg Med*, 22:370–3.

Basu S, Qayyum H, Mason S (2016). Occupational stress in the ED: a systematic literature review. *Emerg Med J*, 34:441–447.

Berger E (2013). Physician Burnout. *Annals Emerg Med*, 61:A17–A19.

Bledsoe BE et al. (2006). Helicopter scene transport of trauma patients with nonlife-threatening injuries: a meta-analysis. *J Trauma*, 60:1257–65; discussion 1265–6.

Blunt I (2014). *Focus on: A&E attendances*. London, Nuffield Trust.

Boden DG et al. (2016). Lowering levels of bed occupancy is associated with decreased in-hospital mortality and improved performance on the 4-hour target in a UK District General Hospital. *Emerg Med J*, 33:85–90.

Butler DP, Anwar I, Willett K (2010). Is it the H or the EMS in HEMS that has an impact on trauma patient mortality? A systematic review of the evidence. *Emerg Med J*, 27:692–701.

Cameron PA (2014). International emergency medicine: past and future. *Emerg Med Australas*, 26:50–5.

Celso B et al. (2006). A systematic review and meta-analysis comparing outcome of severely injured patients treated in trauma centers following the establishment of trauma systems. *J Trauma*, 60:371–8; discussion 378.

Collins A (2015). View from Canberra: telephone advice no substitute for GP care. *NSW Doctor*, 7:10.

Cone D et al. (eds.) (2015). *Emergency Medical Services. Vol 2*. Chichester, John Wiley & Sons.

Delgado MK et al. (2013). Cost-Effectiveness of Helicopter Versus Ground Emergency Medical Services for Trauma Scene Transport in the United States. *Annals Emerg Med*, 62:351–364.e19.

Department of Health and Social Care (2013). *Planning and designing accident and emergency departments (HBN 15-01)* (Online). Available at: https://www.gov.uk/government/publications/hospital-accident-and-emergency-departments-planning-and-design (accessed 7 March 2018).

Design Council (2011). *Reducing violence and aggression in A&E*. London, Design Council.

Dyer W, Steer M, Biddle P (2015). Mental health street triage. *Policing: A Journal of Policy and Practice*, 9:377–87.

Edwards N (1996). The growth in emergency admissions – a challenge for health services research. *J Health Serv Res Policy*, 1:125–6.

European Association for Injury Prevention and Safety Promotion (Eurosafe) (2013). *Injuries in the European Union*. Amsterdam, Eurosafe.

European Society for Emergency Medicine (2007). *Policy statement on emergency medicine in Europe*. Brussels, EuSEM.

Eurostat (2017). *Accidents and injuries statistics* (Online). Available at: http://ec.europa.eu/eurostat/statistics-explained/index.php/Accidents_and_ injuries_statistics#Main_statistical_findings (accessed 7 March 2018).

Filippatos G, Karasi E (2015). The effect of emergency department crowding on patient outcomes. *Health Science Journal*, 9:1–6.

Forster AJ et al. (2003). The effect of hospital occupancy on emergency department length of stay and patient disposition. *Acad Emerg Med*, 10:127–33.

Gaieski DF et al. (2017). The impact of ED crowding on early interventions and mortality in patients with severe sepsis. *Am J Emerg Med*, 35:953–60.

George J, Wilkinson I (2016). Moving patients to create bed capacity. *J R Soc Med*, 109:172–3.

Guttmann A et al. (2011). Association between waiting times and short-term mortality and hospital admission after departure from emergency department: population-based cohort study from Ontario, Canada. *BMJ*, 342:d2983.

International Federation for Emergency Medicine (2018). *About us* (Online). Available at: https://www.ifem.cc/about-us/ (accessed 7 March 2018).

Jones S, Wallis P (2013). Effectiveness of a geriatrician in the emergency department in facilitating safe admission prevention of older patients. *Clin Med (Lond)*, 13:561–4.

Kehoe A et al. (2015). The changing face of major trauma in the UK. *Emerg Med J*, 32:911–15.

Larsson A, Greig-Pylypczuk R, Huisman A (2015). The state of point-of-care testing: a European perspective. *Upsala J Med Sci*, 120:1–10.

McCullough AL et al. (2014). II. Major trauma networks in England. *Br J Anaesth*, 113:202–6.

Moulton C, Mann C, Tempest M (2014). Better data, better planning: the College of Emergency Medicine sentinel sites project. *Br J Hosp Med (Lond)*, 75:627–30.

National Audit Office (2017). *NHS Ambulance Services*. London, National Audit Office.

Nick H et al. (2015). Telemedicine in care homes in Airedale, Wharfedale and Craven. *Clinical Governance: Int. J*, 20:146–54.

Oredsson S et al. (2011). A systematic review of triage-related interventions to improve patient flow in emergency departments. *Scand J Trauma Resusc Emerg Med*, 19:43.

Parenti N et al. (2014). A systematic review on the validity and reliability of an emergency department triage scale, the Manchester Triage System. *Int J Nurs Stud*, 51:1062–9.

Parker L (2004). Making see and treat work for patients and staff. *Emerg Nurse*, 11:16–17.

Purdy S (2010). *Avoiding hospital admissions: What does the research evidence say?* London, King's Fund.

Ramsay AI et al. (2015). Effects of Centralizing Acute Stroke Services on Stroke Care Provision in Two Large Metropolitan Areas in England. *Stroke*, 46:2244–51.

Reed M et al. (2005). Care-Seeking Behavior in Response to Emergency Department Copayments. *Medical Care*, 43:810–16.

Sakr M et al. (2003). Emergency nurse practitioners: a three-part study in clinical and cost effectiveness. *Emerg Med J*, 20:158–63.

Selby JV, Fireman BH, Swain BE (1996). Effect of a copayment on use of the emergency department in a health maintenance organization. *N Engl J Med*, 334:635–41.

Siddiqui M, Roberts ET, Pollack CE (2015). The effect of emergency department copayments for Medicaid beneficiaries following the Deficit Reduction Act of 2005. *JAMA Intern Med*, 175:393–8.

Sivarajasingam V et al. (2016). Trends in violence in England and Wales 2010–2014. *J Epidemiol Community Health*, 70:616–21.

Sophia R, Bashir WA (2014). A geriatrician in the emergency department. *GMJ*, 44:32–4.

Sun BC et al. (2013). Effect of Emergency Department Crowding on Outcomes of Admitted Patients. *Annals Emerg Med*, 61:605–11.e6.

Swann G et al. (2013). An autonomous role in emergency departments. *Emerg Nurse*, 21:12–15.

Tadros G et al. (2018). Impact of an integrated rapid response psychiatric liaison team on quality improvement and cost savings: the Birmingham RAID model. *Psychiatrist*, 37:4–10.

Tang N et al. (2010). Trends and characteristics of US emergency department visits, 1997–2007. *JAMA*, 304:664–70.

Totten V, Bellou A (2013). Development of emergency medicine in Europe. *Acad Emerg Med*, 20:514–21.

Turner J et al. (2013). Impact of the urgent care telephone service NHS 111 pilot sites: a controlled before and after study. *BMJ Open*, 3:e003451.

Whittaker W et al. (2016). Associations between Extending Access to Primary Care and Emergency Department Visits: A Difference-In-Differences Analysis. *PLoS Med*, 13:e1002113.

Wilson A et al. (2009). The clinical effectiveness of nurse practitioners' management of minor injuries in an adult emergency department: a systematic review. *Int J Evid Based Healthc*, 7:3–14.

8 | *Advances in perioperative medicine*

MARC WITTENBERG[1], HARRY THIRKETTLE[2], MICHAEL
GROCOTT[3]

[1] Consultant in Anaesthesia & Perioperative Medicine, Royal Free
London NHS Foundation Trust
[2] Honorary Fellow, Medtech Campus, Anglia Ruskin University
[3] Professor of Anaesthesia and Critical Care Medicine, University of
Southampton

The scope of perioperative medicine

Perioperative medicine describes the practice of patient-centred, multi-disciplinary, and integrated medical care of patients from the moment of contemplation of surgery until full recovery (Grocott & Mythen, 2015). This encompasses the three stages of surgical care: preoperative, intraoperative, and postoperative.

This definition covers a wide range of patients with many different conditions, ranging from a low-risk, young, healthy person undergoing minor surgery in an ambulatory care setting to a high-risk older person with multiple co-morbidities undergoing major and complex surgery.

Perioperative care also involves a range of settings and disciplines. For the purpose of this chapter, it is taken as encompassing the period after a person with a possible surgical condition is referred to hospital by a primary care provider or ambulatory specialist, through traditional perioperative care, most commonly undertaken within a hospital, to their discharge and full recovery, as shown in Figure 8.1.

Historically, the care provided to the surgical patient has been focused on the type of procedure being undertaken and the immediate recovery period, under the responsibility of an individual practitioner, a surgeon. It has typically been viewed in isolation from other elements of the patient's experience, with little coordination and communication either within or beyond the hospital setting. However, reflecting a number of emerging factors that will be explored in this chapter, this model of care is being transformed to one that is individualized, coordinated, and delivers high quality care centred on the needs of the patient. This

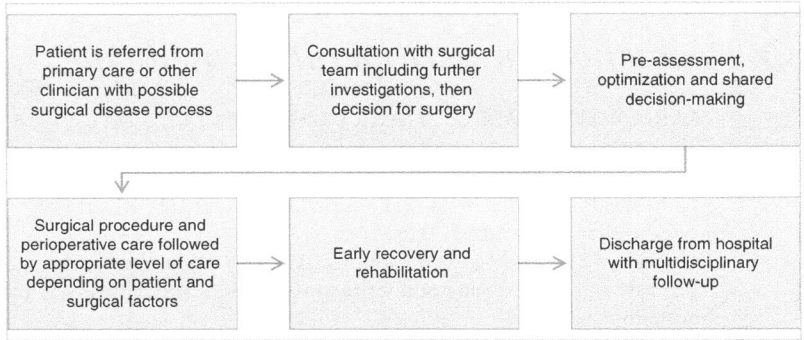

Figure 8.1 Patient pathway for elective surgery

Source: Authors' compilation

is particularly the case for high-risk patients with complex medical and social needs, undergoing major elective or emergency surgery. A major driver of the evolving model of perioperative care is the fact that patients with significant co-morbidities are increasingly being referred for surgical treatment. In the past these people would have been considered too high risk, or would have had a shorter life expectancy as a result of their medical conditions.

Over the last 10 to 20 years there has been a paradigm shift in the way that surgical patients are managed, driven by a mix of wider societal and clinical factors. During this time demand for surgery has risen considerably. According to OECD data, for example, in Denmark the rate of hip replacements was 140 per 100 000 population in 1996 but rose to 215 per 100 000 population in 2010 (OECD, 2015). A similar increase was observed in other western European countries, such as the Netherlands, but the increase was more pronounced in some of the southern European countries such as Greece, where it rose from 33.6 per 100 000 population in 1996 to 152 per 100 000 population in 2010.

During this time productivity has increased, driven in part by the increase in day-case surgery. The average length of stay (ALOS) (all causes) decreased across many European countries between 2000 and 2010. For example, the decline in the Netherlands was from 8.5 to 5.6 days, in the United Kingdom from 9.5 to 7.4 days, and in Greece from 8 to 6.6 days.

There is, however, considerable inter-country variation in length of stay. For example, the ALOS (for all types of patient) in Sweden was 15% lower than in the United Kingdom in 2011, with France having an ALOS 20% lower and Norway 36% lower. There are many reasons for this, reflecting different health system structures, organizations and economic contexts; however, the variation suggests that there may be opportunities to reduce length of stay in some settings, thereby potentially increasing productivity and making better use of available capacity. For example, widespread uptake of enhanced recovery programmes which combine a range of techniques to facilitate early discharge, and improvements in surgical techniques and care pathways which allow ambulatory surgery to be performed, both have the potential to dramatically impact productivity and efficiency. The impact of these changes could be significant; if ALOS in England fell by 15% by 2023, for example, with no further reductions in beds and all other things being equal, the NHS could treat around 18% more acute patients than it did in 2013/14 – an average annual increase of around 1.6% (Alderwick et al., 2015). However, as the cost of a patient recovering in a hospital bed is much less than that of undertaking a surgical procedure, the total cost would increase, possibly substantially.

Currently about 10 million patients undergo a surgical procedure in the English NHS each year, with consistent rises year on year, with a 27% increase seen in the number of surgical admissions between 2003/4 and 2013/14 (Royal College of Surgeons of England, 2017). The cost of elective (non-emergency) surgical care to the system is £16 billion (€20 billion). Out of these, around 250 000 patients are characterized as high risk (see below for a discussion of risk), representing 15% of all those who require inpatient surgical care and 80% of post-operative deaths (Royal College of Anaesthetists, 2016). Much of this risk is due to pre-existing long-term conditions and complex care needs, with the number of people living with multiple long-term conditions increasing steeply with age (Barnett et al., 2012) and thus growing with an ageing population. For example, the 1.25 million people in the United Kingdom aged 85 or older are expected to treble in number over the next 35 years, and across Europe to rise from 5.1% of the population in 2014 to 12.2% by 2070 (Wilkinson et al., 2012; Eurostat, 2017). In England the number of people with multiple long-term conditions was expected to reach 2.9 million out of a population of 53 million by 2018 (5.5%) (Department of Health, 2012).

Improvements in perioperative management and surgical techniques have increased the numbers of people with pre-existing conditions deemed eligible for surgery and have, paradoxically, also been driven by the need to reduce the risk of complications. However, in many countries there is evidence of implicit ageism, with older people less likely to receive surgical interventions (Margulies et al., 1993). For example, a 2014 report showed that in England there was a 37-fold difference in rates of breast excision in patients with breast cancer over the age of 65, depending on where they live (Royal College of Surgeons & Age UK, 2014). This has led to calls to focus on physiological rather than chronological age (Kowdley et al., 2012). However, among those who do receive surgery, older physiological age may be associated with a greater risk of complications which, when superimposed upon their already compromised physical state, mean that they may experience significant reductions in survival in the medium and longer term, and in their ability to return to their pre-operative function. Consequently, it is increasingly important that the scope of perioperative care extends beyond the immediate period of recovery from the acute effects of surgery.

This calls for a model of care that extends across specialties and professional groups and over time. Although the concept of perioperative medicine has been in use for more than a decade, until recently it has been applied only in a few selected areas and, even then, often incompletely. One area where it has been used is in cardiac surgery, where many facilities have established mechanisms to deliver efficient, multidisciplinary, patient-centred care. In contrast, most surgical specialties lack a unified approach to the prevention and management of perioperative surgical, medical, psychological, and social complications.

This is changing, with new models of perioperative care that emphasize improvement and consistency of outcomes for patients after surgery (Kehlet, Delaney & Hill, 2015). These are fundamentally multidisciplinary, led by professionals who can take a system-wide approach and who can be drawn from a range of medical specialties, but most often anaesthesia, surgery, geriatric or internal medicine. This chapter will explore these models in detail and suggest opportunities and barriers to their future development.

The role of perioperative care

Perioperative medicine aims to deliver the best, multidisciplinary, person-centred care before, during and after surgery. There is a natural tendency to focus on major surgical interventions for the highest risk patients; however, the evolving models of care can be of benefit to the entire surgical population. As the vignettes in Box 8.1 reveal, there is huge variation in the perioperative care provided.

Box 8.1 Patient stories: traditional versus integrated care

Patient story: traditional non-integrated care
Stan is 72 years old with a history of high blood pressure and diabetes. He is a heavy smoker. He goes to his primary care provider as he has been losing weight recently and suffering with stomach pains. His GP refers him urgently to a surgeon, who does some further tests and confirms that Stan has bowel cancer. He recommends that he undergoes surgery and a few days later Stan comes back to the hospital to the pre-assessment clinic (PAC) and sees an anaesthetist, who is concerned that he may have chronic airways disease and that his diabetes is poorly controlled. The anaesthetist refers the patient back to the GP for further investigations but due to the urgent need for surgery, Stan arrives on the day of the operation without record of these tests. The surgery goes well and the cancer is removed; however, two days later Stan develops a chest infection and spends three days in the high dependency unit. His recovery is further complicated by a wound infection. After six weeks Stan is discharged from hospital to a rehabilitation facility and then home, where he requires carers three times per day.

Patient story: integrated care
Ruby is 81 years old with a history of cardiac disease and chronic kidney impairment. Following her complaints of symptoms of abdominal pain and bloating, her GP orders some blood tests and scans which raise the suspicion of ovarian cancer. She is referred to a "one-stop shop" clinic which takes place in a local health centre; there, she has a consultation with a surgeon and cancer specialist who offer her surgery and chemotherapy. On the same day she has further tests to assess her fitness for surgery, followed by a consultation with a cardiologist and an anaesthetist, where a shared decision is made to proceed to surgery. Records are kept electronically and shared with Ruby's care providers. She is supported by a specialist cancer nurse who provides her with a single point of contact and

---

Box 8.1 (cont.)

coordinates her care. The operation goes well and she is electively cared for in the high dependency unit in order to provide early detection and treatment of any complications. Ruby's recovery is uneventful and she returns home 10 days after the surgery, to begin chemotherapy shortly afterwards.

Perioperative care is often poorly coordinated, with weak systems of communication, focused on the individual practitioner and existing organizational structures. At worst, vital information about the patient is not shared between practitioners, resulting in untimely or delayed care and errors. Also, patients may undergo procedures in circumstances where they have not been made fully aware of the implications, resulting in dissatisfaction, poor outcomes, and a worsening of their general health status. However, where good perioperative medicine exists, the care provided is focused on the needs of the patient, employing individualized care pathways. The care is well coordinated and timely, and patients share in the decision-making process. Models of care vary (as explored below) but have common themes:

- Multidisciplinary: involving doctors (both primary and secondary care), nurses, allied health care professionals, such as physiotherapists, occupational therapists, speech and language therapists and dieticians, social workers and administrative staff.
- Crossing organizational interfaces: particularly primary care, secondary care and social care (Johnson et al., 2013).
- Well led: this could be by doctors from different specialties, including anaesthesia, surgery, acute medicine, cardiology, geriatrics and others. Most commonly, anaesthetists lead perioperative teams since they are the most numerous hospital specialty and their current training model makes them natural candidates to do so. However, the interdisciplinary nature of good care means that there should be an emphasis on deploying the skills and expertise available in order to achieve optimal patient outcomes.
- Robust communication: through the provision of a single point of contact for patients, surgeons and primary care providers, facilitated where possible by technology that enables the secure collection and exchange of patient data.
- Evidenced-based with continual improvements in quality driven by robust audit data.

- Patient-centred: respecting patients' autonomy, listening to and respecting their wishes, and keeping them informed and involved with their care are the key tenets of patient-centred care which is now widely seen as an essential component of gold standard practice (Epstein & Street, 2011). This model of care is gradually superseding its antiquated predecessors – doctor- and disease-centred care – and represents a paradigm shift from the patriarchal style of medicine which was practised for much of the 20th century.
- Using appropriate technology: at present the majority of perioperative care is delivered in a visit-based system with the patients travelling to a hospital/clinic to be reviewed by the health professional who provided the index treatment. With the rise of digital health platforms and the ever-increasing availability of technology, there is potential for increasing amounts of perioperative care to be delivered remotely in a home-based system.

Multidisciplinary assessment and optimization – models of care

Geriatrician-led

Pre-operative CGA provided by a consultant geriatrician-led MDT involves multidomain assessment and optimization of the condition of the high-risk or older surgical patient (Partridge et al., 2014; Moug et al., 2016). This is particularly important given the increased frequency of risk factors and adverse post-operative outcomes in the older patient. The MDT can also support the surgical teams with post-operative medical care, focusing on functional optimization and discharge planning for both emergency and elective patients.

There is growing evidence that CGA is associated with improved process and outcomes such as decreased length of stay, reduction in delays and cancellations, and reduction in medical complications. One example is the Proactive care of Older People undergoing Surgery team (POPS) at Guy's and St Thomas' NHS Foundation Trust in London (Dhesi, 2012). The POPS team was designed to improve perioperative care and planning, address problems with poor rehabilitation and delayed discharges, and reduce the high rates of post-operative medical complications in elderly patients.

The Medical Research Council framework for complex interventions (Craig et al., 2008) was used to create, implement, and evaluate the

POPS team. It is a geriatrician-led MDT which includes anaesthetic and surgical teams, therapists, social workers, and nursing staff. Patients with multiple co-morbidities, frailty and/or cognitive impairment are identified and referred to the POPS team. A CGA is then performed and a personalized perioperative care plan generated. Pre-operatively, risk factors and co-morbid conditions are identified and optimized, discussions are held with the patient, their family and the MDT to aid shared decision-making, and the appropriate level of post-operative care is determined. Post-operatively, regular geriatrician reviews and ward rounds take place and cases are discussed at POPS MDT meetings; there is also close communication between the POPS team and community/social services, facilitating quick and effective discharge to the community.

Around 1000 elective patients are seen by the POPS team annually, and the team also reviews any appropriate patients admitted to the surgical wards as an emergency. The impact of this service has been impressive, with significant reductions in medical complications, including pneumonia and delirium, pressure sores and delayed mobilization, and in length of stay in hospital (Dhesi & Swart, 2016). Similar findings were obtained with the Systematic Care Older Patients undergoing Elective Surgery (SCOPES) service at Nottingham University Hospitals NHS Trust in England (Dhesi & Swart, 2016).

Anaesthetist-led

Patients are triaged (based on estimated perioperative risk of mortality), with higher-risk patients attending an anaesthetist-led clinic. The clinician employs a range of clinical assessment and physiological testing (e.g. cardiopulmonary exercise testing) to provide an objective assessment of the risks and benefits of surgery. The clinic is supported by a range of health care professionals to provide expert advice and support (including organ specialists, therapists, and allied health care professionals).

Assessment of fitness for surgery

The assessment of fitness for surgery, and therefore risk of post-operative complications, is fundamental to perioperative care. There is strong evidence for an association of objectively measured fitness with outcomes from major surgery: in general, fitter people do better and this is perhaps even more important than chronological age (Snowden et al., 2013).

Assessing fitness allows an assessment of risk, thereby facilitating a discussion leading to a shared decision about whether and how the patient should proceed to treatment. Simple methods have been used to gauge cardiorespiratory fitness, for example using patient questionnaires to ascertain the person's maximal level of daily activity and the 6-Minute Walk Test where the distance walked by the person predicts morbidity and mortality.

Reliably and objectively testing and quantifying fitness is increasingly becoming a prerequisite for major elective surgery, particularly in those patients known to have risk factors such as chronic diseases or obesity. Cardiopulmonary exercise testing (CPET) uses an incremental exercise test (usually on a treadmill or exercise bike) to generate safe, accurate, and repeatable data that correspond with the demands of major surgery on the body (Carlisle & Swart, 2007).

Barriers to greater use of CPET include the costs of setting it up, the routine operation of the equipment, and the need for skilled expertise to conduct the assessments and interpret the test results. Often the test is conducted by physiologists, supported by clinicians. Many anaesthetists are now trained to make these assessments and there is growing recognition that the cost of managing post-operative deterioration in patients who have not been thoroughly assessed and their condition optimized often outweighs the costs of providing the tests.

Assessment of fitness can be done as part of comprehensive pre-operative screening. This can be nurse-led and most hospitals in England also have consultant anaesthetist-led clinics to assess more complex patients. At this point in the patient journey blood investigations and assessments of the function of other body systems (heart, lungs and kidneys) are also done and patients may be referred for specialist opinions.

Historically, pre-operative testing was largely performed on the day before surgery and it was left to the admitting junior doctor to decide which tests should be performed, leading to significant variability in pre-operative testing and creating the potential for significant patient harm. With the shift towards PACs this process has become more rigorous and standardized, with significant improvements to patient care. PAC is now widely accepted as the gold standard of care across Europe, exemplified by a law passed in 1994 in France which stipulates that a PAC visit must be completed at least two days before any admission for elective anaesthesia (Flynn & Silvay, 2012). However, the PAC approach has its own pitfalls as there is a tendency towards over-testing and delays to treatment as incidental abnormalities are followed up and investigated further. The recognition of risk of patient harm due to unnecessary investigations, and delayed definitive treatment of the initial pathology, have led to a trend of more selective pre-operative testing (Feely et al., 2013; Bohmer, Wappler & Zwissler, 2014).

This is exemplified by the joint recommendations from the German societies of Anaesthesiology, Internal Medicine, and Surgery (DGAI, DGIM, and DGCH), published in 2010. These recommendations highlight the importance of precise medical history and examination, and suggest a standardized scheme to identify factors which may necessitate further testing. If there are no such factors and the procedure to be performed is low risk, the authors claim that no further testing is needed. The recommendations address patient- and procedure-specific indications for pre-operative testing such as laboratory tests, electrocardiogram, X-ray, echocardiogram, pulmonary function and extended cardiac testing. The aim is to reduce unnecessary investigations which have been shown to have no beneficial effect on perioperative patient safety, thereby streamlining the pre-operative assessment process and reducing costs and delays to treatment. A national survey of German anaesthesiologists performed in 2013 suggests that the recommendations have been effective, with 39.1% of anaesthetists stating that they now conduct fewer ancillary tests (Dhesi & Swart, 2016).

Risk optimization and lifestyle modification

Once a comprehensive assessment of risk has been undertaken, and as part of the multidisciplinary approach, measures to optimize the chances of a good outcome from surgery can be decided in collaboration with the patient. Through liaison with other professionals, control of chronic diseases such as diabetes, asthma and heart disease can be optimized. In addition, lifestyle advice can be given and other services can be signposted, including smoking cessation (McKee, Gilmore & Novotny, 2003), alcohol reduction, weight loss, and dietary and nutrition advice.

Recently, the concept of "prehabilitation" has been adopted; this consists of a group of interventions that are introduced into the patient pathway pre-operatively, aimed at enhancing a person's ability to withstand the stress of major surgery and achieving lasting beneficial effects on recovery (Gillis et al., 2014). Although the choice of timing must be balanced with the risk of delaying surgery (particularly in cases where cancer is suspected or diagnosed), it is evident that improvement in pre-operative fitness will optimize the chances of a successful outcome from surgery.

One major intervention, with increasing evidence of benefit (although not consistently), is exercise therapy (Snowden & Minto, 2015). There is overwhelming evidence that physical activity improves the health of people with chronic conditions and also prevents many common diseases (Academy of Medical Royal Colleges, 2015). This is also true in the context of the pre-operative phase but it is important that an exercise programme achieves a high level of adherence, with support from the appropriate health professionals. Several studies have shown significant improvements in length of stay and reductions in post-operative complications following cardiac surgery in patients who have used prehabilitation programmes (Hoogeboom et al., 2014). There is also some evidence that prehabilitation can benefit patients undergoing thoracic, abdominal and major joint surgery, particularly in high-risk patients with poor pre-operative condition (Hoogeboom et al., 2014).

Unfortunately, the current body of evidence surrounding prehabilitation is skewed towards low-powered randomized controlled trials in healthy individuals, whereas the greatest benefit is likely to be seen in high-risk patients. Furthermore, there is a lack of consensus regarding the most efficacious exercise programme, for example whether it should be resistance or aerobic training, and whether it should be delivered in a hospital or home-based environment (Hoogeboom et al., 2014).

Pre-operative risk assessment and shared decision-making

The concept of shared decision-making (SDM) is attracting increasing attention in many countries (Blanc et al., 2014). It represents a shift from antiquated paternalistic medicine to a patient-centred model, and is especially pertinent in the field of perioperative medicine as decisions surrounding surgeries can have life-changing consequences.

SDM is defined as "a broad term that describes [a] collaborative effort between the physician and patient to make an informed clinical decision that enhances the chance of treatment success as defined by each individual patient's preferences and values" (Slover, Shue &

Koenig, 2012). It involves the provider offering information on possible treatment modalities, including risks, benefits and alternatives, and the patient sharing their relevant values and preferences. A mutual decision can then be made on a treatment plan most likely to deliver the best outcome with respect to these factors, whether it is a choice between different types of surgery, or a choice between surgery and conservative management. This type of patient empowerment has several benefits, including decreased indecision and decisional conflict, and improved patient knowledge and participation in treatment decisions. It allows for care to be tailored to the needs of individual patients and can increase patient satisfaction.

Box 8.2 Patient story: shared decision-making

Anil is 78 years old and undergoes routine screening for abdominal aortic aneurysm (AAA). This reveals that he has an 8cm aneurysm and so is referred to a vascular surgeon. Since the risk of it rupturing is around 50% per year, Anil is offered an open surgical repair and is then seen in a PAC. Anil also has heart failure and emphysema, and his health has been deteriorating for a while. In the clinic he undergoes a CPET, among other tests, which reveals that he has a poor physiological reserve. Following this, he has an hour-long discussion with an anaesthetist, where the risks and benefits of having surgery are discussed. Anil understands that he is at high risk of complications if he has surgery, and will be unlikely to get back to his pre-operative level of function. Following a period of time to reflect and discuss with his family, he returns to the clinic and decides, along with his care providers, not to proceed with surgery and instead to adopt a conservative approach.

SDM has been shown to affect patient decision-making, with a tendency to choose more conservative therapeutic options, particularly in orthopaedic patients (Slover, Shue & Koenig, 2012). It has also been postulated that it can improve equity in health care, as the physician is beholden to explain alternative treatments that may have been unknown to certain groups of patients (Elwyn et al., 2010).

Although SDM is increasing and is seen as the gold standard of patient care, uptake has been limited, due in part to the perception that it is an expensive and time-consuming endeavour that requires an investment in training. However, the impact on consultation time is usually minimal, and the growth of digital technology means that decision-making aids can be produced and disseminated at relatively low cost (Elwyn et al., 2010).

Box 8.3 Torbay Hospital Clinic shows financial viability

The surgical risk assessment and SDM clinic at Torbay Hospital, South Devon Healthcare NHS Foundation Trust, UK, is an excellent example of SDM in operation. Approximately 900 high-risk patients per annum are referred to the SDM clinic to have a comprehensive risk assessment and an in-depth consultation regarding their treatment options. The aim is to empower patients to make more informed decisions on their care and to allow perioperative care planning including allocation of resources such as high dependency and intensive therapy units. This model has been shown to be financially viable, with an estimated £382 (€480) reduction in total cost of care for high-risk patients undergoing bowel cancer resection.

Source: Carlisle et al., 2012

Care bundles – enhanced recovery

In recent years enhanced recovery programmes (ERP) have become increasingly popular, with a substantial body of evidence demonstrating their ability to improve post-operative outcomes and to reduce length of stay. Common components of ERP include pre-operative counselling, planning, and nutrition, usually delivered in an outpatient clinic setting, and after the patient has been admitted to hospital intra-operative management such as guided fluid therapy, maintenance of normothermia (a normal state of temperature) and use of minimally invasive approaches. Post-operatively, initiatives such as early mobilization, prompt resumption of normal diet, innovative analgesic techniques and proactive discharge planning are employed.

Enhanced recovery after surgery (ERAS) for colorectal surgery was first described by Professor Henrik Kehlet in Denmark during the 1990s (Fearon et al., 2005). The principles of this programme are shown in Figure 8.2. Subsequently the same elements have been applied to other surgical specialties, including orthopaedics and gynaecology, and have developed into the international ERAS society with centres of excellence in Canada, Denmark, France, Spain, Sweden and the United Kingdom.

There have been several studies showing improved outcomes, such as length of stay and morbidity, when ERAS is used (Adamina et al., 2011). Despite this body of evidence, uptake of the programme and adherence to its principles have been relatively low; patient-, staff- and practice-related factors as well as a lack of resources have been suggested as potential barriers to entry which must be overcome if widespread implementation is to be achieved (Segelman & Nygren, 2014). Furthermore, there is a paucity of evidence on the effect of ERAS on patient-related outcomes such as quality of life and cost-effectiveness, and further

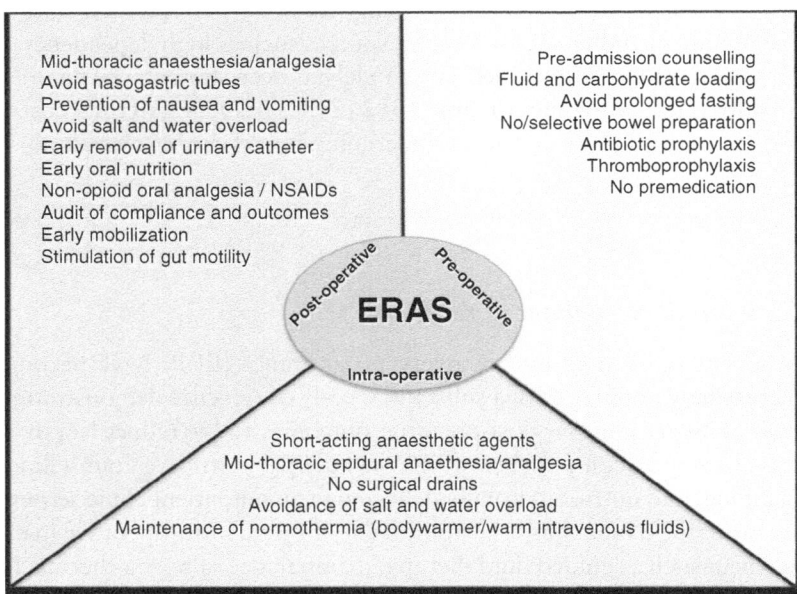

Figure 8.2 Components of enhanced recovery after surgery (ERAS) pathway

Note: NSAIDs: non-steroidal anti-inflammatory drugs
Source: Recreated from Dorcaratto, Grande & Pera, 2013

research is indicated in these areas to quantify the true value of ERAS and other ERPs.

Research on post-operative outcomes in orthopaedic patients after use of ERPs has been promising; however, there is a wide variation in the components of the programmes evaluated, with substantial variations in results (Ibrahim et al., 2013). Development and widespread implementation of a standardized enhanced recovery protocol would help in disseminating best practice. Stowers et al. (2014) suggested a protocol for enhanced recovery after hip and knee arthroplasty described in Table 8.1 below, which shares many features and principles of the ERAS protocol for colorectal surgery while being tailored towards the needs of patients undergoing orthopaedic surgery.

Table 8.1 *A proposed enhanced recovery protocol for elective total hip and knee arthroplasty*

Pre-operative care
• Education, and expectation management
• Discharge planning by MDT, e.g. occupational therapist and social worker
• Nutrition screening using the Malnutrition Universal Screening Tool, with appropriate referral to dietician as required
• Premedication: cyclo-oxygenase-2 selective inhibitors, gabapentin, dexamethasone
Intra-operative care
• Spinal anaesthesia + regional (femoral/saphenous) nerve block or high-volume local anaesthetic
• Liberal perioperative intravenous fluids
• Intravenous prophylactic antibiotics for 24 hours
• Tranexamic acid
• Avoidance of surgical drains
Post-operative care
• Early ambulation
• Early intensive physiotherapy
• Aspirin, thromboembolic deterrent stockings, and intermittent pneumatic compression devices for venous thromboembolic prophylaxis (for those at low risk)
• Multimodal, opioid-sparing analgesia regimen

Source: Recreated from Stowers et al., 2014

Ambulatory surgery

Over the past 20 years there has been a significant increase in productivity driven by the rise in proportion of operations performed as ambulatory cases. Since 2005 England has employed financial incentives to switch to ambulatory surgery, driven by the rollout of a system of payment by results (PbR) for all elective procedures. As day-case patients cost less to treat than patients who stay overnight as inpatients (in 2013/14 the average day-case cost was £698 (€872) and the average inpatient-case cost was £1367 (€1708)), the increasing number and proportion of day cases has helped to reduce overall costs per case. In effect, by treating more patients as day cases, by 2013/14 the NHS had saved around £2 billion (€2.5 billion), equivalent to an average saving over the 15 years since 1998/9 of around 1.4% per year of the total spend on elective day and inpatient care (Appleby, 2015).

Several other factors have facilitated the shift towards day surgery including: cultural change, availability of regional anaesthesia, faster-acting anaesthetic, analgesic (pain-killer) and antiemetic (anti-sickness) drugs, organizational improvements, i.e. day-case units, minimally invasive surgery, and changing patient expectations.

Workforce

Current anaesthetic workforce model

In most countries anaesthetists form the largest single hospital medical specialty and their skills are used in all aspects of patient care (Royal College of Anaesthetists, 2016). While the perioperative anaesthetic care of the surgical patient is the core of specialty work, the scope of anaesthetic practice can extend to:

- The pre-operative preparation of surgical patients
- The resuscitation and stabilization of patients in the ED;
- Pain relief in labour and obstetric anaesthesia;
- Intensive care medicine, although increasingly this is becoming a specialty in its own right with a separate training and accreditation structure;
- Varying age groups: neonatal, paediatric and adult;
- Transport of acutely ill and injured patients;
- Pre-hospital emergency care;

- Pain medicine;
- The provision of sedation and anaesthesia for patients undergoing various procedures outside the operating theatre.

In the main, services are delivered by specialists, placing large demands on the current workforce in some countries. With an ageing population, many with multiple co-morbidities and requiring more complex surgical procedures, there are projections of at least a 25% increase in demand in the United Kingdom by 2033 (Centre for Workforce Intelligence, 2015).

Non-physician anaesthetists

In some European countries anaesthesia is currently delivered by non-physicians, albeit with supervision by consultants (Vickers, 2000). Box 8.4 illustrates some examples.

Box 8.4 Employment of non-physicians to give anaesthetics

Sweden: Anaesthetic nurses (ANs) are all drawn from nursing backgrounds. They may enter AN training directly after graduating as a nurse, although most also have a minimum of two years' practical nursing experience. The AN training programme lasts for one year. Physicians supervise a variable number of theatres and for the most part physicians must be present at the induction and reversal of anaesthesia.

The Netherlands: Anaesthetic nurses are drawn from either nursing backgrounds or straight from school with good exam results; the former group undergo two years' training and the latter three years' training. Physicians normally supervise two operating theatres and must be present at the induction and reversal of anaesthesia. An AN must be present at every anaesthetic.

The United Kingdom: The main groups eligible to commence training as a physician's assistant (anaesthesia) or PA(A) are registered health care professionals with at least three years' clinical experience and/or degree level studies, or graduates with a biomedical science or biological science degree. Typically PA(A)s work in a 2:1 model where there is one consultant anaesthetist supervising two PA(A)s or a trainee anaesthetist and a PA(A) simultaneously

---

Box 8.4 (cont.)

in two operating theatres. PA(A)s are also used to reduce theatre downtime, leading to increased throughput on lists and theatre utilization, pre-operative assessment, exercise testing, provision of sedation to other specialties, cardiac arrest teams, and for regional and local anaesthetic provision. This model has not, however, been widely adopted, with only around 120 PA(A)s trained by 2015, but this is projected to increase with plans by the Department for Health and Social Care to fully regulate PA(A)s.

Perioperative care workforce model

As has been outlined above, optimal perioperative care is delivered by a well led MDT, focused around the patient. In many acute care settings the components of the team already exist but are often fragmented and exist in isolation with poor communication between them. Members of the perioperative MDT include:

- Doctors (both primary and secondary care), including:
  - ➤ Anaesthetists
  - ➤ Surgeons
  - ➤ General practitioners
  - ➤ Care of the Elderly physicians
  - ➤ Specialist physicians such as diabetologists, cardiologists and respiratory physicians
  - ➤ Radiologists
  - ➤ Intensivists
- Nursing staff
- Physicians' assistants
- Allied health care professionals such as:
  - ➤ Physiotherapists
  - ➤ Occupational therapists
  - ➤ Speech and language therapists
  - ➤ Dieticians
  - ➤ Social workers
- Administrative staff

Training

High quality and well organized training is integral to the future of perioperative care. Clinical training for physician anaesthetists combines the acquisition of clinical knowledge, skills and behaviours, with a broad range of clinical leadership and management skills necessary. In addition, clinicians are now increasingly required to have at least a working knowledge of improvement science, discussed in more detail later in the chapter, and the ability to apply relevant research into their clinical practice.

As has been discussed, good quality perioperative care transcends traditional boundaries in terms of clinical specialties and across organizational forms. This requires that training adapts too, whereby clinicians from different specialties such as anaesthesia, surgery and medicine acquire similar skills and knowledge in order to collaborate more closely. Post-graduate qualifications, such as the UCL Perioperative Medicine MSc, are open to all health care professionals thus promoting true multidisciplinary working (https://www.ucl.ac.uk/surgery/courses/msc-perioperative-medicine).

Barriers to delivery of perioperative care

There is a projected shortfall of physician anaesthetists, as well as other specialties. In the United Kingdom changes to medical and nursing training has resulted in a deficit of applications for training posts, meaning that some roles within the perioperative team are left unfilled. This threatens the sustainability of the workforce and poses safety challenges in terms of rota gaps, unmet service need, and increased requirement for locum or ad-hoc positions. Recently, there has also been difficulty filling positions for higher training in anaesthesia (http://www.rcoa .ac.uk/news-and-bulletin/rcoa-news-and-statements/rcoa-links-low-fill-rates-inadequate-supply-of-trainees). However, this situation may offer an opportunity for the design and implementation of new models of care (as discussed below) and improved patient outcomes.

Good quality perioperative care transcends traditional organizational forms and systems. For example, patients will often be cared for by their primary surgical team in conjunction with other medical and non-medical specialists in primary and secondary care. This demands good communication. Due to difficulties sharing information in health systems, however, information is often not passed on or made available when it is required. This can lead to replication, waste and, at worst, error. In addition, further barriers to the provision of good quality care, as with other health care settings, include inter- and intra-provider variation, processes lacking reliability, and lack of standardization.

Addressing these issues is best done using improvement science principles (see below).

The future

Health care systems are facing challenges from the ageing population with a greater prevalence of chronic co-morbid conditions, and the opportunities to intervene provided by advances in medicine. However, with these challenges comes the opportunity to innovate and implement transformational change to the way that we deliver perioperative care. Consideration also needs to be given to the appropriateness of costly, complex surgical therapies, and whether centrally funded health care systems should be expected to provide these with the possible consequence of less available resources for more established therapies with proven cost-effectiveness. Policy-makers have a responsibility to engage with the public in discussion, and as a society, in order to determine where each health care system's priorities lie within a cost-constrained environment.

For the vast majority of patients undergoing a surgical procedure, the episode is uncomplicated with good outcomes. However, increasing numbers of patients are being exposed to greater risk through a combination of their pre-existing condition, the surgical treatment itself, or issues regarding the delivery of care. The development of the perioperative care model offers a solution that can optimize the chances of a good outcome, particularly for high-risk patients.

Excellent perioperative care is, in part, already being offered in an individualized manner with the ability to draw on expertise and resource, as and when the patient needs it. This is described in Figure 8.3.

There are a number of enablers to the provision of quality, coordinated perioperative care including: technology, research and improvement science, and improved models of care.

Technology

Although the use of technology in medicine is growing, we have yet to truly tap into its full potential. Advances in genomics, telemedicine, robotics, virtual and augmented reality, artificial intelligence and electronic medical records have the potential to cause a paradigm shift in the delivery of perioperative care. As these advances in computing

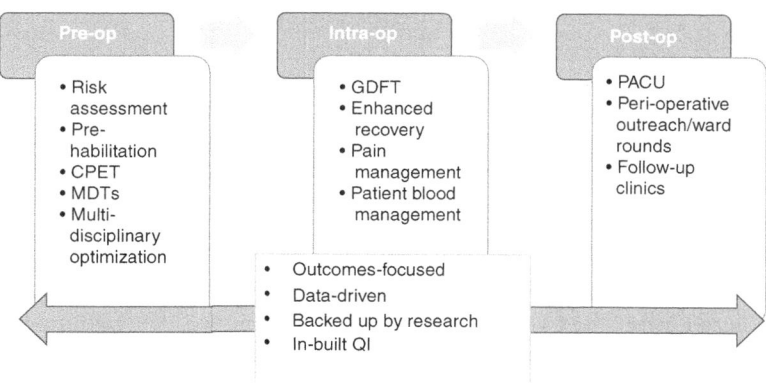

Figure 8.3 Individual perioperative care pathway

Source: Authors' compilation

Notes: CPET: cardiopulmonary exercise testing; MDT: multidisciplinary team; GDFT: goal directed fluid therapy; PACU: post-anaesthesia care unit; QI: quality improvement

continue at an exponential rate, the challenge for perioperative care providers is to find new and effective ways to harness technology to improve outcomes for their patients. However, this is often costly and demands front-loaded funding. Even if this results in cost-savings and efficiencies in the medium to longer term, financial cuts mean that technology programmes face significant challenges.

Increasingly data are being digitized, which can then be analysed, shared and used to drive quality improvement. For example, powerful machine-learning algorithms could be applied to ascertain which patient, provider and procedural characteristics will impact most on their post-operative outcomes, or be used to supply live decision support to PACs enabling selection of appropriate pre-operative tests and a bespoke prehabilitation package. Digitized data can be seamlessly and securely transferred between stakeholders, including hospitals, primary care providers, research and academic institutions, and patients themselves. This increased availability of information presents manifold opportunities for research and identification of best practice, allows for safer and more efficient delivery of care through the avoidance of repetitive data gathering, and can empower patients by giving them ownership of their medical records.

Innovation in anaesthesia in the past 10 years has centred on a number of aspects:

- Airway equipment, for example video laryngoscopy.
- Ultrasound machines, which are now in widespread use in anaesthesia for use in diagnosis, vascular access and regional anaesthesia where needles are inserted under direct vision and local anaesthetic drugs are deposited around nerves.
- The increasing profile given to human factors and systems design, particularly in the management of clinically challenging, time-sensitive situations. The Clinical Human Factors Group (CHFG), founded by Martin Bromiley, a pilot whose wife died as a direct result of medical error, is at the forefront of this (Clinical Human Factors Group, 2018); mitigation of these important sources of error and risk to patients has been increasingly recognized as having a significant impact in perioperative care. Techniques implemented to help control human factors include: application of learning from other sectors, such as the aviation industry, human factors design and engineering, and improved simulation and team working techniques (Weinger & Gaba, 2014).
- Drugs, especially those that enable enhanced recovery; for example, sugammadex is a novel reversal agent for some muscle relaxant drugs, although its use is limited by its relatively high cost.
- Increasing awareness around the environmental impact of anaesthesia, particularly that of the volatile agents and nitrous oxide, which are greenhouse gases, is driving increased use of total intravenous anaesthesia (TIVA). There is also increasing evidence that TIVA with propofol is associated with decreased reoccurence of malignancy following cancer surgery, the mechanism of which is unclear.

Research and improvement science

The evolution of perioperative medicine needs to occur in parallel with the development of the research agenda, with a particular focus on translating discoveries and advances into meaningful changes in care delivery and outcomes for patients more rapidly. At present, basic scientists are directing their efforts at understanding the biological mechanisms underlying postoperative morbidity, and why its impact should be so sustained. Clinical triallists are evaluating interventions to mitigate adverse outcomes in pragmatic studies involving tens of thousands of patients. It is recognized that unplanned variations in structures and processes between health care providers have a significant impact on outcomes after surgery; thus initiatives within the field of improvement science are focusing on this area.

Improvement science in health care is a concept that has been generating increasing interest over the past few years, as health care providers, academics, and front-line staff look to improve care delivery and generate practical real-life learning and approaches to aid development and dissemination of best practice. However, it is still in what some authors call the "pre-paradigm phase of emergence", which in part means there is an absence of an agreed definition (Marshall, Pronovost & Dixon-Woods, 2013). Commonly the term is used to describe the application of the principles of W Edwards Deming to health care. A broader definition of improvement science is that it is a coordinated approach to quality improvement (QI), which aims to create practical learning that can make a timely difference to patient care (Marshall, Pronovost & Dixon-Woods, 2013).

Improvement science is built around the robust scientific assessment of QI projects, including the design, deployment, and assessment of complex multifaceted interventions. If applied correctly, it adds considerable external validity to the results of these interventions, allowing them to be taken up more rapidly by other institutions and health care systems, and breaking down silos of best practice. The process of rapid testing and improvement helps to generate confidence in the proposed changes among the stakeholders.

Furthermore, this approach helps to mitigate the risks caused by poorly planned and unscientific QI projects, which are not evidence-based, nor appropriately monitored to ensure positive impact on patients. Therefore improvement science is critical to maximizing the impact of QI interventions and effective use of resources as health care systems adjust to the demands of modern and future medicine (Varkey, Reller & Resar, 2007).

There has been a lot of research looking at QI interventions in perioperative care. This is because although significant advances have been made in recent years, there are an estimated 234 million surgical procedures performed annually around the world with considerable risk of patient harm. A recent systematic review of QI research in perioperative care using techniques such as audit and feedback, Plan-Do-Study-Act (PDSA) cycles, and methodologies such as Lean Six Sigma which are used to remove waste and reduce variation, demonstrated that although there were many studies in this field, the reporting was suboptimal, leading the authors to conclude that we need to orientate research towards QI and improvement science in perioperative care and develop a comprehensive, coherent, and valid framework for the design and reporting of QI interventions in this field (Jones et al., 2014).

Recognition at all levels of health care from policy-makers, commissioners, and organizational boards to front-line staff that QI should be part of an organization's daily business is essential in order that a culture of continuous improvement is sustained. Improvement work performed as part of teams is most effective but in order for this to occur, it is important that time and resources are dedicated to it; however, in many instances, in part due to the sustained pressures of delivering against rising demands, QI is regarded as a non-mandatory activity.

Fundamental to developing a supportive and nurturing culture that encourages innovation and improvement is the adoption of coaching. An example of an effective health care system that has embedded coaching into its systems is the Sheffield Microsystem Coaching Academy (Sheffield Microsystem Coaching Academy, 2018).

Collaboration between academics and clinicians is flourishing with the recognition that "big data" and nationally funded audits of processes and outcomes can be used to study and deliver improvements in these outcomes.

Developing evidence can be combined with significant advances in technology, digital health, patient empowerment and anaesthetic techniques to produce gold standard models of care. These models of care and existing examples of best practice should be scaled across health care systems in order to reduce variability in standards of care delivered and to improve patient outcomes.

Improved models of care

In the immediate future efforts to improve perioperative care should include the dissemination of existing best practice – for example, enhanced recovery programmes have been shown to improve post-operative outcomes; however, their use has remained sporadic. This is a prime example of where best practice, validated by research, could be scaled to positively impact the lives of vast numbers of patients. These programmes have the potential to bring greater improvements by taking a more holistic approach, including nutrition and prehabilitation, and by utilizing the power of technology to improve patient engagement.

Perioperative care could also be rapidly improved by the uptake and dissemination of shared decision-making principles, empowering patients to take more charge of their care journeys, and putting patient preference at the centre of perioperative care. Where digital patient information resources are created, these should, where possible, be made open source and widely disseminated to spread best practice in a cost-effective manner.

As we redesign our services and meet the demands of 21st-century medicine, it is important to embrace the truest form of disruption, which is taking techniques and learning from different sectors and applying it in innovative ways to solve the problems we face. One good example of this would be the application of engineering and manufacturing principles such as lean methodology to health care systems. This would develop superior, more efficient processes, with fewer delays for the patient and higher productivity for the hospital, and consequently free up capacity to treat more patients and generate more funding (Dahlgaard, Pettersen & Dahlgaard-Park, 2011), which could then be reinvested in order to fund the array of technologies discussed elsewhere in this chapter. Furthermore, when we are implementing new models of care or improving existing ones, it is important that we utilize the improvement science techniques described above in order to ensure maximum efficiency and continuous improvement, and create data with external validity.

When health care providers look further ahead and plan delivery of perioperative care in the mid-21st century, it is important that they embrace the shift towards patient-centred, home-based care, and integrate the necessary infrastructure to utilize the myriad of technological advances that are already presenting themselves (Rosen et al., 2016).

It is possible that much preoperative assessment could be completed remotely through the use of telemedicine consultations, at home diagnostic equipment, and digital educational resources to deliver prehabilitation and relevant information for the patient. This type of remote working will free up space in hospitals and will allow health care professionals to work more efficiently, but it also require substantial staff training, organizational culture change, and investment in the necessary equipment and software to make it a reality.

The operating theatres of the future should allow for advanced surgical equipment such as robotics and imaging devices. Digital connectivity will be paramount to allow incorporation of remote multidisciplinary input, access to electronic health records, and integration of machine learning and artificial intelligence clinical decision-making and technical assistance tools. Robotic surgery has also created the interesting concept of remote operating; conceivably the principal surgeon could operate from a console thousands of miles away from the patient, allowing their expertise to be shared on a global scale. Fully autonomous robotic operating devoid of any requirement for human input is viewed by many authors as being the future of surgery, with the potential to become the standard operative modality and revolutionize perioperative care (Moustris et al., 2011).

The transition to these improved models of care will be challenging and, due to the level of infrastructural improvements required, will be likely to require substantial up-front investment. However, there are some favourable societal trends emerging, for instance the general public are increasingly becoming digitally connected, with most households in developed countries now having internet access, and smartphones and other devices being readily available. This technological environment is perfectly primed to connect patients and health care providers and can facilitate the patient-centric and home-based care of the 21st century.

Furthermore, the previously discussed challenges that health care is currently facing, with rising demand for services and financial constraints, represent significant drivers for change; the need to innovate in order to improve efficiency and modernize care delivery has never been greater. This is well demonstrated in the United Kingdom by the NHS five-year forward view policy document (NHS England, 2016), which puts innovation and new models of care at centre stage.

References

Academy of Medical Royal Colleges (2015). *Exercise: the miracle cure and the role of the doctor in promoting it.* London, AoMRC.

Adamina M et al. (2011). Enhanced recovery pathways optimize health outcomes and resource utilization: a meta-analysis of randomized controlled trials in colorectal surgery. *Surgery*, 149:830–40.

Alderwick H et al. (2015). *Better value in the NHS. The role of changes in clinical practice.* London, King's Fund.

Appleby J (2015). Day case surgery: a good news story for the NHS. *BMJ*, 351:h4060.

Barnett K et al. (2012). Epidemiology of multimorbidity and implications for health care, research, and medical education: a cross-sectional study. *Lancet*, 380:37–43.

Blanc X et al. (2014). Publication trends of shared decision making in 15 high impact medical journals: a full-text review with bibliometric analysis. *BMC Med Inform Decis Mak*, 14:71.

Bohmer AB, Wappler F, Zwissler B (2014). Preoperative risk assessment – from routine tests to individualized investigation. *Dtsch Arztebl Int*, 111:437–45; quiz 446.

Carlisle J, Swart M (2007). Mid-term survival after abdominal aortic aneurysm surgery predicted by cardiopulmonary exercise testing. *Br J Surg*, 94:966–9.

Carlisle J et al. (2012). Factors associated with survival after resection of colorectal adenocarcinoma in 314 patients. *Br J Anaesth*, 108:430–5.

Centre for Workforce Intelligence (2015). *Anaesthetics and intensive care medicine in-depth review*. Web page. Available at: https://assets.publishing .service.gov.uk/government/uploads/system/uploads/attachment_data/ file/507348/CfWI_Anaesthetics_ICM_main_report.pdf (accessed 8 February 2020).

Clinical Human Factors Group (2018). *About us*. Web page. Available at: http://chfg.org/about-us/ (accessed 7 March 2018).

Craig P et al. (2008). Developing and evaluating complex interventions: the new Medical Research Council guidance. *BMJ*, 337:a1655.

Dahlgaard JJ, Pettersen J, Dahlgaard-Park SM (2011). Quality and lean health care: a system for assessing and improving the health of healthcare organisations. *Total Quality Management & Business Excellence*, 22:673–89.

Department of Health (2012). *Long Term Conditions Compendium of Information*. Available at: https://www.gov.uk/government/publications/ long-term-conditions-compendium-of-information-third-edition (accessed 2 February 2020).

Dhesi J (2012). *Case study – Proactive Care of Older People undergoing Surgery (POPS) service*. British Geriatrics Society web site. Available at: https://www.bgs.org.uk/resources/proactive-care-of-older-people- undergoing-surgery (accessed 8 March 2016).

Dhesi JK, Swart M (2016). Specialist pre-operative assessment clinics. *Anaesthesia*, 71(s1):3–8.

Dorcaratto D, Grande L, Pera M (2013). Enhanced recovery in gastrointestinal surgery: upper gastrointestinal surgery. *Dig Surg*, 30:70–8.

Elwyn G et al. (2010). Implementing shared decision making in the NHS. *BMJ*, 341:c5146.

Epstein RM, Street RL Jr (2011). The values and value of patient-centered care. *Ann Fam Med*, 9:100–3.

Eurostat (2017). *Population structure and ageing* (Online). Available at: http://ec.europa.eu/eurostat/statistics-explained/index.php/Population_structure_and_ageing#Past_and_future_population_ageing_trends_in_the_EU (accessed 7 March 2018).

Fearon KC et al. (2005). Enhanced recovery after surgery: a consensus review of clinical care for patients undergoing colonic resection. *Clin Nutr*, 24:466–77.

Feely MA et al. (2013). Preoperative testing before noncardiac surgery: guidelines and recommendations. *Am Fam Physician*, 87:414–18.

Flynn BC, Silvay G (2012). Value of specialized preanesthetic clinic for cardiac and major vascular surgery patients. *Mt Sinai J Med*, 79:13–24.

Gillis C et al. (2014). Prehabilitation versus rehabilitation: a randomized control trial in patients undergoing colorectal resection for cancer. *Anesthesiology*, 121:937–47.

Grocott MP, Mythen MG (2015). Perioperative Medicine: The Value Proposition for Anesthesia?: A UK Perspective on Delivering Value from Anesthesiology. *Anesthesiol Clin*, 33:617–28.

Hoogeboom TJ et al. (2014). Merits of exercise therapy before and after major surgery. *Curr Opin Anaesthesiol*, 27:161–6.

Ibrahim MS et al. (2013). An evidence-based review of enhanced recovery interventions in knee replacement surgery. *Ann R Coll Surg Engl*, 95:386–9.

Johnson JK et al. (2013). What can artefact analysis tell us about patient transitions between the hospital and primary care? Lessons from the HANDOVER project. *Eur J Gen Pract*, 19:185–93.

Jones E et al. (2014). Describing methods and interventions: a protocol for the systematic analysis of the perioperative quality improvement literature. *Syst Rev*, 3:98.

Kehlet H, Delaney CP, Hill AG (2015). Perioperative medicine – the second round will need a change of tactics. *Br J Anaesth*, 115:13–14.

Kowdley GC et al. (2012). Cancer surgery in the elderly. *Scientific World Journal*, 303852.

Margulies DR et al. (1993). Surgical intensive care in the nonagenarian. No basis for age discrimination. *Arch Surg*, 128:753–6; discussion 756–8.

Marshall M, Pronovost P, Dixon-Woods M (2013). Promotion of improvement as a science. *Lancet*, 381:419–21.

McKee M, Gilmore A, Novotny TE (2003). Smoke free hospitals. *BMJ*, 326:941–2.

Moug SJ et al. (2016). Frailty and cognitive impairment: unique challenges in the older emergency surgical patient. *Ann R Coll Surg Engl*, 98:165–9.

Moustris GP et al. (2011). Evolution of autonomous and semi-autonomous robotic surgical systems: a review of the literature. *Int J Med Robot,* 7:375–92.

NHS England (2016). *Five Year Forward View.* London, NHSE. Available at: https://www.england.nhs.uk/five-year-forward-view/ (accessed 2 February 2020).

OECD (2015). *Health Care Utilisation.* OECD Health Statistics (Online). Available at: https://stats.oecd.org/Index.aspx?DataSetCode=HEALTH_PROC (accessed 3 March 2016).

Partridge JS et al. (2014). The impact of pre-operative comprehensive geriatric assessment on postoperative outcomes in older patients undergoing scheduled surgery: a systematic review. *Anaesthesia,* 69 (s1):8–16.

Rosen JM et al. (2016). Cybercare 2.0: meeting the challenge of the global burden of disease in 2030. *Health Technol (Berl),* 6:35–51.

Royal College of Anaesthetists (2016). *What do anaesthetists do?* Web page. Available at: http://www.rcoa.ac.uk/considering-career-anaesthesia/what-do-anaesthetists-do (accessed 8 March 2016).

Royal College of Surgeons & Age UK (2014). *Access All Ages 2: variations in access to surgical treatment among older people.* London, Royal College of Surgeons.

Royal College of Surgeons of England (2017). *Surgery and the NHS in numbers* (Online). Available at: https://www.rcseng.ac.uk/news-and-events/media-centre/media-background-briefings-and-statistics/surgery-and-the-nhs-in-numbers/ (accessed 7 March 2018).

Segelman J, Nygren J (2014). Evidence or eminence in abdominal surgery: recent improvements in perioperative care. *World J Gastroenterol,* 20:16615–9.

Sheffield Microsystem Coaching Academy (2018). Web page. Available at: http://www.sheffieldmca.org.uk/ (accessed 7 March 2018).

Slover J, Shue J, Koenig K (2012). Shared decision-making in orthopaedic surgery. *Clin Orthop Relat Res,* 470:1046–53.

Snowden CP, Minto G (2015). Exercise: the new premed. *Br J Anaesth,* 114:186–9.

Snowden CP et al. (2013). Cardiorespiratory fitness predicts mortality and hospital length of stay after major elective surgery in older people. *Ann Surg,* 257:999–1004.

Stowers MD et al. (2014). Review article: Perioperative care in enhanced recovery for total hip and knee arthroplasty. *J Orthop Surg (Hong Kong),* 22:383–92.

Varkey P, Reller MK, Resar RK (2007). Basics of quality improvement in health care. *Mayo Clin Proc*, 82:735–9.

Vickers MD (2000). Non-physician anaesthetists: can we agree on their role in Europe? *Eur J Anaesthesiol*, 17:537–41.

Weinger MB, Gaba DM (2014). Human factors engineering in patient safety. *Anesthesiology*, 120:801–6.

Wilkinson K et al. (2012). *An age old problem – a review of the care received by elderly patients undergoing surgery*. London, National Confidential Enquiry into Patient Outcome and Death (NCEPOD).

9 | *Advances in imaging*

PETER CAVANAGH

The scope of imaging

Radiology is constantly evolving in its clinical application, playing a central role in numerous patient pathways in health care. Advances in sophisticated technologies have extended the scope of its application to every organ, offering not only essential services in diagnosis, monitoring treatment, and predicting outcomes but more recently therapy in the form of interventional radiology. The result of these developments is that the volume of activity is continuing to grow in all imaging techniques (often referred to as imaging modalities).

The term "imaging" encompasses a number of diagnostic tests, some of which may be performed outside a radiology department. There is great variation among countries and by specialty in how these processes are undertaken and where.

Imaging was originally founded on the plain X-ray. Despite the development of newer techniques towards the latter part of the 20th century, the plain X-ray still plays an important role in diagnosis (although its role is often to rule out pathology, rather than for primary diagnosis) and its uses continue to grow. However, the newer modalities of ultrasound, CT and MRI are increasing at a more rapid rate. Figure 9.1 shows the increased activity in England in the last 20 years. This demonstrates a 3.6% compound growth in the last five years.

Major growth can be observed in the more complex cross-sectional imaging techniques, with compound annual growth rates (CAGR) in the last 10 years of 10% for CT and 12.3% for MRI (see Table 9.1). There is slightly less growth recorded in ultrasound at 5.3%, but this may be an underestimate as a significant amount of ultrasound is now performed outside imaging departments and would therefore not be recorded in these figures.

Although these figures are specific for England, a similar picture is seen throughout Europe and internationally. This growth is significantly in excess of that expected by demographic drivers and is predominantly

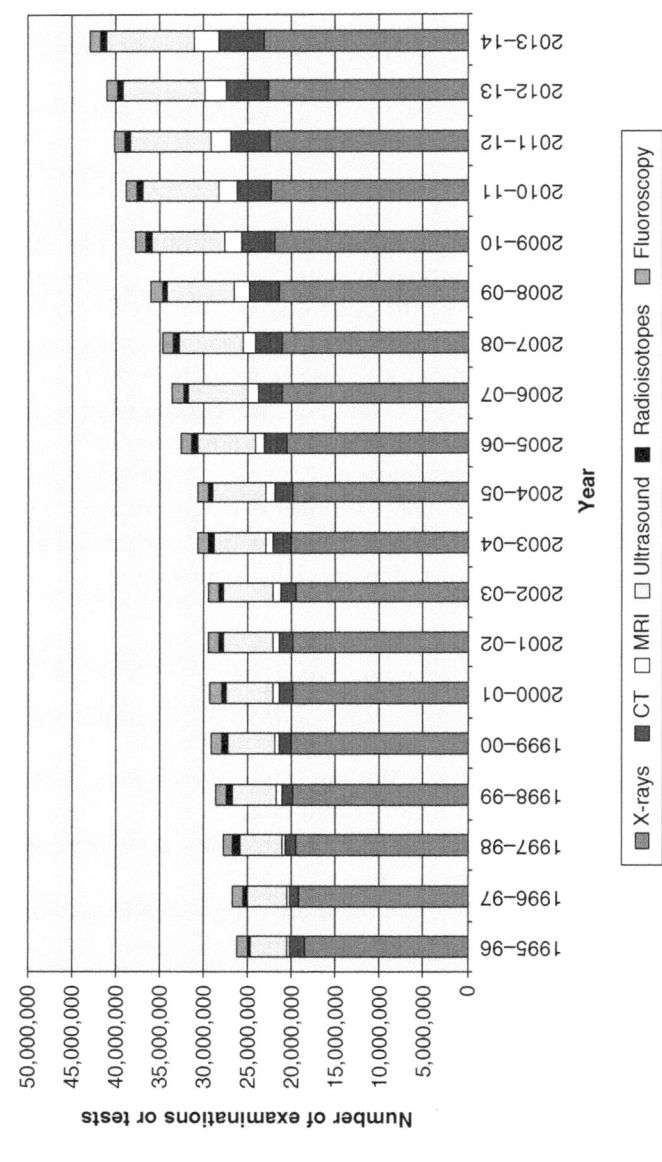

Figure 9.1 Total number of imaging and radiodiagnostic examinations or tests, by imaging modality, England, 1995–96 to 2013–14

Source: NHS England Annual Imaging and Radiodiagnostics Data, 2014

Table 9.1 *Compound annual growth rates (CAGR) for radiology modalities in England*

Modality	CAGR for past 5 years	CAGR for past 10 years
X-rays	1.46%	1.40%
CT	9.13%	10.05%
MRI	9.70%	12.32%
Ultrasound	5.72%	5.32%
Radio-isotopes	0.25%	0.70%
Fluoroscopy	1.23%	0.90%

Source: NHS England Annual Imaging and Radiodiagnostics Data, 2014

due to the increased reliance on imaging particularly in areas such as cancer, vascular conditions (including stroke and cardiac disease), and trauma.

As well as the established diagnostic techniques, imaging continues to expand at pace particularly focusing on the concept of molecular imaging utilizing ultrastructural diagnostics, nanotechnology, and functional and quantitative diagnostics. The main example of this in current practice is the use of fusion imaging, which combines the structural information gained from CT (or MRI) with the functional information from positron-emitting radiopharmaceuticals in the form of positron emission tomography fused with computed tomography (better known as PET-CT). The result is the depiction of the spatial distribution of specific metabolic or biochemical activity with clear anatomical localization.

This improved image clarity and tissue differentiation in a number of situations has dramatically increased the range of diagnostic information, in many cases providing increased confidence in terms of underlying pathology. These fused images are vital tools in a number of clinical areas, notably cancer diagnosis and treatment, but they are also used in neuroimaging and cardiac imaging (Box 9.1).

One of the most significant changes in radiology in the last 20 years has not come from developments in imaging techniques. Rather, the technological advances in information technology (IT) have had a major impact on the way that radiology is currently practised. The days of viewing X-rays on sheets of film are in the past. These days, when images are acquired, they can be post-processed, manipulated and also

---

Box 9.1 Molecular imaging

Molecular imaging is rapidly gaining recognition as the future direction of imaging providing information of what is happening at the molecular/cellular level in terms of both structure and function. The main techniques currently in clinical practice utilize radio-pharmaceuticals to provide functional information combined with traditional scanning techniques to provide structural information. However, there is active research into other techniques utilizing optical imaging for instance. The current research suggests that this form of imaging combined with genomics may be able to provide more personalized focused imaging in terms of earlier diagnosis, particularly in the field of cancer care, and allow more selective, effective treatment management.

---

transmitted rapidly not just within a hospital but also anywhere in the world as soon as they have been acquired. This technology, referred to as picture archiving and communication systems (PACS), has challenged the traditional model of patient, scanner and radiologist all located in the same site (Box 9.2). Images can now be reviewed and reported from remote locations, opening up options for different delivery models.

Box 9.2 Picture archiving and communication systems

PACS (picture archiving and communication systems) is a health care technology for the short- and long-term storage, retrieval, management, distribution and presentation of medical images. PACS allows a health care organization (such as a hospital) to capture, store, view, and share all types of images internally and externally.

A PACS has four major components:

- imaging systems, such as MRI, CT or X-ray equipment
- a secure network for distribution and exchange of patient information
- workstations or mobile devices for viewing, processing, and interpreting images
- archives for storage and retrieval of images and related documentation and reports.

Box 9.2 (cont.)

PACS has been a major driver for changing the way imaging services are delivered. The electronic storage and transfer of images facilitates quick and easy access to images and reports. In addition it has allowed the radiologist to review the images at a site remote from their acquisition, giving rise to teleradiology as a new concept.

So far in this chapter, the emphasis has been on the diagnostic role of imaging. However, imaging can also be used to guide therapy, a specialty referred to as interventional radiology (IR) (Box 9.3). This is now established as an alternative to conventional surgery in numerous conditions, offering less invasive alternatives with improved outcomes, safety, and cost-effectiveness, as well as more patient-focused care. As such, IR is a vital component of hospital medicine, providing life-saving care, both in and out of hours. IR services have replaced or enhanced many surgical procedures as well as allowing new treatments for patients which were not previously feasible. Interventional radiologists are part of the multiprofessional teams treating a wide range of pathologies and working closely with surgical colleagues.

Box 9.3 Interventional radiology

The impact of interventional radiology

Aortic aneurysm: Rupture of the abdominal and thoracic aorta can be prevented and treated by the insertion of covered stents, which have largely replaced conventional surgery for this condition. In some cases these procedures are now carried out under local anaesthesia.

Gastrointestinal haemorrhage: Embolization therapy is increasingly performed by interventional radiologists for the control of uncontrolled bleeding from the lower and upper gastrointestinal tract. This life-saving procedure carries a much lower risk to the patient and in many cases is the treatment of choice.

Postpartum haemorrhage: Bleeding after childbirth remains the most common cause of maternal death and the role of IR in managing this emergency is well established.

Box 9.3 (cont.)

Cancer: By using minimally invasive techniques, early cancers can be destroyed using radiofrequency or cryotherapy. Patients avoid the need for major surgery and long-term outcomes are very favourable. Newer techniques allow selective radiotherapy or chemotherapy for the treatment of liver lesions. Embolization can be used to devascularize tumours prior to surgical resection with resulting improvements in safety.

Early management of stroke: In the early stages of stroke the infusion of thrombolytic agents dissolves the clot and mechanical removal of blood clots can be performed to minimize disability and reduce the risk of death. Patients who suffer stroke from subarachnoid haemorrhage (bleeding around the brain) are now most frequently treated by interventional radiologists using embolization techniques.

Renal obstruction: Obstruction of the outflow from the kidney is frequently complicated by infection, which leads to septicaemia (infection in the bloodstream) and risk of death. Interventional radiologists are able to bypass the obstruction, for example through percutaneous nephrostomies.

The interconnections of imaging in the hospital setting

Imaging plays a significant role in most hospital-based specialties. The exact workload of an imaging department depends, to a certain extent, on the clinical specialties available within the hospital (e.g. neurosurgery, oncology).

In UK hospitals, A&E and general practice (direct access) are the specialties with the highest radiology demand, followed by Trauma and Orthopaedics, and this makes up approximately 50% of the activity. There is further demand from other specialities such as general surgery, general medicine, obstetrics and gynaecology, rheumatology, geriatrics, gastroenterology, cardiology, thoracic medicine, vascular surgery, ophthalmology, ENT, neurosurgery, neurology, paediatrics, oncology, psychiatry and intensive care.

The model of imaging provision varies throughout Europe. In many countries the hospital-based imaging department remains the main provider of imaging for emergency and urgent care, as well as planned care and community services. As discussed in the next section, in some countries the demand from primary care and from office-based practice is met by imaging services based off-site from acute hospitals.

In looking at new models of delivery, it may be more useful to consider where imaging plays a role in patient pathways and at what stage in this pathway imaging is best accessed. Table 9.2 is not exhaustive but lists the more common pathways and presentations relying on imaging.

Diagnostic radiology does not just offer an image acquisition and reporting service. Radiologists work closely with their clinical colleagues to ensure that patients get the most appropriate investigation and that

Table 9.2 *Common pathways and presentations relying on imaging*

Suspected or diagnosed cancer	Breast, brain and neuro-axis, head and neck, lung, oesophagus and stomach, colon and rectum, liver, pancreas, kidney and ureter, bladder, prostate, testes, ovary, uterus and cervix, lymphoma, musculoskeletal, melanoma
Cardiovascular disease	Chest pain, heart failure, pulmonary embolism, venous thromboembolism, aortic aneurysm, peripheral vascular disease
Respiratory disease	Chest infection/pneumonia, chronic obstructive pulmonary disease, restrictive lung disease
Head and neck	Deafness, balance disorders, tinnitus, sinus disease, thyroid disease, visual disturbances incl. field defects
Neurological conditions	Acute stroke, transient ischaemic attack, headache, epilepsy, multiple sclerosis, dementia, Parkinson's disease and other movement disorders
Trauma	Head injury, fractures, chest and abdominal injury
Musculoskeletal	Back pain, myelopathy and radiculopathy, joint pain, osteoarthritis, rheumatoid arthritis
Pregnancy	
Genito-urinary	Renal failure, renal stone disease, renal tract obstruction, pelvic mass, pelvic pain, haematuria
Endocrinology	Hypertension, Cushing's disease, adrenal disease
Surgical	Acute "surgical" abdomen, paediatric surgical conditions

the interpretation of the report is understood in relation to the clinical context. In this role, the radiologist plays an important part in the MDT approach to patient care, which has been acknowledged as a significant factor in improving outcomes, particularly in cancer care (Morris et al., 2006; Stephens et al., 2006; Coory et al., 2008). This has led to the development of MDT meetings where clinical radiologists (who usually lead the meetings) with their diagnostic pathologist colleagues work alongside their clinical colleagues to decide the correct clinical plan for each patient. These diagnostic specialists aid surgeons and oncologists in developing appropriate care plans based on the staging of the cancer. In this function it is now common for the biopsy of the primary tumour to have been performed by a radiologist under imaging guidance aided by the pathologist's interpretation. Figure 9.2 illustrates the extent of these MDT meetings in a typical large hospital.

IR also interacts with a large range of clinical services, as illustrated in Figure 9.3. The patients treated by interventional radiologists may be inpatients on wards in the hospital, but more frequently are treated as day cases. Larger imaging departments may have their own day-case facilities, but if not, the IR service needs access to such a resource.

Links with services outside hospitals

Patients access imaging services from a number of different situations, including:

- hospital inpatients
- outpatient services based in hospitals
- consulting rooms outside hospitals
- primary care doctors/health care professionals
- self-referral.

Imaging activity referrals from outside the hospital setting are increasing significantly. This is influenced by a number of factors including a drive to earlier diagnosis of conditions such as cancer and heart disease (Independent Cancer Task Force, 2015), as well as the increasing capability to support patients to manage their health care outside the hospital. In areas such as plain X-ray and ultrasound the workload from primary care can often amount to over 50% of the imaging activity.

Although imaging is usually thought of as a tool to confirm a diagnosis, it is important to emphasize the role of the negative test in

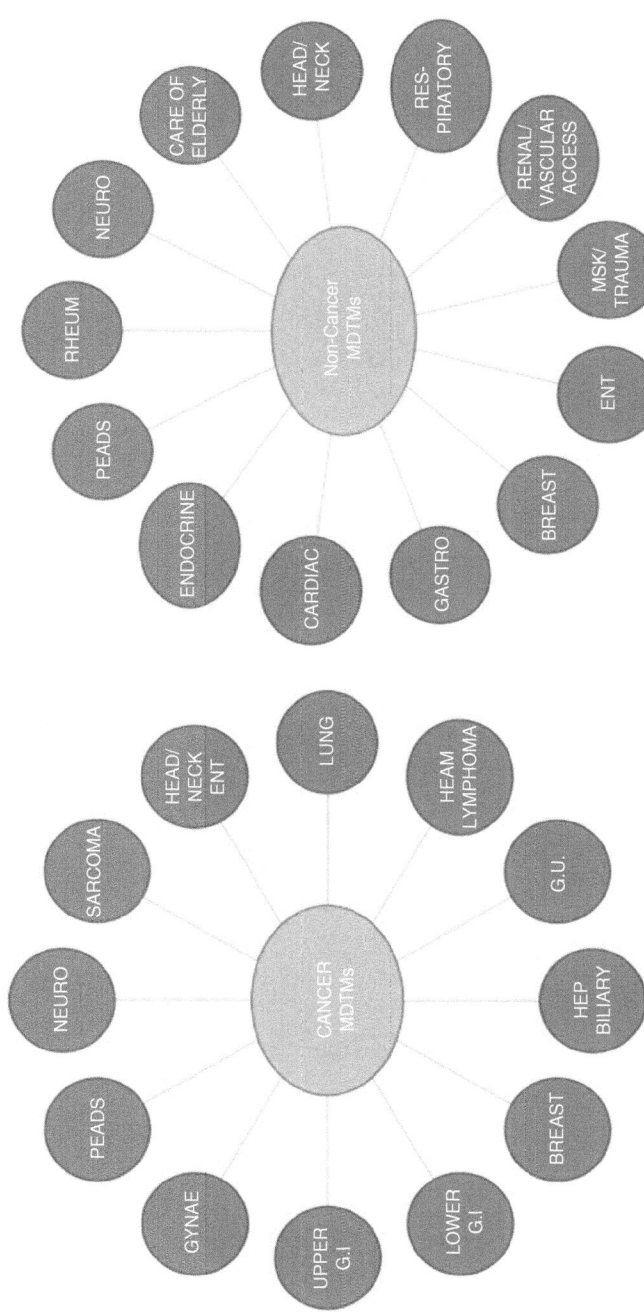

Figure 9.2 Multidisciplinary team meeting (MDTM) participants

Source: Royal College of Radiologists, 2012

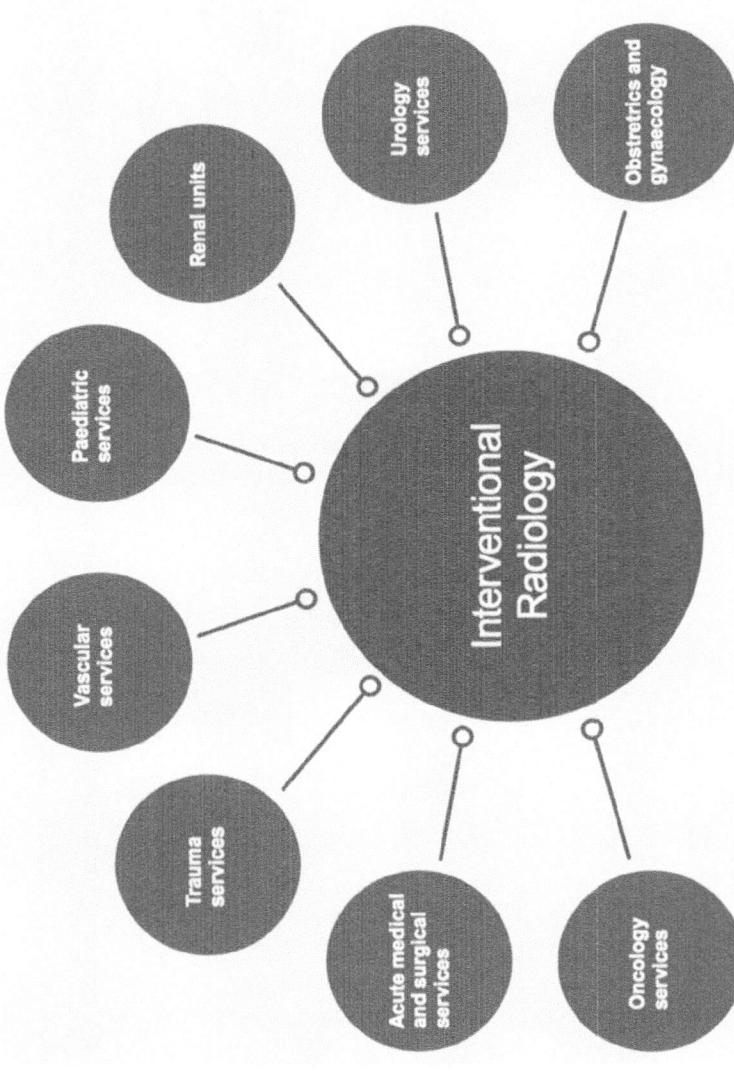

Figure 9.3 Interventional radiology interactions with hospital departments

Source: Royal College of Radiologists, 2014

excluding significant disease. In many pathways early access to imaging can avoid unnecessary hospital outpatient appointments and, more importantly, unnecessary hospital admissions.

In many European countries there is direct access to imaging from primary care for all main modalities (i.e. CT, MRI, ultrasound and plain X-ray). This applies particularly to the field of musculoskeletal problems where there is high demand for MRI in the management of back pain and joint pain.

There are varying delivery models across Europe to meet these demands. In some countries the hospital imaging service also provides imaging services for referrals from outside the hospital, while in other countries much of this activity is provided in centres located outside hospitals either linked to or independent of the hospital departments. These centres may also provide services for "outpatient" imaging from specialists who work in office practice, notably in insurance- or private-based health care systems.

Workforce

There are two main clinical professions that deliver imaging in Europe: radiologists and radiographers.

A radiologist is a doctor who is also an imaging expert with special-ized training in obtaining and interpreting medical images. As mentioned already, radiologists can also treat diseases by minimally invasive, image-guided surgery (interventional radiology). Like other doctors, a radiologist must first qualify as a doctor from an accredited medical school and spend a variable period in clinical practice. Following this, they will undertake further postgraduate training before qualifying as a radiologist (usually for a further five years in most European countries).

A radiographer (or medical imaging technologist) is a trained health professional whose primary role is to produce medical images that assist radiologists and other doctors to diagnose or monitor a patient's injury or illness. In most European countries they have undergone training at degree level or equivalent followed by in-post further subspecialization. Some radiographers extend their role beyond that of image acquisition. This practice is more common in the United Kingdom than in most other European countries. Such activities include interpretation of ultrasound tests, mammography screening, and trauma plain film reporting.

Box 9.4 The four-tier radiographer structure in the United Kingdom

The United Kingdom is probably the most advanced European country in developing a career progression in its radiology workforce through the development of four tiers of radiographer training and professional development. These include:

- *Assistant practitioner* (not a trained radiographer): an assistant practitioner performs protocol-limited clinical tasks under the direction and supervision of a registered practitioner (radiographer).
- *Practitioner* (state registered, degree educated): a practitioner autonomously performs a wide-ranging and complex clinical role, and is accountable for his or her own actions and for the actions of those they direct.
- *Advanced practitioner* (state registered): an advanced practitioner, autonomous in clinical practice, defines the scope of practice of others and continuously develops clinical practice within a defined field.
- *Consultant practitioner* (state registered): a consultant practitioner provides clinical leadership within a specialism, bringing strategic direction.

A smaller workforce of nurses, health care assistants, and physicists as well as administrative and clerical roles supports these two professional groups. The development of PACS is creating a key role for IT support.

The legislative and regulatory framework varies, particularly with ultrasound. For example, in many countries (including the United Kingdom), radiologists have little involvement in performing and interpreting obstetric ultrasound. The obstetric ultrasonographers may be radiographers who have trained specifically in this practice, but may also be obstetricians and midwives.

A similar picture can be seen, to varying degrees, in other specialties where clinicians have acquired their own ultrasound equipment and provide a focused ultrasound service to support their specialty interest, e.g. urology, orthopaedics, or vascular surgery. This practice is most advanced in cardiology, where the cardiologists have developed their own expertise to acquire and interpret images as well as carry out interventional procedures under radiological guidance. In the United Kingdom, for instance, the term echocardiography refers to ultrasound of the heart and is usually performed within the cardiology department by separately trained technicians under the supervision of cardiologists, while cardiologists, rather than radiologists, often report CT and MRI of the heart and great vessels. This may be carried out on separate dedicated scanners in large centres, but more commonly the radiographers in the main imaging department acquire the images.

Existing barriers to delivering optimal imaging services

As the role of imaging has gained greater importance in health care, there is a real challenge to respond to the increased demand due to a number of factors, which has led to significant variation in the use of radiology in Member States across Europe. Figure 9.4 illustrates the variation in CT and MRI activity across Europe.

The following challenges and barriers are thought to be the major influences on the current usage and effectiveness of imaging in Europe.

Evidence-based access to imaging

It is difficult to draw conclusions from a comparison of imaging activity between different countries, as there is a lack of evidence to indicate what the appropriate level should be and this will anyway vary with patterns of disease. In France and the United Kingdom, for example, national societies have developed evidence-based guidelines to encourage referring doctors to use imaging appropriately. These guidelines have been adopted by a number of other European countries with varying effectiveness (Remedios et al., 2014; Royal College of Radiologists, 2016). The use of imaging tests involving radiation (CT, plain X-ray and nuclear medicine) is governed by European legislation in the form of the newly updated European Directive 2013/59/Euratom. This states, among other things, that all requests for such tests are "justified" by a responsible trained health care professional. The goal is to protect patients from unnecessary exposure to radiation. Despite this, there is evidence of an inappropriate over-usage of radiology in certain clinical situations. There is also likely to be overuse of MRI and ultrasound, although as these do not involve exposure to ionizing radiation, they are not governed by this regulation.

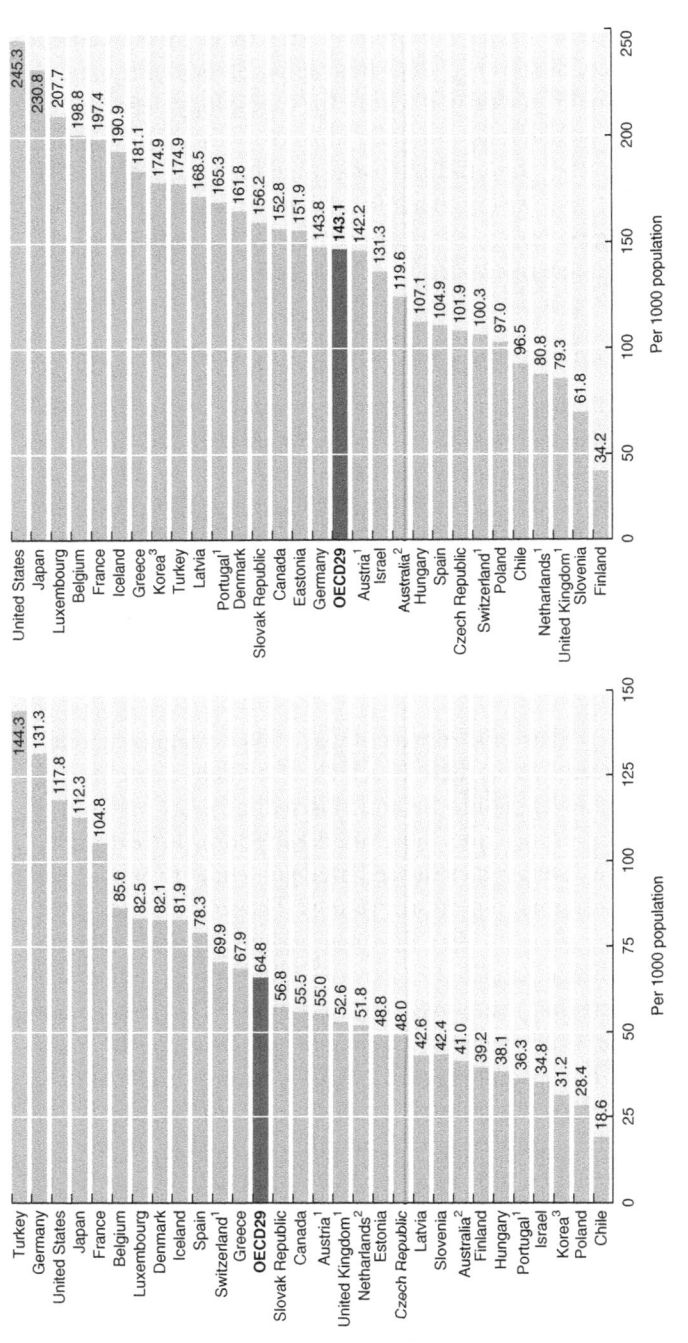

Figure 9.4 MRI and CT exams per 1000 population, 2015 (or nearest year)

Source: OECD (2018)

However, the concern does not just relate to possible over-usage of imaging. There is evidence suggesting the variation in cancer outcomes in Europe is partly due to variation in early access to imaging for diagnosis in suspected cancer.

Workforce issues

The marked growth in imaging activity in the last 10 years has been met with differing degrees of workforce expansion across Europe, but in most countries the increase in radiologists and to a lesser extent radiographers has lagged behind the growth in activity. The situation is most acute in those countries that started from a low base of radiologist per head of population. Figure 9.5 illustrates the variation in a number of European countries.

The situation with radiographers is not as acute, although in the United Kingdom, for instance, radiographers and ultrasonographers are included with radiologists on the government shortage occupational list for immigration purposes. This situation is mitigated somewhat by the United Kingdom approach to skill-mix, described earlier.

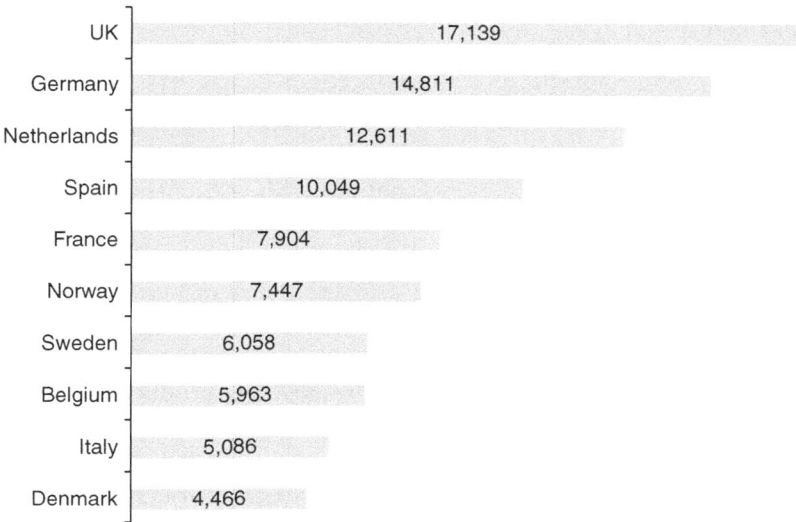

Figure 9.5 Number of inhabitants per radiologist, 2011 (including residents in training)

Source: Kamalasekar, 2011

This shortage of radiologists is further compounded by the fact that they have developed additional roles, for instance in interventional radiology, the performance of biopsy techniques, and in their role in the MDT mentioned earlier. A recent survey from the European Society of Radiology found that 58% (out of 31 respondents) reported having too few radiologists for their current needs and 55% (out of 30 respondents) replied that they would not have enough radiologists in training to serve their respective nations.

In addition, there has been a drive to subspecialization with the increasing complexity of imaging techniques. This is creating a real challenge, particularly in smaller hospitals/services where it is proving increasingly difficult to provide an expert specialized opinion over seven days a week, throughout the year. Networking between hospitals is seen as a partial solution to this.

Equipment

There is also considerable variation in the equipment base across Europe. This is illustrated in Figure 9.6, which compares the provision of CT and MRI scanners in a number of European countries and international comparators.

The international economic crisis has coincided with the recent rapid increase of imaging activity described earlier. This has significantly constrained the previous regular turnover of imaging equipment, resulting in a higher than usual amount of aged equipment, at a time when technological developments continue. This is leading to increasing levels of obsolescence.

This slow-down in equipment replacement is not only the direct result of shrinking budgets, but also the consequence of adaptive strategies leading to better use of resources. Radiology, based on highly technical hardware and diagnostic pathways, offers a fertile ground for workflow standardization resulting in productivity gains. Efficiency plans focus on a variety of measures including: merging of departments/hospitals, sharing of equipment, closing down excess capacity, policies for equipment upgrade, patient throughput optimization, and extension of opening hours. New equipment often offers improved imaging quality and reduced radiation exposure, due to the improvement of X-ray technology or to the substitution of non-ionizing technologies (e.g. MRI).

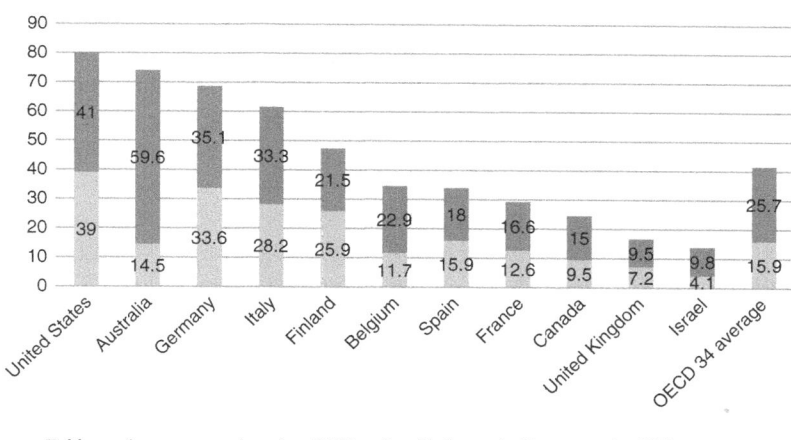

Magnetic resonance imaging (MRI) units ■ Computed tomography (CT) scanners

Figure 9.6 Scanner equipment per million people in selected OECD countries, 2015 (or nearest year)

Source: OECD (2018)

Funding issues

Within Europe, there are many different types of funding models for health care, mostly based on revenues from taxation or social insurance. There is also great diversity in how imaging is reimbursed. However, in the current economic climate, many facilities have faced substantial budgetary pressures, forcing reorganization of facilities, staffing arrangements, and equipment.

The reduction in budgets for radiology departments can give rise to a biphasic effect on volumes within a fee-for-service model. There can be an initial tendency to increase the volumes to compensate for the reduction in revenues resulting from the reduced procedural reimbursements, followed by a trend to reduce the volume of procedures requested, due to the attention paid to appropriateness.

In systems where there are global budgets, there is a tendency to increased utilization of low-cost techniques, such as ultrasound and plain radiography, to attempt to substitute for the higher costs of higher tech procedures, such as MRI and CT. This is one of the explanations for the disproportionate place of ultrasound and radiography in some countries, in comparison with more sophisticated imaging techniques.

Organizational constraints

As mentioned previously, there are varying models of imaging provision, which are influenced by a number of national and local drivers. The traditional model is that of imaging departments as part of an acute hospital and from this central base services are provided to the hospital and local community in terms of access to primary care requests. This has the advantage of centralization of high-cost equipment and skilled staff. However, the disadvantages include poor access for non-hospital patients and dealing with the competing agendas of acute/emergency care and planned/community care through one department. In many countries alternatives to this model have developed, ranging from provision of ultrasound services in primary care facilities, through mobile ultrasound, X-ray, CT and MRI services, to fully comprehensive planned care diagnostic centres (non-emergency) offering a full range of imaging services often alongside other health care activities (e.g. laboratory testing, consultation rooms, day-case procedures).

Hospital design and imaging service location

A key constraint to providing appropriate, responsive imaging services within a hospital is the location and design of the imaging department. Historically, the imaging department has usually been in one location with the possible exception of A&E, where there was provision for plain X-ray examinations.

As the role of imaging has developed as an integral part of the examination of the patient, the need to co-locate imaging equipment with certain clinical services has become essential. This can be solved relatively easily in the case of ultrasound but, in the absence of a new building, the relocation of MRI and CT scanners provides a considerable challenge. This is not just due to the problem of finding an appropriate space but is compounded by the specific radiation protection considerations for CT and equivalent safety considerations for MRI with its high magnetic field.

CT scanning should now be an integral service within an emergency department to deal with conditions such as acute trauma and stroke. In addition, as most inpatient scanning occurs within the first few hours of admission, it makes sense from both a patient-centred and efficiency approach to locate ultrasound, CT and MRI close to the admissions unit.

The problem is that many hospitals do not have a centralized admissions function and therefore the challenge of delivering this approach is often too great. This results in considerable movement of patients around the hospital, which at best results in a poor experience for the patients and at worst can delay management and in some situations raise safety issues.

There are similar drivers of patient-centredness and efficiency within the outpatient setting with an impetus to offer one-stop clinics, which include consultation, investigations, and sometimes treatment in one visit. Thus in certain specialties that are high users of diagnostics (e.g. orthopaedics, gastroenterology, gynaecology), it makes sense to ensure that imaging facilities are either in the clinic area or adjacent to it.

This need for co-location creates the challenge of ensuring an appropriate level of staffing for such equipment. To a certain extent the development of PACS has solved this problem for radiologist support, but there can still be considerable challenges for radiographer and technologist staffing with potential for redundancy of scanning time.

The future of imaging services

There is no evidence that the current increase in demand for imaging services is likely to reduce in the next five years. Recent work commissioned by Cancer Research UK suggests that the current increase in demand for CT, MRI and ultrasound will continue at the current rates (Cancer Research UK, 2015). Although there is less reliance on plain X-rays in certain areas of medicine, trauma and orthopaedics will continue to rely on skeletal plain films while the chest X-ray is unlikely to reduce in usage.

Research into the effectiveness of screening in ovarian and lung cancer will shortly be published. It is likely that this will suggest the introduction of screening programmes for at-risk patients. In lung cancer this would result in a further marked increase in CT of the chest.

One of the limiting factors to the expansion of the use of CT has been the risk of repeated radiation exposure, but the new generation of scanners has markedly reduced radiation levels. This is one of the drivers behind calls to evaluate lung cancer screening programmes and is likely to increase the use of CT in other presentations.

The usage of PET-CT will further increase in the next five years, predominantly in the area of cancer management, but the role of fusion imaging is likely to expand beyond cancer. One such area of expansion appears to be in neurological conditions, particularly dementia. Other forms of molecular imaging are most likely to remain as research tools in the next five years with no immediate plans for widespread use in clinical practice.

The scope of interventional radiology continues to expand. A proportion of IR has focused in the area of vascular disease. This will continue to expand with further applications in areas such as thrombectomy in the treatment of acute stroke. There is also likely to be a further major expansion in the use of interventional image-guided therapy in cancer care. This will extend beyond its established use in symptomatic relief and palliation. There are already a number of indications for its primary use in treatment (e.g. neo-adjuvant embolization, image-guided ablation and brachytherapy, trans-arterial chemo-embolization (TACE), selective internal radiation therapy (SIRT), and isolated perfusion chemotherapy).

The implication of current and future developments in imaging for the organization, management and design of the hospital in the mid-21st century

Although some of the functions of hospitals may change in the future, the management of emergency and urgent care will remain their primary focus. Imaging will continue to play a vital role in supporting this activity, with an increasing reliance on CT particularly for trauma and the acutely ill patient.

It is therefore important that the planning of imaging facilities is part of any planning of new emergency and admission departments in order to deliver timely, safe and efficient services. Imaging will also be required in high dependency areas such as intensive therapy units, high dependency units and certain wards. Thus, great thought needs to be put into hospital design to avoid inappropriate siting or unnecessary duplication of imaging facilities with resultant unnecessary redundancies.

It is likely, therefore, that imaging will no longer be housed in one department and consideration will need to be made in terms of staffing, particularly in facilities that need to be accessible 24/7. With the challenges of workforce supply, described earlier, it is essential that the efficient flow of patients through imaging is a key consideration in hospital design.

The challenge that imaging departments face in balancing the demands of emergency and urgent care with planned care could be addressed, but this is dependent on two main factors. The first of these relates to the future role of the acute hospital in dealing with planned care, particularly in the form of outpatient facilities. If these remain on the main hospital site, then there will need to be imaging provision alongside them, particularly where the concept of the one-stop visit is to be achieved.

The second factor is the demand for access to imaging from primary care. In this situation there is no need for the patient to attend the hospital and in fact there are definite advantages both to the patient and to the hospital if such visits can be avoided. This could be achieved by further development of imaging services outside hospitals. To make these cost-effective, they may need to be centralized in diagnostic centres for modalities such as CT and MRI, while ultrasound could potentially be delivered in GP surgeries if there is appropriate demand.

If such diagnostic centres were to be developed, they would also have the potential to provide an alternative facility for hospital outpatients, particularly if the diagnostic centres had facilities for consultations and minor procedures.

All hospitals that deal with emergency and acutely ill patients need access to interventional radiology. As with radiology, this must be available 24/7. Although the emergency work will require inpatient beds with full clinical support, there will also be a demand for planned procedures which can be performed on a day-case basis. Consequently, a facility that can deliver this should be located adjacent to the interventional suite. Although all hospital emergency Should this be 'hospital emergency departments' or 'hospital emergency patients'? and inpatients will need access to interventional radiology services, it is unlikely that all acute hospitals of the future will have enough demand for such work to justify their own comprehensive funded service. The solution to this will be the development of various forms of network where either the patient is transferred to the experts (or possibly the experts travel between hospitals).

For radiology to continue to play a key role in health care it must be able to respond to the workforce needs and therefore adequate provision must be made for education and training.

Likewise for imaging to continue to develop and support health care in the future, adequate provision and funding of research involving imaging is essential and this is likely to be concentrated in larger hospitals. The provision of imaging is essential to much of medical research, particularly in the monitoring of new therapies. However, there is a need to carry out primary imaging research if the true potential of new technologies is to be achieved.

At present the radiology department remains predominantly the domain of the radiologist, but this is changing and there is no specific reason why other clinical specialists trained in imaging should not use imaging facilities (if possessing appropriate skills). If the case for this is established, then a coordinated imaging resource is far preferable to the growth of isolated services often with unused capacity and challenges of equality of access.

The opportunities and barriers to making this vision of the future a reality

As imaging continues to develop, it will remain heavily dependent on appropriate levels of workforce and equipment, but IT solutions have the potential to improve the efficiency of services. There are already electronic requesting systems in existence that are linked to evidence-based resources to aid the clinician in requesting the most appropriate test first time and avoiding unnecessary investigations and delays.

There is considerable interest and research into the use of artificial intelligence (AI) in the interpretation of imaging investigations. Although this is not yet at the stage of routine practice, it is likely that this will prove significant and may eventually substitute for radiologists in certain investigations.

As radiology increases in its complexity, it will be even more challenging for every hospital imaging department to employ enough radiologists to provide a comprehensive service throughout the week. One partial solution to this is the provision of efficient comprehensive PACS systems. This opens up options for transferring images in real time to radiologists outside the acquiring hospital. If used appropriately, this can facilitate the development of networks of expertise, which will support smaller hospitals and enable them to provide appropriate comprehensive services in a timely fashion. This can be particularly effective in the emergency situation, avoiding onerous rotas for small numbers of radiologists. An example where PACS can be used to provide support to such hospitals is that commonly seen in neuroradiology where a hub and spoke model often exists, with neuroradiologists supporting local radiologists with second opinions. There are also examples of network solutions where a group of subspecialized radiologists provide a service across a number of hospitals. In the emergency situation services now exist that offer radiologist reporting "out of hours", removing the need for onerous on-call rotas for the local radiologists.

These solutions will not overcome the need for a significant increase in the radiologist workforce, but will help to ensure the effective use of radiologists.

There is an obvious need for this subspecialization radiological expertise within the hospital setting to provide expertise to the various clinical specialties that imaging supports. However, a great deal of radiology provision to primary care is of a relatively general nature and it will be important that adequate expertise remains to deal with this relatively large workload in a timely manner. Thus it will be important that radiology departments ensure that the development of subspecialization does not leave this important element of their work under-provided for. This is an area where the extended role of the radiographer may be a solution in some areas, particularly in the interpretation of the plain X-ray and in the performing and reporting of general ultrasound by sonographers. Some of their current work may be replaced by non-radiographer technologists working under their supervision.

Another challenge already mentioned is appropriate levels of imaging equipment. As there will be an increase in competition for space in existing hospitals, PACS also offers the solution to consider locating imaging equipment off the main site. This equipment, if sited effectively, could give better access to patients who do not require hospital facilities (e.g. outpatients and primary care patients). By decanting this work off the main site, it could have the added benefit of improving efficiencies in delivering inpatient imaging support.

Another issue to be considered, particularly in cross-sectional imaging (CT and MRI), is the increase in obesity in the European population. This has added another challenge to manufacturers who now have to consider increasing both the size of the machines and their weight limitations to accommodate the increasing number of patients who would not physically fit in the traditional scanners.

Finally, whatever innovative solutions are explored, these will not be effective unless an appropriate funding system is in place. This is obviously challenging in the current economic climate; however, there is no doubt that inadequate or inappropriate funding mechanisms have the potential to significantly hold back the effective use of imaging in the hospital of the future. It has to be realized that in many circumstances effective imaging services will deliver higher quality health care with efficiency savings elsewhere in the system, for example in reduced length of stay, avoidance of hospital admission, and reduction of unnecessary outpatient appointments.

Thus, it is essential that imaging services are an integral part of the planning of the hospital of the future to ensure that resources are used effectively and the potential improvements in both quality and efficiency of patient care are realized.

References

Cancer Research UK (2015). *Horizon Scanning – an evaluation of imaging capacity across the NHS in England.* Written by 2020 Delivery. Available at: https://www.cancerresearchuk.org/sites/default/files/horizon_scanning_-_final.pdf (accessed 26 September 2016).

Coory M et al. (2008). Systematic review of multidisciplinary teams in the management of lung cancer. *Lung Cancer*, 60:14–21.

Independent Cancer Task Force (2015). *Achieving World Class Cancer outcomes – a Strategy for England 2015–2020.* Available at: www.cancerresearchuk .org/sites/default/files/achieving_world-class_cancer_outcomes_-_a_strategy_for_england_2015–2020.pdf (accessed 26 September 2016).

Kamalasekar S. (2011). *Teleradiology – An Integral Part of eHealth Agenda in Europe.* Frost & Sullivan.

Morris E et al. (2006). The impact of the Calman-Hine report on the processes and outcomes of care for Yorkshire's colorectal cancer patients. *Br J Cancer*, 95:979–85.

NHS England Annual Imaging and Radiodiagnostics Data (2014). Web page. Available at: https://www.england.nhs.uk/statistics/statistical-work-areas/diagnostics-waiting-times-and-activity/imaging-and-radiodiagnostics-annual-data/ (accessed 10 March 2015).

OECD (2018) *Health at a Glance 2017.* Available at: https://www.oecd-ilibrary.org/social-issues-migration-health/health-at-a-glance-2017_health_glance-2017-en (accessed 20 September 2018).

Remedios D et al. (2014). European survey on imaging referral guidelines. *Insights Imaging*, 5(1):15–23. doi: 10.1007/s13244-013-0300-6.

Royal College of Radiologists (2012). *Investing in the clinical radiology workforce – the quality and efficiency case.* Available at: https://www.rcr .ac.uk/sites/default/files/RCR_CRWorkforce_June2012.pdf (accessed 26 January 2020).

Royal College of Radiologists (2014). *Investing in the interventional radiology workforce: the quality and efficiency case.* Available at: https://www.rcr .ac.uk/publication/investing-interventional-radiology-workforce-quality-and-efficiency-case (accessed 26 January 2020).

Royal College of Radiologists (2016). *About iRefer.* Web page. Available at: https://www.rcr.ac.uk/clinical-radiology/being-consultant/rcr-referral-guidelines/about-irefer (accessed 26 September 2016).

Stephens MR et al. (2006). Multidisciplinary team management is associated with improved outcomes after surgery for esophageal cancer. *Dis Esophagus,* 19:164–71.

10 | *Advances in laboratory medicine*

RACHAEL LIEBMANN[1], DIGBY INGLE[2]

[1] Consultant Histopathologist, Queen Victoria Hospital
NHS Foundation Trust; Vice President, Royal College of
Pathologists,United Kingdom
[2] Former Regional Coordination Manager, Royal College of
Pathologists

Acknowledgements

Dr Niall Swan, Faculty of Pathology, Royal College of Physicians, whose presentation slides helped script the National Framework for Quality Assurance in Cellular Pathology Case Study.

Professor Tim Helliwell, Consultant Histopathologist and Clinical Director for Cellular Pathology, Liverpool Clinical Laboratories, Royal Liverpool University Hospital, for writing the Genomics Case Study.

Angus Turnbull, Medical Student, Imperial College London, and Dr Michael Osborn, Consultant Histopathologist, Imperial College & Imperial College Healthcare NHS Trust, Department of Cellular Pathology, for co-writing the Decline of Consented Autopsy Following Hospital Death in Europe Autopsy Case Study.

Introduction

Advances in laboratory medicine are happening at an uneven rate. On the one hand there has been a rapid expansion in innovative rapid molecular diagnostic techniques, but on the other hand translation into clinical impact has often been slow. Pathology services in many parts of Europe are undergoing modernization and reform but in some places this can be slow and patchy.

In this chapter, the terms pathology and laboratory medicine are used as synonyms to indicate cellular pathology, microbiology, virology, chemical pathology, immunology and haematology, molecular pathology, genetics and histocompatibility, and other laboratory-based medical specialties. As important as it is diverse, pathology is poised to become a key medical specialty, central to the development of stratified and personalized medicine, but it needs to overcome several challenges, not least the huge increase in complexity of tests, demand for digital data, the expectation of ever-reducing test costs, and shortages of trained staff. These issues as they impact upon European pathology are outlined with some specific national case studies.

The points below illustrate some of the emerging trends:

- **An unprecedented velocity of technological advance.** Pathology services will continue to lead the transformation of medical care through, for example, genomics, proteomics, tandem mass spectrometry, and microarrays. These advances will have significant impact not only in the delivery of diagnostic and therapeutic services, but also in the workflow and ethos of patient care. Advances in technology, however, come at increased costs to organizations and health care consumers.

- **Self-testing and near-patient testing will proliferate.** In parallel with advances in large-scale technology within laboratories there will be a proliferation in self-testing and single use devices to perform pathology tests outside the laboratory. The accuracy and reliability of these devices need to be vigorously examined, and capturing and storing the data generated by these devices might be problematic. There is a need to coordinate results from self-testing and point-of-care devices with the results from formal laboratories. The increased use of "wearable IT" with a health care purpose will raise expectations for seamless transmission of information to and from patients, and primary and secondary care providers, including pathologists. However, these devices, part of the "Internet of things", raise concerns about data security, including both unauthorized access and commercial exploitation by software providers. Resolution of the confidentiality, privacy and security concerns will be led by patient or consumer demand.

- **Increasing collaboration and partnership is key.** Greater interdisciplinary contact within medical specialties and subspecialties and between organizations is an inevitable consequence of the requirement to ensure high quality. For example, an integrated diagnostic service between pathologists and radiologists could speed up diagnoses, increase accuracy, and improve patient outcomes. Ensuring that pathology services are adjacent to clinical teams will be important to minimize risks to patients, but there is a need to understand better the options for remote working arising from videoconferencing and telepathology so that the right balance is achieved between clinical adjacencies, reducing unnecessary specimen transport, and achieving economies of scale.

- **Digital pathology is a disruptive technology.** This development has great potential to make pathologists' working lives more efficient, facilitate intra- and inter-departmental consultations, improve the efficiency and documentation of research, and enhance education and training. However, the adoption of digital pathology requires resolution of some longstanding issues. The time taken to scan slides, the significant storage required for the images, the capital cost of slide scanners and the variable costs associated with storage space, and sufficient data security will all need to be addressed as a priority.

- **The laboratory is a translational environment.** For example, as clinical genomics moves from research to a routine diagnostic, prognostic and predictive method, this presents numerous challenges in terms of sample processing, quality control, and service developments in management and reporting. The knowledge base of pathologists trained and experienced in traditional methods will be tested by the need to provide and interpret the new reports. It is difficult for established pathologists, mostly based in traditional laboratories that do not provide the new tests, to add interpretation of these new tests to their repertoire. This may well require a new approach to learning which can integrate knowledge of clinical genomics into everyday practice. The implementation of new technologies tends to follow the Gartner Hype Cycle (Figure 10.1).

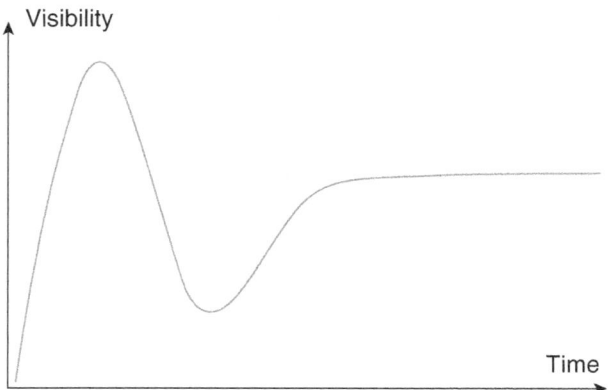

Figure 10.1 Gartner Hype Cycle

Source: Gartner, 2015

What do these advances mean for the role of the hospital in the future?

Laboratory medicine is the bridge between analysis and interpretation of clinical data and care delivery. Pathologists order, conduct, and interpret the results of hundreds of individual tests to support clinical decisions that enable good patient care. The laboratory's role as a centre of diagnostics within the hospital of the future, however, may need to be redefined in the light of pressures for cost efficiencies, greater effectiveness and improved performance, and the impact of emerging technologies.

A common theme in European pathology is the quest for greater efficiency. In this respect, laboratories have looked towards increased automation to improve productivity and meet increased demand. Automation of the laboratory can lead to better task integration and quicker turnaround times. The argument follows that patients benefit as quicker clinical decisions can be made with the potential to shorten hospital stays.

Across Europe the modern laboratory environment is increasingly being organized to create networks based on large consolidated centres (hubs) and smaller local testing centres (spokes). A key driver for service reconfiguration has been cost pressures. In some countries laboratories face a bleak ultimatum: restructure or lose all your work. The key question, as Lord Carter put it in his Review of NHS Pathology Services in England (Carter et al., 2008), "What is the right level of consolidation?"

Another driver for change is the desire to reduce variation of diagnostic tests across countries both in test investigation costs and the over/under-requesting of tests. The United Kingdom Atlas of Variation, for example, shows that cancer patients who received an early-stage diagnosis – a critical factor in treatment outcome – ranged from 22.7% to 60.8% between the United Kingdom's best- and worst-performing areas (Public Health England, 2015).

Major advances in diagnostic laboratory medicine may be disruptive, as technical advances have the potential to provide a more efficient and cost-effective pathology service. For example, molecular diagnostic technologies are being utilized in a wide range of medical specialties including genetics, infectious disease, oncology and haematology. Their advantages have been well documented and allow for the simultaneous sequencing of many millions of individual DNA molecules. Using this technology, pathologists and researchers are provided with increased sensitivity and specificity for the detection of abnormal DNA in solid tissues and body fluids, as well as a wide range of metabolites and signalling molecules and immune system responses to drug therapies. Technological innovation in pathology appears to be accelerating the paradigm shift to precision or stratified medicine, an approach that takes into account individual variability in genes, environment, and lifestyle for each person.

A plethora of other technological advances are impacting on the pathology laboratory, including liquid and gas chromatography and plasma mass spectrometry, conventional and next-generation sequencing, point-of-care testing (POCT) and "lab-on-chip" devices prompted by miniaturization of molecular assay steps, biochips and microfluidics, and digital pathology systems which allow the scanning, imaging, and storage of histological slide data for analysis by pathologists.

The adoption of these emerging technologies across Europe, however, is varied and this is a fundamental challenge for pathology. The impact of new technologies on the hospital in the future will be difficult to predict but tough to ignore in terms of investment decisions. Technology has provided pathology with a unifying narrative and the vision of the laboratory as an aggregate of preventative, diagnostic, predictive, prognostic, and interpretative roles will become key to the development of the future hospital.

Some of the reasons for varied adoption or "technology diffusion" include: length of time the technology has been available; a hospital's culture of embracing innovation (e.g. a large teaching hospital may find it easier to adopt new technologies because a translational research culture pervades); at national level there could be incentives and a supportive infrastructure to speed up the rate of adoption – or conversely nothing at all; it could be that some hospitals are simply better at measuring the impact of technology adoption in terms of patient health outcomes; in the case of POCT diagnostics, it is often the case that costs are accrued in a different area from the gains. The Review on Antimicrobial Resistance (2015) provides an example where a primary care facility may invest in a diagnostic device that could reduce the number of hospital admissions. While this is desirable, the costs saved are not only hard to quantify, but the money saved might not be passed on to the facility even though it has paid for the test.

Pathology departments are increasingly presented with opportunities to form translational research networks within hospitals, universities and biomedical research centres, and with industry. Several laboratories do not have the organizational resilience to translate research technologies to a clinical environment. In turn, this may prompt the need for new workforce capabilities aligned to the most desired patient outcomes within each European country.

As an endpoint, there is growing evidence to support the emergence of "population health systems" as a means of meeting future health care needs. A population health system is defined by the American-based Institute for Healthcare Improvement (2015) as a framework for improving patient experience, improving the health of populations, and reducing the costs of health care. Approaches to population health have long been enshrined in many tax-financed health care systems, forming the basis of the purchaser/provider split in the United Kingdom, Italy and some other countries since the 1990s, and in Scandinavian countries where health care is organized by local government, but are now gaining increased traction in other parts of Europe, as identified by the United Kingdom King's Fund (Alderwick, Ham & Buck, 2015). The Kaiser Permanente model in America is often seen as a prime innovator in this regard. Making the shift towards effective population health commissioning will require collaboration across a range of sectors and wider communities and may intensify further change for the pathology laboratory in the hospital of the future.

Box 10.1 Case Study – Genomics England and the 100 000 Genomes Project

Context

- Whole genome sequencing technology is sufficiently advanced to rapidly provide vast amounts of information on the nature of diseases and predisposing factors.
- The technology is likely to impact on the delivery of a wide range of health care services, from inherited diseases, through infections, to cancer.

Challenges

- By 2017 to sequence 100 000 genomes from NHS patients with rare diseases (and their families) and those with cancer.
- To link genome sequences with high quality clinical and pathological information.

Box 10.1 (cont.)

- To accelerate the availability and uptake of advanced genomic practice into the NHS through better diagnostics, devices, and treatments.
- To improve public understanding and support for genomic medicine.

Responses

- Genomics England Limited created to drive the project, to inform training, and to develop partnerships with industry.
- Eleven Genomics Medicine Centres created in 2014/15 with the remit to deliver against a specification and under strict performance management.

Achievements to date

- Detailed protocols with research standards for the identification and recruitment of patients and families, sample collection and processing, and the validation of results and feedback of information to participants.
- NHS Genomic Medicine Centres have developed local partnerships with the public, patients, and a range of local NHS organizations and universities.
- Laboratory processes underpinned by an external quality assurance scheme.
- The information technology required to support this complex process has been developed and implemented locally so that data collection is efficient and comprehensive. Data are transmitted securely to a central data hub.
- Recruitment of patients and families to the rare diseases pathway started in April 2015.
- Recruitment of patients to the cancer pathway began in September 2015.
- Genomics England Clinical Interpretation Partnerships have been created as topic-specific groups of clinicians and researchers from universities and the NHS to analyse the data from the project. These will be integral to helping front-line clinicians and pathologists formulate the genomic data useful for managing patients in the context of personalized medicine.

Source: Written by Tim Helliwell with information from Genomics England, 2015

Where does pathology sit within wider hospital activity?

Pathology is the largest diagnostic service in hospitals as measured by the number of requests it responds to annually, in expenditure, and in the proportion of clinical decisions it affects. For example, in the United Kingdom over 50% of biochemical tests are related to chronic disease management and pathology is involved in 70% of all diagnoses made in the NHS (Right Care, 2011). Pathology is part of the clinical governance of public hospitals and the wider health system, playing an important role in monitoring and managing disease, infectious agents, and public health.

The development of subspecialties in pathology is well developed to meet the needs of patients: cytopathology, dermatopathology, chemical pathology, haematology, medical microbiology, virology, endocrine pathology, forensic pathology, immunology, cytogenetics, blood transfusion, neuropathology, ophthalmic pathology, to name but a few. However, these subspecialties are not uniform across Europe.

Depending on the urgency of tests, pathology investigations can take place in what are often termed "hot" or "cold" laboratories. Hot laboratories process pathology tests requiring a fast turnaround and clinical support. Cold laboratories process less-urgent high volumes of routine tests. Because there is less urgency to receive the results of these tests, cold laboratories can be located further away from the patient. As the technical complexity of test methods increases, so does the complexity of reporting.

Pathology services are closely integrated with other clinical services, to support patient care by providing information and expertise to facilitate diagnosis and treatment decision-making. This is particularly true with cancer, a disease process whose complexity is increasingly recognized, with a detailed understanding of the pathological characteristics essential for targeted treatment. The complex pathway undertaken by what might appear superficially to be the simple process of taking a tissue biopsy is set out graphically in an illustrated web page: http://www.journeyofatissuebiopsy.com

Adjacency to clinical teams is important if pathology is to be integrated as a valued "companion diagnostic" and to move away from having a passive service role to taking on an active one. Adjacency to molecular diagnostic centres will also become important in order to benefit from genomic (gene expression), proteomic (protein expression) and metabolomic (metabolite profile) data and to hasten the shift to personalized medicine.

Pathologists are core members of MDTs and provide essential inputs for patient management. Laboratories are used to working across primary and secondary care organizations and will often serve several secondary and tertiary care providers. Providers of pathology services in public hospitals also play a leading role in the education and training of pathologists, clinical scientists and researchers. They are increasingly required to provide specialist input for translational research including involvement with clinical trials and evaluation of new technologies.

The wider and extended role of pathology is demonstrated by the range of other clinical services provided, which includes:

- specialist information and advice to health care professionals in primary and secondary care as well as public health
- mandatory surveillance of disease
- infection prevention and control
- guidance and advice, quality assurance and support for POCT in a range of hospital settings (e.g. outpatient clinics)
- specialist advice on blood transfusion
- mortuary services, including post-mortem examinations.

Box 10.2 Case Study – a national framework for quality assurance in cellular pathology

The Irish National Cancer Control Programme

Context

- Irish population = 4.5 million.
- 23 000 new cases of cancer annually.
- 7500 cancer-related deaths annually.

Challenges

- Projected doubling of new cases by 2020.
- High-profile cancer misdiagnosis cases in 2007 and 2008.
- National histopathology workload increasing each year.

Box 10.2 (cont.)

- No formal measures to assure the public that pathologists practise to the highest international standards.
- No national standards or benchmarks for key aspects of diagnostic service.

Responses

- Development of a National Quality Improvement Programme within each Irish pathology department to review performance routinely and drive improvement against intelligent targets.
- Programme initiated in 2008 with strong collaborative commitment from Irish Health Service Executive Quality Improvement, Service Management and Information and Communication Technology Divisions, National Cancer Control Programme, Independent Hospitals Association of Ireland, Department of Health and Faculty of Pathology, Royal College of Physicians of Ireland.

Achievements to date

- A unique national programme across: 27 public and 7 private laboratories; 8 different laboratory information systems; and small and large hospitals with different levels of resourcing.
- Robust clinical governance including monitoring and key indicator reviews.
- Development of a central repository National Quality Assurance Intelligence System for Histopathology.
- Collection of national data for histopathology which has never before collected on this scale.
- Confidence in the data to understand in real time workload and extent of quality activities.
- Ability to set national targets based on accurate and locally owned data.

Source: Swan, 2015

How does pathology link with services located outside the hospital?

The interface between pathology and services located outside the hospital is well established but may not be well understood. The health care services based outside hospitals are described as primary and community care sectors, which lie between self-care and hospital care. Hospital pathology has a long history of working with outside services (i.e. primary care doctor practices and health clinics).

In Europe primary care differs considerably and several categories of organization exist. Meads (2009) provides a valuable typology of primary care organizations in Europe. To add to the complexity, European countries will have different arrangements for registration with a primary care doctor or GP. This may be financially encouraged, compulsory, voluntary or free.

Pathology is a touch point across the patient's lifecycle from pre-natal to post-mortem. The diagram below illustrates where pathology sits regarding screening, diagnostic, and monitoring functions.

Laboratories are often located in or near hospitals to meet demand for a 24/7 service. Many hospital departments are highly pathology-dependent and need to respond rapidly to the clinical needs of busy emergency medicine departments and intensive care units. This means that extensive networks of transport, IT and management links between laboratories have evolved outside the hospital to provide quick turn-around times for tests and equitable access to services over defined geographical areas.

There is also the wider reach of pathology services and diagnostic products into local populations. "Smart pathology" is emerging in the

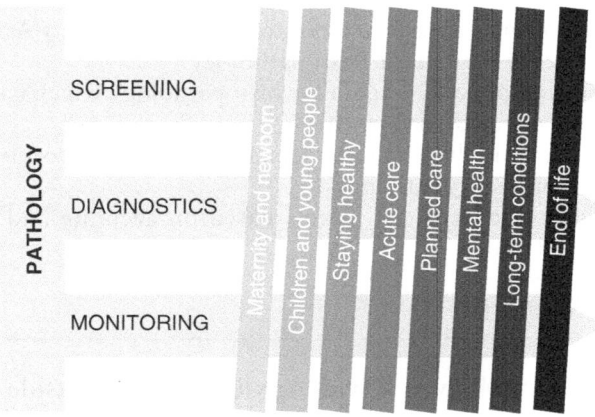

Figure 10.2 Pathology touch points

Source: NHS England National Pathology Programme, 2014

form of new-generation POCT devices. The availability and use of these have steadily increased in Europe. They have been used in primary care, diabetic and sexual health clinics, and care homes for over 40 years, but are now being assimilated into high street retail outlets as well as the home. The rapid test turnaround time provided by POCT potentially allows for accelerated identification and classification of patients into high-risk and low-risk groups (Larsson, Greig-Pylypczuk & Huisman, 2015). There are, however, regulatory and quality assurance challenges which need to be overcome. The proliferation of so many additional users and devices in operation make the maintenance of acceptable quality levels problematic (St John & Price, 2014).

The future relationship between hospital pathology and primary care needs to be shaped by value expectations and whether value of service can be demonstrated through improved patient outcomes and managed costs. Insights could also be gleaned as to how a laboratory could better manage demand on its services and how this might benefit the local health community. Some examples could include the use of data for comparing testing rates to emergency admissions, number of tests requested, length of hospital stay, and cost of emergency readmissions for relevant conditions.

An example of this type of work was the INvestigation of ThE Root Causes of Excessive RepliCatE Pathology Testing (INTERCEPT) study, which involved over 115 000 patients from North Staffordshire, England, and aimed to reduce the burden of unnecessary pathology requesting. It used HbA1c testing (a test for monitoring blood sugar control in people with diabetes) as a model by assessing adherence to national guidelines and recommendations for retesting intervals. Results from the study found over half of key blood test requests from doctors for patients with diabetes were inappropriate and that guidance on monitoring diabetes patients was not being followed by the majority of primary care and hospital doctors. Further work by this research team found major incentives to establish systems that provided timely HbA1c tests in terms of fewer diabetes-related emergency admissions per 1000 patients, fewer hospital bed days, and reduced costs of emergency admissions for diabetes-related illnesses (Driskell et al., 2012).

The key message for health commissioners and policy-makers is that primary care engagement with pathology professionals and wider use of this type of data can change requesting behaviour and produce better patient outcomes.

The pathology workforce

Pathology is a combination of medically trained pathologists, clinical scientists and biomedical scientists together with essential support from staff occupying a wide range of laboratory roles. Each European country uses different pathology specialty taxonomies. The European Union of Medical Specialists identifies 43 specialist sections, with the sections relevant to pathology including clinical genetics, infectious diseases, laboratory medicine, medical biopathology, medical microbiology, and pathology. The workforce is therefore extensive and heterogeneous in its composition.

Across Europe demand for diagnostic services continues to rise year on year both in terms of the number of samples and the increasing complexity of test requests. This puts considerable pressure on the workforce as the emergence of new tests steadily drives up case volume. Europe's ageing population and the increased incidence of cancer, chronic diseases, and other co-morbidities continue to add pressure.

Advances made in molecular-based diagnostics offer new approaches and the number of variants generated that have as yet unknown medical significance will require clinical interpretative support. Since the time of Hippocrates all medicine has been "personalized" at the point of diagnosis and treatment, but genomics and molecular-based diagnostics bring the potential for personalized prevention strategies based on the inherent likelihood of future disease for each individual. Also these new technologies will require the monitoring of the effects of ever more complex individually tailored drug treatments. Technologies that are part of molecular diagnostics are far reaching and rapidly being developed for genetic testing, infectious diseases testing, blood screening, oncology testing, cardiovascular testing, and others. Continued growth is expected. It is anticipated that a constant stream of test kits for the newest molecular targets will become commercially available requiring pathology staff to expand their understanding of these techniques to provide the services and interpret the results. Far from being replaced by new technology, it seems likely that demand for most "traditional" pathology tests will increase due to increased uptake of molecular-based diagnostics. This must be borne in mind when considering workforce requirements.

Pathologists now perform complex investigations to determine the phenotype, prognosis and likely response to treatment of a variety of diseases. The potential clinical significance of these data frequently cannot be encompassed in simple reports but require detailed interpretation and simultaneous communication to clinicians and to patients in order that appropriate management strategies might be formulated, agreed, and reviewed as response to treatment becomes apparent. There will be a need for pathologists to provide more interpretative and advisory services directly to patients as they obtain the right to access their own results directly. Pathologists increasingly find themselves making significant and important contributions as to how diagnostic testing can improve the whole patient pathway. This may include guidance, explanation, and interpretation provided to other health care professionals less able to deal with the complexity of modern diagnostic medicine.

Chemical pathologists, as a direct consequence of the increasing prevalence of diabetes, obesity, and lipid disorders, are pivotally involved in the provision of direct specialist patient care. This will inevitably lead to more involvement in community provision of pathology services and the support of patients to reduce morbidity. As microbiologists, haematologists, and biochemists become more clinically involved in providing direct patient-facing care, they have less time available to provide traditional laboratory oversight. The oversight of laboratory services is intrinsically linked to the quality of the service provided and to patient outcomes and so the importance of external quality assurance monitoring will increase.

The increasing use and dependency on POCT will continue to expand, not just in primary and secondary care, but also in the high street and in patients' homes. There will be vital input required from pathology professionals to ensure that the technical aspects of such POCT is carried out to an adequate quality-assured standard in the correct clinical context.

Pathologists make significant contributions to research, both directly via their own research activity, but also by providing essential and important collaboration and diagnostic support to many other studies and trials. However, a worrying trend in some European countries is the demise of clinical research roles in pathology.

Scientific and medical staffing levels in pathology services are declining in most countries and a detailed analysis of the workforce crisis in the United Kingdom in relation to cancer services is highlighted in a Nuffield Trust report (Imison, Castle-Clarke & Watson, 2016) and in a Cancer Research UK review (Bainbridge et al., 2016). One possible solution is improved training and broader roles for scientific staff traditionally not involved in detailed microscopic cancer diagnosis, as illustrated in the case study in Box 10.3.

Box 10.3 Case Study – extending the roles of scientists in cellular pathology

Biomedical Scientist Histopathology Reporting Pilot in the United Kingdom

Context.

- Clinical scientists are an accepted facet of clinical provision in some pathology disciplines.
- In 2011 the NHS Information Centre found only 17 consultant clinical scientists in cytology and histopathology in the United Kingdom.
- Some extended roles for scientists already exist in cytology, macroscopic dissection, and molecular pathology.
- There is no formal clinical scientist training programme in cellular pathology.

Challenges

- Projected increase in new cases of cancer.
- Increased quality-assurance scrutiny and national key performance indicators.
- Inability to fill consultant vacancies in many parts of the country.
- Large backlogs of patients' biopsies and resections awaiting reporting or being outsourced.
- Career opportunities limited for scientists in cellular pathology.
- Predicted reduction in demand for cervical cytology as a primary screening modality.

Responses

- Development of an RCPath-led nationwide pilot of new ways of working in cellular pathology.
- Participants trained to report cellular pathology in clinical context.
- High volume, low complexity and low litigation areas of practice initially chosen to prove concept.
- Pilot participants recruited in 2012, 2013 and 2014.
- Curriculum and assessment tools developed with RCPath approval and strong collaboration with the Institute of Biomedical Scientists.

Box 10.3 (cont.)

Achievements to date

- An innovative national training programme across 37 NHS hospitals.
- Robust educational standards and clinical assessments.
- New Conjoint Board established with the Institute of Biomedical Science to move the pilot onto a permanent footing.

For the future hospital

- Expansion of areas of reporting practice planned with the introduction of new curricula and training programmes.
- Expansion of the recruitment into cellular pathology reporting to wider health care scientist population.
- Formal clinical scientist training programme in cellular pathology.

Source: Liebmann et al., 2015

Barriers to optimal pathology services

Barriers impeding the delivery of an efficient and effective pathology service include those related to service configuration, demand management, workforce, finance, quality, attitude, IT, and innovation adoption. These are discussed in turn.

Service configuration barriers

In some European countries there are too many laboratories carrying out specialist tests on too small a scale. Reconfiguration can be seen as a way to optimize pathology and to attain economies. However, consolidation, such as joint ventures and mergers, must be compliant with national and European competition law, which can constrain reorganization, as well as the undesirability of creating commercial monopolies that can lead to higher costs, worse performance, and reduced innovation.

The impetus for transformation can be slowed or blocked because pathology is not high enough on hospitals' priority lists. Many hospitals are evaluating options to develop new models of care within social, community, primary, and secondary care and this may push pathology modernization further down the chain of importance.

Demand management barriers

Most laboratories across Europe have experienced significant increases in workload year on year and the capacity of a service to manage demand is stretched, especially without a commensurate rise in staffing levels. Workload, measured in terms of crude sample numbers or test requests, is increasing and this probably belies actual workload because greater sophistication of diagnosis is now needed.

For example, increasing numbers of cases now require consensus reporting and referral for specialist opinion, demonstrating increasing sophistication of diagnostic processes and an increasingly risk-averse culture. Equally, more objective assessments are now required, whether it is a lead to provide reproducible assessments that determine patient treatment (e.g. quantitative immuno-histo-chemistry results which act as a threshold for breast cancer oncotherapy).

Where pathology is excluded from strategic planning processes and investment decisions, there is a risk that there will be unexpected, unplanned, and unfunded demands on those pathology services in the future.

Increased expectations will contribute to demand pressures in the following areas: providing ongoing clinical advice to doctors in training and primary care doctors, direct interpretative and advisory liaison work with patients who can access their test results directly, and provision of direct specialist outpatient care in diabetes, obesity, lipid disorders, and metabolic diseases.

Medical microbiology has seen an increased requirement for ward-based consultation with patients with suspected or proven infection, as a means to facilitate earlier discharge from hospital. Increasing antimicrobial resistance has placed greater emphasis on antimicrobial stewardship, with pathologists working alongside pharmacists specializing in antimicrobials.

There is a need for payment systems to take account of these rapid changes, with regular revisions that recognize new ways of delivering care. The regular reviews of the system for paying providers in Germany offers such an example.

Workforce barriers

Wider training issues, such as the trend in some countries to expand general medical training before specialization, could lead to a shorter time for pathologists to acquire specialist competencies. Recruitment to particular pathology specialties has been problematic. Outsourcing tests or using locum staff may alleviate workload but this only represents a short-term and expensive solution. There is uncertain capability to undertake some emerging techniques and technologies. The ability of pathologists, for example, to understand the disease phenotype (the detailed characteristics of the patient) is essential for interpretation of the current explosion in "-omics" data, i.e. genomics, proteomics, metabolomics, and transcriptomics.

Financial barriers

Traditionally, diagnostic tests in pathology have seemed cheaper than, for example, the costs of imaging. However, with many pathology services increasing their repertoire to include molecular testing, costs are increasing. A test costing €1000 could be perceived as being expensive but this has to be seen in context, such as whether the test is used to determine the use of a drug treatment which may cost more than 10 times as much. Unfortunately there can be a focus on the unit cost of pathology rather than looking more holistically at the "downstream" value for money that pathology contributes to the whole health care economy.

Establishing a transparent tariff for pathology tests could be beneficial, as is the case in many countries, such as Germany. Having tariff transparency would enable business cases for service transformation to be built up more easily.

Quality barriers

Many pre- and post-laboratory processes remain outside laboratory control, even though they impact significantly on the value of the service. End-to-end quality depends on others (e.g. requesting clinicians) over whom pathology has less control. The quality of the clinical pathology service will be impacted where there are areas of differential influence and control.

Appropriate ordering and commissioning of relevant laboratory tests and having timely access to the tests and test results are central to the provision of quality care for patients and patient flows through the hospital system. There is considerable variability in awareness and understanding, which leads to suboptimal and inappropriate use.

ISO 15189 accreditation may have value in assessment of laboratory quality management systems but is highly expensive to maintain and is entirely focused on processes within the laboratory and not on the end-to-end pathology contribution to health care.

Attitudinal barriers

Van Krieken, President of the European Society of Pathology, identified a lack of collaboration between pathologists and other stakeholders such as the pharmaceutical sector. His idea is to move towards a system in which tests and drugs are integrated, so that payment for a drug includes all necessary testing (van Krieken, 2015).

It is frequently observed that pathologists themselves need to take on more of a clinical leadership role and move out of the shadows. Risk-averse over-requesting of tests can prevail due to perceived threats of medico-legal liability and a monetary incentive may exist for over-requesting in some systems.

If testing is perceived as a cost-free service as far as requestors are concerned, there is little incentive to avoid waste and duplication. The most effective method of managing demand and promoting new technology is to ensure appropriate recovery of cost to the laboratory budget from other clinical budgets.

IT barriers

Within many European countries a wide range of IT systems are in use and this creates problems of interoperability between service users and pathology. In radiology the Digital Imaging and Communications in Medicine (DICOM) standard has achieved a near-universal level of acceptance among medical imaging equipment vendors and health care IT organizations but such a standard does not yet exist in pathology.

The lack of end-to-end IT connectivity in pathology limits the opportunity to achieve effective communications between laboratories and those ordering tests, as well as decision support, both of which minimize inappropriate or unnecessary repeat testing. There is a widely held perception that results data are not being fully leveraged by pathology service users and providers, and this is a key obstacle to cost and service improvement.

Innovation adoption barriers

At a national level delays in approval processes can constrain innovation. At a local level many test sites will be required by ISO 15189 to perform their own evaluation of a new test and duplicate many of the assurances already fulfilled by the test developer.

Aggressive national pathology cost saving plans may discourage adoption of new techniques. A complex cost–benefit relationship often underpins decisions to use new devices. Point-of-care devices are a good illustration and highlight how costs and benefits are often accrued in different areas. A primary care group may have funded a diagnostic device and reduced the need for patient hospital visits but may not receive the benefit of saving money for the health system because of opaque reimbursement mechanisms.

Investment in innovation for some pathology specialties has been limited. For example, many drug companies have no commercial interest in the development of rapid diagnostics for determining antibiotic sensitivity because of low commercial returns. The uptake and adoption of diagnostic tests across Europe shows significant variation. For example, C-reactive protein (CRP) tests have been used for some time in the Netherlands and Scandinavia to indicate whether an infection is bacterial or viral, and these countries have some of the lowest rates of prescribing antibiotics in Europe (Review on Antimicrobial Resistance, 2015).

In recent years there has been growing interest in using more accurate, efficient and reliable technologies such as mass spectrometry. Despite the important scientific advantages of such technologies, many clinical diagnostics services have continued to use traditional immunoassays, facing barriers such as the need for investment and expertise in mass spectrometry.

The future of pathology

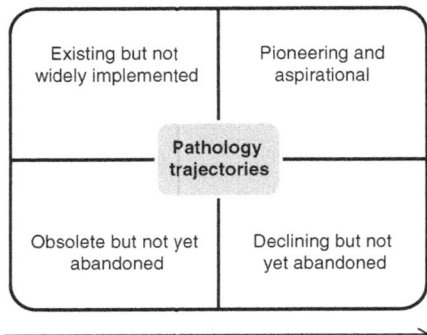

Figure 10.3 Quadrant highlighting pathology trajectories

Source: Authors' compilation

Obsolete but not yet abandoned

Obsolete ways of working include: laboratory standard operating procedures existing in isolation from patient pathways, single-handed pathologists, and old methods and out-of-date technologies.

Declining but not yet abandoned

Some aspects of hospital laboratory medicine are in decline but have not yet been abandoned. In some instances this is because there is a hope that the importance of these activities will be recognized. Notably, research capacity in pathology is in a steady decline and academic pathology is small scale and disjointed in all but a few major teaching centres where huge efforts are being made to keep up this aspect of the service.

In the United Kingdom there was such widespread concern about the loss of research capacity in 2015 that the National Cancer Research Institute, together with the ECMC Pathology Network Group, funded the Cellular Molecular Pathology initiative (CM-Path) – a five-year project which was awarded £635k. It aims to reinvigorate pathology research by building the change needed to support academic cellular molecular pathology. A report on the Experimental Cancer Medicine Centre Initiative (2015) gives more details.

Also, most pathology services are making great efforts to retain the interpretive and clinical advice aspects they provide, which is threatened by low-cost, dumbed-down "results-only services" which sacrifice patient-centred care and close working relationships between pathologists and clinical requestors. Importantly, hospital autopsies are in decline all over Europe (Box 10.4).

Box 10.4 Case Study – decline of consented autopsy following hospital death in Europe

Context

- Consented autopsy rates have fallen significantly in Europe over the past half century to the verge of extinction (Turnbull, Osborn & Nicholas, 2015).
- The benefits of autopsy are established and include: clinical audit, patient safety, public health in a time of global antibiotic resistance, epidemiology, research, education, improved mortality statistics, improved diagnostics, improved resource allocation, comfort and explanation to grieving families.
- The priority of the autopsy in modern health and social care is highlighted by the Francis report and in the United Kingdom will be crucial to the work of Medical Examiners of the Cause of Death due that was due to be implemented in England in 2018.

Challenges

- The main reasons for the decline are: perceived difficulties in obtaining consent; a limited role given current diagnostics ("autopsy is pointless in modern medicine – we know the diagnosis"); and religious objection.
- In some countries legislation is thought to have had an impact on hospital autopsies, such as the Human Tissue Act in the United Kingdom.
- A change in attitude is required so that autopsy is considered an altruistic act similar to organ donation.

Responses

- Most religions contain no objection to autopsy and most families would consent to autopsy if appropriately asked.
- The number of diagnostic discrepancies would decline with an increase in autopsies.
- Diagnostic discrepancies may be due to co-morbidities or atypical clinical presentation.

Box 10.4 (cont.)

- Despite technological progress, autopsy still has an important role in the assessment and improvement of the quality of surgical practice.

Achievements to date

- The European Critical Care Foundation (ECCF) held a conference in 2015 on the decline of the hospital autopsy to raise awareness among health care professionals.
- The idea to establish a pan-European anonymized autopsy database ("Europsy") was proposed at the ECCF meeting.

For the future hospital

- Autopsy should be offered to families across Europe upon the death of a relative to demonstrate willingness to discuss the patient's last episodes of care.
- Pathologists need to clarify and simplify the consent process to design a simple, yet effective, autopsy consent form.
- Alternative autopsies such as digital autopsies could be encouraged but their limitations should be understood and they are currently expensive and do not allow tissue to be obtained for in-depth diagnostic and research purposes.
- Medical research requires accurate causes of death. Autopsy should be used as a gold standard end-point for any deaths occurring in clinical trials.
- Specialist hospital professionals could be trained in consent, such as a pathology liaison nurse whose role would be to gain consent, to provide feedback to clinicians and to families, and to teach hospital staff about death.
- Teaching opportunities should be exploited so that students and junior doctors gain greater exposure to autopsy practice.

Source: Turnbull, Osborn & Nicholas, 2015

Existing but not widely implemented

Exciting new ways of providing pathology testing are not always implemented widely. For example, expansion of POCT and self-testing into the high street and homes has begun but in some instances is limited by patient acceptability (for a more detailed exposition see Larsson, Greig-Pylypczuk & Huisman, 2015). There are many other barriers to take-up of these devices, including the test devices themselves, patients' use of and interaction with the devices, providers' understanding of their uses, and the health systems in which they are used. Successful uptake usually requires integration of knowledge at these levels, which in turn can lead to trust and confidence.

The implementation of digital autopsies is limited by the diagnostic limitations of the technique. Standardization of units of measurement, reference ranges, coding and methods is required to enable results data to be of benefit in monitoring long-term conditions and in disease prevention, and implementation is limited by failure to implement national developments such as the National Laboratory Medicine Category in the United Kingdom.

Pioneering and aspirational

Some aspects of pathology service provision are envisioned but not yet in place. A key reason for this may be the traditionally slow rate of uptake of new technologies in pathology. The following technological innovations are discussed:

Wearables

Wearables are devices with sensors that monitor physiology. They can be integrated into devices such as smart phones, fitness bands, and clothing to track health and fitness. It is conceivable that these devices are able to generate self-monitored health data which could then be streamed directly into cloud-based data repositories or patient electronic health records. From here, general practitioners and hospital clinicians could access the data. However, several questions arise, including whether these devices are fit-for-purpose in bypassing an initial patient diagnosis and whether they can be used to triage a problem and direct the patient to relevant specialists. The accompanying growth of related apps could also facilitate transfer of data across different platforms and devices and lead to greater interoperability but it is too early to know whether patients would actually want this to happen. It also raises some regulatory issues as the devices would have to be cleared to use the same biomarkers which are used in clinical laboratory tests.

The challenge for pathologists and laboratory managers is that if wearables become mainstream, strategies will need to be developed for data collection, understanding what utility these data will have and how to manage such data in conjunction with conventional laboratory test data.

Biosensor point-of-care devices

A biosensor is a compact analytical device that detects, records, and transmits information regarding a physiological change or process. The use of biosensors is well established in the management of chronic illnesses, such as blood glucose monitoring in diabetes and cholesterol monitoring in cardiovascular disorders. Biosensors have also shown potential for in vivo sensing of disease-specific biomarkers such as cancer. Here, sensors with nanoscale dimensions have been developed for effective diagnostics purposes (Hasan et al., 2014). Biosensors have many advantages: they are easy to use and yield fast results; there is no need to use labelled reagents; the cost per test ratio is low (although initial investment in the device is needed); and only a small sample is required. Challenges which need to be overcome focus predominantly on sensor accuracy and their minimum detectable levels. Additionally, it could be argued that some biosensors are "pseudo-portable" because their detection platform relies on bulky fluidic and detection systems.

Undoubtedly the next-generation whole-cell biosensors will see continued miniaturization of components, improved computing power, enhanced amplification capacity, and applications made further afield. The migration of some pathology tests from laboratories to point-of-care devices will continue and it is hoped that concerns about quality assurance and reliability, and their integration into a locally managed pathology network, will be fully addressed.

The promise of using POCT devices as an effective diagnostic in other contexts such as general practice is under review in many European countries. In the United Kingdom the National Institute for Health and Care Excellence (2014) issued draft guidance which recommended that GPs should consider using a POCT (CRP) to help decide whether patients presenting with mild pneumonia need antibiotics. A narrative review of primary care POCT and antibacterial use in respiratory tract infection was undertaken by Cooke et al. (2015). The researchers drew attention to a survey of Dutch general practitioners who reported that the most common POCTs currently used by family physicians were: blood glucose

(96%); urine leucocytes or nitrite (96%); urine pregnancy (94%); hae-moglobin (58%); and CRP (48%). The most commonly desired POCTs were: D-dimer (70%); troponin (65%); brain natriuretic peptide (BNP) (62%); chlamydia (60%); and International Normalized Ratio (INR) (54%). In terms of wider scalability for POCT devices, agreed protocols would have to be in place for data sharing across connected diagnostic networks within constituent countries as well as across Europe.

New technologies in pathology are sometimes heralded as game changers that will bring significant benefits to patients and providers alike. However, caution is needed over claims made by new technologies. The Theranos company is a case in point. Theranos was an American company founded in 2003 which successfully raised capital to stream-line and standardize blood tests by creating a hand-held device using a few drops of blood obtained via a finger-stick "nanotainer" vial. It developed its own proprietary analyser to test blood samples. However, there were allegations against Theranos about discrepancies between a number of their specific blood tests when compared with traditional quality-assured methods. This resulted in a formal complaint to US regulators, which led to a finding that several clinical standards had been violated. A review of Theranos' systems, processes, and procedures resulted in Ms Holmes being charged by the Securities and Exchange Commission with widespread fraud, accusing her of exaggerating – even lying – about her technology while raising $700 million from investors said to include some of the world's richest people (*New York Times*, March and May 2018). There is a cautionary tale in the adoption of new technologies in pathology service. It is essential that the clinician is at the centre of technological adoption in the interests of patient safety and quality of care.

Conclusion

The tree of medicine diagram below provides a reminder of the centrality of pathology in medicine, as the trunk of the tree that links all aspects together is pathology.

Pathology in European hospitals is at a crossroads, with the future contingent on a willingness to address the barriers discussed in this chapter. There are many opportunities for pathologists to play a cen-tral clinical role. Despite operating under unrelenting fiscal constraints in some countries, pathology is entering into the "genome era" and pathologists must acquire and demonstrate visionary leadership.

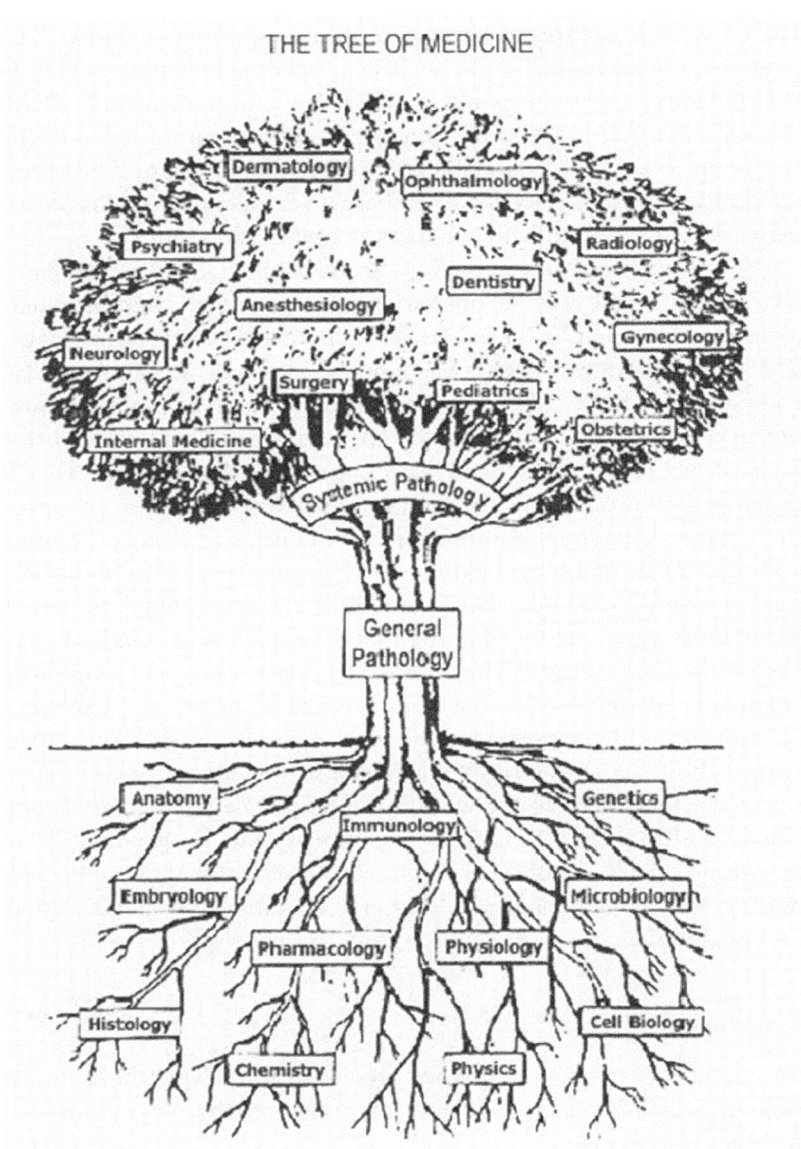

Figure 10.4 The tree of medicine (date of publication unknown)

Pathology services tend to be ignored by policy-makers and managers, and a key challenge will be to demonstrate how high quality pathology provision improves accuracy of diagnosis and effectiveness of monitoring or treatment, so creating better patient health outcomes. Quality in pathology reduces patient pathway costs as well as providing key health care data and impacting on all other health care interactions. The redesign of pathology so that it becomes part of an integrated patient pathway should be explored and communicated so that a clear demonstration of its value can be evidenced. This would enable pathology to be delivered where it is required while operating within an integrated quality framework (Myers, 2014).

References

Alderwick H, Ham C, Buck D (2015). *Population health systems. Going beyond integrated care*. Available at: https://www.kingsfund.org.uk/sites/default/files/field/field_publication_file/population-health-systems-kingsfund-feb15.pdf (accessed 1 October 2016).

Bainbridge S et al. (2016). *Testing times to come? An evaluation of pathology capacity across the UK*. London, Cancer Research UK.

Carter L et al. (2008). *Report of the Second Phase of the Review of NHS Pathology Services in England*. London, Department of Health. Available at: http://webarchive.nationalarchives.gov.uk/20130107105354/http:/www.dh.gov.uk/prod_consum_dh/groups/dh_digitalassets/@dh/@en/documents/digitalasset/dh_091984.pdf (accessed 1 March 2016).

Cooke J et al. (2015). Narrative review of primary care point-of-care testing (POCT) and antibacterial use in respiratory tract infection (RTI). *BMJ Open Respir Res*, 6, 2(1):e000086. Available at: http://bmjopenrespres.bmj.com/content/2/1/e000086.full (accessed 14 January 2016).

Driskell OJ et al. (2012). Inappropriate requesting of glycated hemoglobin (Hb A1c) is widespread: assessment of prevalence, impact of national guidance, and practice-to-practice variability. *Clin Chem*, 58(5):906–15.

Experimental Cancer Medicine Centre Initiative (2015). *New funding for pathology is keeping cancer research at the cutting edge*. Available at: https://www.ecmcnetwork.org.uk/news/announcement/new-funding-pathology-keeping-cancer-research-cutting-edge (accessed 24 October 2016).

Gartner (2015). *Gartner hype cycle*. Web page. Available at: http://www.gartner.com/technology/research/methodologies/hype-cycle.jsp (accessed 1 October 2015).

Genomics England (2015). *The 100,000 Genomes Project*. Web page. Available at: https://www.genomicsengland.co.uk/the-100000-genomes-project/ (accessed 1 October 2015).

Hasan A et al. (2014). Recent Advances in Application of Biosensors in Tissue Engineering. *BioMed Res Int*, 2014:307519. Available at: http://dx.doi .org/10.1155/2014/307519 (accessed 14 January 2016).

Imison C, Castle-Clarke S, Watson R (2016). *Reshaping the workforce to deliver the care patients need*. Research report. London, Nuffield Trust.

Institute for Healthcare Improvement (2015). *IHI Triple Aim Initiative*. Web page. Available at: http://www.ihi.org/engage/initiatives/TripleAim/Pages/ default.aspx (accessed 1 October 2015).

Larsson A, Greig-Pylypczuk R, Huisman A (2015). The state of point-of-care testing: a European perspective. *Ups J Med Sci*, 120(1):1–10. Available at: http://www.ncbi.nlm.nih.gov/pmc/articles/PMC4389002/ (accessed 1 October 2015).

Liebmann R et al. (2015). Breaking new ground in histopathology: report from the pilot of BMS histopathology reporting. *Bulletin of the Royal College of Pathologists*, 169(1):27–30. Available at: https://www.rcpath .org/profession/publications/college-bulletin/january-2015/breaking-new-ground-in-histopathology-report-from-the-pilot-of-bms-histopathology-reporting.html (accessed 1 October 2015).

Meads G (2009). The organisation of primary care in Europe: part 1 trends – position paper of the European Forum for Primary Care. *Qual Prim Care*, 17(2):133–43. Available at: http://www.ncbi.nlm.nih.gov/pubmed/19416606 (accessed 1 October 2015).

Myers M (2014). *International Keynote Address: Pathology in the United Kingdom, a road less travelled*. Presentation at the National Pathology Forum 2014, Australia. Available at: http://www.slideshare.net/informaoz/ dr-martin-myers-lancashire (accessed 1 October 2015).

National Institute for Health and Care Excellence (2014). *Pneumonia*. Web page. Available at: http://www.nice.org.uk/guidance/indevelopment/GID-CGWAVE0607 (accessed 14 January 2016).

New York Times (2018). Elizabeth Holmes, Theranos C.E.O. and Silicon Valley Star, Accused of Fraud. 14 March 2018. Available at: https://www .nytimes.com/2018/03/14/health/theranos-elizabeth-holmes-fraud.html.

New York Times (2018). Caught in the Theranos Wreckage: Betsy de Vos, Rupert Murdoch and Walmart's Waltons. 4 May 2018. Available at: https:// www.nytimes.com/2018/05/04/health/theranos-investors-murdoch-devos-walmart.html.

NHS England National Pathology Programme (2014). *Digital First: Clinical Transformation through Pathology Innovation*. https://www.england.nhs

.uk/wp-content/uploads/2014/02/pathol-dig-first.pdf (accessed 1 October 2015).

Public Health England (2015). *The NHS Atlas of Variation in Healthcare, September 2015.* Available at: http://fingertips.phe.org.uk/documents/ Atlas_2015%20Compendium.pdf (accessed 1 October 2015).

Review on Antimicrobial Resistance (2015). *Rapid Diagnostics: Stopping Unnecessary Use of Antibiotics.* Available at: https://amr-review.org/sites/ default/files/Paper-Rapid-Diagnostics-Stopping-Unnecessary-Prescription-Low-Res.pdf (accessed 24 October 2016).

Right Care (2011).The *NHS Atlas of Variation in Healthcare, November 2011.* Available at: https://fingertips.phe.org.uk/documents/Atlas_2011%20 Compendium.pdf (accessed 1 October 2015).

St John A, Price CP (2014). Existing and Emerging Technologies for Point-of-Care Testing. *Clin Biochem Rev*, 35(3):155–67. Available at: http://www .ncbi.nlm.nih.gov/pmc/articles/PMC4204237/ (accessed 1 October 2015).

Swan N (2015). *A National Framework for Quality Assurance in Cellular Pathology – The Irish Approach,* Presentation on 25 June 2015. Available at: http://www.pathsoc.org/files/meetings/Dublin2015Presentations/QA%20 -%201%20Swan.pdf (accessed 1 October 2015).

Turnbull A, Osborn M, Nicholas, N (2015). Hospital autopsy: endangered or extinct? *J Clin Pathol*, 68(8):601–4.

van Krieken H (2015). The Changing Face of Pathology. *The Pathologist*, issue 0715. Available at: https://thepathologist.com/issues/0715/the-changing-face-of-pathology/ (accessed 1 October 2015).

11 | *Conclusions – Challenges for hospitals of the future*

MARTIN MCKEE, SHERRY MERKUR, NIGEL
EDWARDS, ELLEN NOLTE

Almost every aspect of society today has been shaped by technological developments. Take the nature of the modern state. The historian Philip Bobbitt describes how the introduction of gunpowder to Europe rendered the medieval city states, protected by high walls, obsolete. Gutenberg's invention of the printing press, allowing for the cheap distribution of information to the masses, paved the way for the Reformation and later for revolutions. The discovery of magnetism, and thus the compass, made it possible to establish global networks, enabling exchange of people and ideas and, ultimately, the system of international trade that prevails today. The invention of the steam engine, powering both railways and mines, paved the way for the industrial revolution and, with it, the growth of major cities. These examples illustrate how technological advances have created huge societal changes that rippled out into further cycles of innovation, driving the shift from local feudalism to a global post-industrial society.

Health care has similarly been influenced by technological change. As described in the first chapter, the modern hospital owes its origins to the need to concentrate resources around laboratories, operating theatres, and X-ray facilities. Safe anaesthetics, antibiotics, and the concept of asepsis changed hospitals from places where patients increased their risk of dying simply by entering to ones that could cure or, if this was not possible, alleviate symptoms. Yet, as also noted in that chapter, many of the assumptions that underlie the concept of the modern hospital are now being challenged. Numerous examples throughout this book show how technological advances are changing the way that health care is provided. In some cases these advances are specific to health care, such as desktop kits that take over many of the functions once reserved for the laboratory, or mobile monitoring systems, such as those that can track physiological changes in patients as they go about their everyday life. For example, it is now possible to attach an ultrasound probe to a smart phone that will allow a health professional to look inside the

288

body of their patient even in the remotest of areas. Patients can also have their chronic conditions managed without the need to regularly travel to hospital appointments, as in the case of COPD where specialist expertise can be obtained at a distance.

Other technological advances are generic, such as advances in communications technology. The smart phone that most people carry has the computing power of a supercomputer of the 1960s. Information and images can be transmitted rapidly between teams of health professionals, ensuring that all have up-to-date information on the patient they are managing and giving access to specialist advice from experts across the world and in future to artificial intelligence to support image analysis and decision support. In some cases, in future, sophisticated image analysis software will outperform skilled clinicians.

These developments have several characteristics. First, most were not anticipated or, if they were, the consequences were often very different from what was first predicted. For example, while the discovery of insulin had, as expected, a transformational effect on the survival of young people with diabetes, it took many years before the long-term complications of diabetes, and with them the need for new models of care, became apparent. The same was true of the introduction of antiretrovirals for HIV. It is only now that the long-term complications of infection with the virus and the accompanying immunosuppression, as well as the side-effects of the medicines, are being recognized, such as increased risks of cardiovascular disease and certain cancers. Fleming's discovery of penicillin transformed the management of many common infections but within a few years the problems of antimicrobial resistance were being recognized.

Second, many have required significant changes in ways of working. The survival of patients with noncommunicable diseases has given rise to the challenges of multimorbidity, which in turn has stimulated the creation of MDT working. Advances in diagnostics and treatment have allowed many patients who once would have had to attend hospital to be managed in the community. Many technologies require the development of staff with new skills and some have led to the emergence of new disciplines – for example, interventional radiology and cardiology. Some have allowed tasks previously undertaken by highly trained professionals to be delegated to other staff and in some cases to the patient or their carers, for example monitoring blood sugar for diabetes or clotting to manage anti-coagulation. It is worth noting that much of this change has been in advance of, rather than in response to, changes in policy to payment systems and that policy-makers and payers have often struggled to keep up with the pace of change. Regulations, payment systems, and directives can inhibit and support changes but they are only part of the story of how these technologies are adopted. There are also lessons about the way that poorly designed incentives can create over-adoption: such as the multiplication of cardiac facilities in Bulgaria due to very high profit margins that were unintentionally created by the payment system.

Third, while some of these changes have been transformational, their development and spread have generally been incremental. For example, new, safer, and more effective medicines in the same class provide clear benefits, but do not demand new models of care. Others are more disruptive, such as the earliest developments in minimally invasive surgery, the development of endoscopy, interventional radiology and angioplasty in some cases challenging established ideas about by whom and where care is provided. Another more structural example is stroke units, which have revolutionized stroke treatment over the last quarter of a century. They both improve survival and reduce long-term dependency. Moreover, the delivery of early supported discharge, which involves patient care and therapy in their own home following stroke, has been shown to shorten length of hospital stay and improve long-term recovery, thus challenging old treatment pathways.

The clear message from the history of technological advances is that they cannot be ignored. Just as in the past, they will continue to shape the nature of health care and, with it, the roles of those who provide it and the ways in which they work together. To enable the hospital to support these changes rather than obstruct them, attention will need to be given to thinking more creatively and strategically about the workforce, technology, design of buildings, and the wider system in which hospitals operate.

Hospitals will need to be designed in a way that is sufficiently flexible to adapt to these changing circumstances, both in their physical design and their organizational structure. A hospital built today will be unrecognizable to doctors and nurses from the early 20th century. Resistance to change is simply pointless. Yet, too often, it takes years to take full advantage of innovation. Health care often lags far behind developments in other sectors, illustrated when, in 2017, the computer system of large parts of the English NHS were paralysed by a ransomware attack that exploited systems using the obsolete Windows XP software. Nonetheless, health systems also demonstrate many remarkable examples of entrepreneurialism, with individual clinicians and their teams introducing innovative technology and ways of working, despite the system in which they work seemingly doing everything possible to obstruct them. The challenge, for health policy-makers, is how to encourage this entrepreneurialism in ways that maximize health gain, while not destabilizing the overall health system.

Preparing for the future

In the following section, we look briefly at some of the examples of innovation that reflect themes in earlier chapters and the opportunities and challenges that they pose for the hospital now and in the future.

We begin with the multidisciplinary team. As noted above, the growth of multimorbidity and the complexity of the responses to it, involving different groups of professionals, require completely new ways of working. A typical patient aged 75 or above may have five or six different conditions, each requiring long-term medication or other forms of therapy, not all of which may necessarily be compatible. Yet they may still be able to lead a normal life with appropriate input from different professionals. This requires a high level of organization, with seamless transmission of information. These patients are on a journey, and the challenge for the health system is to make it as smooth as possible. Unfortunately, in practice, it can be more like an exploration of an unknown land, moving from point to point almost at random, often getting lost in the process. Advances in technology can improve this process, in particular by ensuring the timely sharing of information. However, much more is needed. In particular, such teams can only operate in a culture characterized by collaboration, with flat hierarchies and mutual respect among all those involved. Creating these teams is not easy and requires deliberate work to develop and maintain them. Research in health care suggests that the appearance of teamwork may often disguise a lack of clear purpose, poorly defined membership, leadership problems, unhelpful hierarchical behaviours, and a lack of support for the team (West & Markiewicz, 2016).

MDTs in cancer care involve coordinated working among different professionals, which is required to synchronize the complex array of interventions and frequent patient contacts. Oncology MDTs can include a broad range of health professionals with different skills including in diagnostics, oncology, pathology, radiology, surgery, nursing, and palliative care, who must work together and also alongside other professionals in psychology and psychiatry. Also professionals involved in new models of perioperative care, which emphasize improvement and consistency of outcomes for patients after surgery, are fundamentally multidisciplinary. Health professionals are drawn from a range of medical specialties, including anaesthesia, surgery, geriatric, and internal medicine, and should be led by those who can take a system-wide approach.

A related issue is the tension between generalists and specialists among health professionals. Unfortunately, in many health systems the specialist occupies a privileged position in the medical or nursing hierarchy, making it difficult to attract and retain generalists. Patients with multimorbidity will from time to time require highly specialized inputs. For example, a patient with diabetes, among other conditions, may need laser treatment on their retinas. This is a highly skilled task. They may also have kidney failure requiring dialysis, again a task requiring considerable expertise. But at the same time, they need someone who can take a holistic view of their health problems, ensuring that a treatment initiated for one problem does not exacerbate another. The growth of multimorbidity and polypharmacy as populations age presents a significant challenge to the model of narrow specialism. Patients increasingly fail to fit neatly into the way that medical specialisms have been organized.

As a consequence the fastest-growing area in hospital medicine in the USA has been in the specialism known as "hospitalists" (Wachter & Goldman, 2016). These are often internal medicine specialists (although they can be drawn from other disciplines) and are now appearing in paediatrics and other areas. Their role is to act as coordinators of patient care within the hospital and to co-manage cases with some specialties. Social complexity and difficulty in discharging patients as a result are also problematic and the hospitalist movement has been criticized for not paying sufficient attention to these issues (Gunderman, 2016). The chapter on frailty offers a similar model of a general physician with specialist skills for managing complexity, but shows the importance of services that can cross the boundary between the hospital and other types of care and address patients' wider needs. Although this has been focused on older people, these issues of complexity are not confined to the old. The question of the optimal balance between specialist and generalist care has not been answered.

In countries where primary care is the main provider of care for chronic diseases, the increasing levels of demand and the large and growing body of scientific knowledge involved in managing chronic conditions mean that there is a need to help primary care doctors, nurses, and other clinicians in their work and in keeping up to date. Hospital specialists in areas such as endocrinology, respiratory medicine, nephrology, cardiology, rheumatology, etc., have a key role in supporting the management of conditions such as diabetes, heart failure, and asthma, overseeing the administration of complex treatments and providing feedback and help with activities such as quality improvement and process redesign. This may require new skills, different approaches to patient consultations, and a change in the relationship between hospitals, primary care, and patients. The key aspects of this include:

- Rethinking the traditional outpatient model based on referral to a specialist.
- Improving case management skills of health professionals to ensure that the patient's problem is dealt with or that the patient is quickly referred to another professional who can deal with that problem.
- Health professionals working proactively to identify risks for the patient and engaging with them to address these. Often these may require action to deal with non-medical problems in the patient's life that are making compliance with treatment plans difficult.
- Considering and developing strategies for population health and prevention. This will include specialists taking a more direct interest in these areas, including secondary prevention for their existing patients and more active involvement in health promotion for the wider population.
- Specialists acting as consultants and overseers of networks of care and supporting other professionals. This means that the type of patient they deal with will often be more complex.

These challenges have led to a great deal of interest in the creation of various types of integrated care organizations that bring together primary and specialist care, and which potentially can deliver care that meets the characteristics described above. Many of these changes to the relationship between the hospital and its wider system will support integrated care but it is easy to underestimate the scale of the changes in work processes and operating models for hospitals and the staff who work in them that the full development of these models will require. If integrated care systems can deliver on their promise of reducing the use of hospitals, then there are some major challenges as to how to reduce fixed costs if there are reductions in the use of hospital facilities.

The growth of specialism and the narrowing of many specialist fields mean that all but the largest hospitals will not be able to have the full range of expertise on site. The growth of digital technology means that laboratory and imaging expertise does not necessarily need to be in the same location, or even the same country, as the patient. The development of communications technology also offers the opportunity to spread expertise across distances. This can support the growth of specialist referral networks with escalation criteria and standardized protocols. These networks are increasingly common in cancer, neonatal care, neurosurgery, and many rare diseases where there is already a strong trend towards centralization because of a strong body of evidence that for certain types of care – particularly complex care, some types of surgery, and cancer care – higher volumes are associated with improved outcomes.

Referral networks are also found in high volume areas such as maternity services, where different parts of the network will have rules for accepting or transferring patients relating to the level of risk involved. Sometimes these may include retrieval services to ensure the safe transfer of critically ill patients. The organizational arrangements to allow for rapid transfer and return of patients need to be agreed across the network and properly managed or will be a cause of some tension.

The development of hospital networks run by groups such as Helios and Asklepios in Germany, and IHH, Apollo and Parkway in Asia, and which are also increasingly found in other European countries, partly reflects a growing idea that there are economies from both scale and standardization. Agreeing a common approach to a procedure, such as hip replacement, allows for procurement savings but also creates the potential for benchmarking and improvement across a wide network with managed processes to make this happen, as opposed to relying on hospitals joining such approaches voluntarily.

The growth of technology and a strong emphasis on efficiency have had the effect of shortening lengths of stay and increasing the intensity of work in hospitals. This trend will continue and will put increased demands on staff, facilities, and engineering and means that the proportion of beds run as critical or high dependency care is likely to rise.

A second effect has been to move work and specialists, who have been traditionally based in hospitals, to ambulatory settings, creating new ways of delivering care and requiring different approaches to giving specialist advice for inpatient care.

While advances in technology have brought many benefits, they have also created new challenges. One relates to the challenge of providing effective health care to people living in remote areas. As has been noted, the management of conditions such as myocardial infarction, gastro-intestinal bleeding, stroke, and major trauma have been transformed by the introduction of new methods to intervene actively to tackle the fundamental problem, whether it be a blocked artery or catastrophic bleeding. Yet for this to be achieved, there is a need for rapid diagnosis, followed, equally rapidly, by definitive treatment. If these are delayed, the treatment is simply ineffective. Yet in some places, where the population density is low, it will never be possible to provide such definitive diagnosis and treatment sufficiently close to where people live. This will require new and imaginative solutions involving the training of multiskilled doctors and other clinical staff, technology for remote advice and support, and rapid transfer or retrieval services. Remote areas tend to be more explicit with their local population about the limits and capabilities of local services and what will happen in the event of a serious emergency than those in more populous areas.

There are challenges as well as opportunities from the increasing role played by information technology. There is a danger that feeding the system with data can take priority over interacting with the patient. Patients frequently complain that the health professional spent the encounter looking at a screen rather than at them. Health professionals complain that they spend so much time entering data that they are unable to engage in conversation with the patient. Yet in other sectors this challenge has been addressed. There are many new means of entering data, ranging from barcodes to the use of voice recognition software. Unfortunately, in the health sector these appear to be difficult to implement and are significantly under-exploited.

The way forward

We conclude with four recommendations. In producing this book, we have been struck by the lack of fora within which those working in hospitals, those responsible for their design and operation, and those responsible for the policy environment in which they operate can come together to exchange ideas. There are many innovative models of care around Europe but far too few have been evaluated and, where they have been, the findings are not easily available. There is now clear expectation that those responsible for introducing therapeutic innovations, such as new medicines or surgical procedures, should evaluate them and share the results. This is not the case with innovative models of care. There is a clear need to create mechanisms that would enable this to happen.

The second relates to the hospital workforce. The roles and responsibilities of health professionals have changed remarkably over the past few decades. They will continue to do so. In many cases these transitions are managed easily and effectively. Yet in others, they are not. There are sometimes legal and regulatory barriers to change, as well as financial incentives that act as barriers to effective working. There is a danger in sweeping all of these away, as they can provide much-needed protection for health workers, who in many countries are inadequately rewarded for their commitment and dedication. But on the other hand, there is a need for sufficient flexibility to allow them to develop as circumstances change.

The third relates to the hospital and its wider environment. It is abundantly clear that the hospital is only one part of the health system and for many patients the boundary between it and the rest of the health system can act as an impenetrable barrier. Many contemporary advances, in particular those that seek to bring sophisticated treatment to patients as quickly as possible, require models of care that reach beyond the hospital into the patient's home. Similarly, there is a need to ensure that the process of being discharged from hospital is as smooth as possible, and is not seen simply as a means of emptying a bed for the next admission. This means that hospitals need to be planned as part of the wider system in which they sit, both in terms of the opportunities to work differently with primary care and community-based services, but also as a part of a wider network with other hospitals and specialist centres. This also means that traditional approaches that use beds as the currency for planning hospitals is now inadequate and potentially misleading or unhelpful.

The final recommendation relates to connectivity. This means connectivity within and beyond the hospital. It means connectivity through information technology but also in person. Indeed, it particularly means in person. Yet it is necessary to recognize that connectivity has a cost as well as benefits. Time spent in meetings is time not spent treating patients. Too often, meetings are organized where those attending see little point. They feel that their time is being wasted, little is relevant to them, and they spend most of the meeting on their tablets and smart phones, engaged not with those in the room but with those outside it. In time, they drift off, finding excuses to stop attending. There is a clear need to find new ways of communicating in which the benefits outweigh the costs.

It is impossible to know what the hospital of the future will look like, just as it was impossible to say what the future of travel would be before the Wright brothers took their first flight. All that can be said is that the future will be different from the present. What is important is that structures and systems are put in place that have sufficient flexibility and ability to learn as circumstances change.

References

Gunderman R (2016). Hospitalists and the Decline of Comprehensive Care. *New Eng J Med*, 375:1011–1103. doi: 10.1056/NEJMp1608289.

Wachter RM, Goldman L (2016). Zero to 50,000 — The 20th Anniversary of the Hospitalist. *New Eng J Med*, 375:1009–11. doi: 10.1056/NEJMp1607958.

West MA, Markiewicz L (2016). Effective Team Working in Health Care. In: Ferlie E, Montgomery K, Pedersen AR (eds). *The Oxford Handbook of Health Care Management*. Oxford, Oxford University Press, pp. 231–52.

Index

Page numbers in *italics* denote figures.